# Total, Subtotal and Proximal Gastrectomy in Cancer

Walter Siquini
Editor

# Total, Subtotal and Proximal Gastrectomy in Cancer

## A Color Atlas

In collaboration with
Raffaella Ridolfo
Pierpaolo Stortoni
Emilio Feliciotti

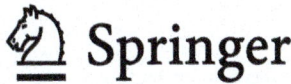 Springer

*Editor*
Walter Siquini
Division of General Surgery
"Madonna del Soccorso" Hospital
San Benedetto del Tronto
(Ascoli Piceno)
Italy

ISBN 978-88-470-3924-7        ISBN 978-88-470-5749-4   (eBook)
DOI 10.1007/978-88-470-5749-4

Springer Milano Heidelberg New York Dordrecht London
© Springer-Verlag Italia 2015
Softcover reprint of the hardcover 1st edition 2015

Printed on acid-free paper

Springer-Verlag Italia Srl. is part of Springer Science+Business Media (www.springer.com)

*To my mother, Antonietta,*
*to my wife, Cristina,*
*and to my daughters, Elisa and Sofia,*
*for their patience, their tolerance and their support…*
*The precious time that I have stolen from them*
*has made this book possible.*

# Preface

The idea of writing this atlas originated 20 years ago, when in the operating room, I was admiring my mentor, Professor Eduardo Landi, while he manually performed a gastro-jejunal anastomosis after subtotal gastrectomy with an accurate technique that was rich in precautions and standardized in every single step. For us young trainees, to be able to reproduce all the surgical steps correctly and succeed in executing gastro-jejunal anastomosis according to the defined technique at our school was, as our mentor said, already sufficient to merit the title of surgeon. Accordingly, for months, I took notes and made sketches of every step in this surgery while it was being performed without ever considering deviations from the rules and with excellent results.

In 2011, the GIRCG (the Italian Research Group for Gastric Cancer) published the monograph *Surgery in the Multimodal Management of Gastric Cancer*, in which I was allocated the chapter 'Total and Subtotal Gastrectomy with D2 Lymphadenectomy: Technical Notes'. The initial draft which I sent to the publisher faithfully reproduced the notes I had taken, but it was written in too much detail for the design of the book. I therefore had to cut the chapter, but the original version was well appreciated by Springer, who asked me whether I would take responsibility for developing a colour atlas which would describe surgery for gastric cancer in detail.

In this way, the present atlas was born. It aims to describe procedures step by step and to guide the surgeon in the performance of both total and subtotal gastrectomy with either manual or mechanical anastomoses and with an open or a laparoscopic approach. A further goal is to describe lymphadenectomy and to explain in detail the timing of proximal gastrectomy with gastric tube reconstruction and intra-thoracic anastomosis for cancers of the oesophago-gastric junction.

In all cases, technical tricks are explained in order to make the procedures easier and more effective and to improve the safety of oesophago-jejunal, gastro-jejunal and esophago-gastric tube anastomoses, minimizing the risk of leakage.

I would like to thank Drs. Giorgio Cutini, Pietro Coletta and Francesco Falsetti, who are responsible for the chapter on laparoscopic subtotal and total gastrectomy.

A large vote of thanks is due to Drs. Raffaella Ridolfo, Pierpaolo Stortoni and Emilio Feliciotti, who supported me in writing and managing this book; without their contributions, it would never have been possible. In addition,

I would like to gratefully acknowledge the contribution of Raffaella and Emilio, who made all the amazing drawings which beautifully enrich this book.

I also owe a debt of gratitude to my colleagues, Drs. Alberto Buonanno, Alessandro Cardinali, Sandro Cognigni, Dezia Fiorelli, Dino Giusti, Raffaele Nigro, Davide Pellegrini and Giulia Tonini, who each day help me to perform the gastric surgery described in this book.

Finally, I would like to thank the operating room nurses, Amelia Faleroni, Teresa Iacoponi, Andrea Liodori, Mauro Marabotto, Simone Mecozzi, Angela Merlonghi, Regina Rosetti, Giuseppe Rossi and Giacomo Sabini, who kindly took the many intra-operative photos shown in these pages.

At the end of this entire hard endeavour, I very much hope that the wealth of intra-operative photographs and drawings in this atlas in conjunction with the explanatory legends will succeed in clearly depicting the individual steps of all the procedures and highlighting tricks and pitfalls and will thereby help the reader to correctly execute this complex and fascinating surgery.

Further, I hope that through this book and the worldwide distribution guaranteed by Springer, the precious technique developed by our surgical school will not be forgotten but instead will be handed down to future generations of young surgeons.

My mentor would definitely be happy about that!

San Benedetto del Tronto, Italy                                                    Walter Siquini
May 2015

# Contents

# Contributors

**Alessandro Cardinali** Division of General Surgery, "Madonna del Soccorso" Hospital, San Benedetto del Tronto, Italy

**Pietro Coletta** Division of General Surgery, "Villa Igea" Private Hospital, Ancona, Italy

**Giorgio Cutini** Division of General Surgery, "Villa Igea" Private Hospital, Ancona, Italy

**Giovanni de Manzoni** Department of Surgery, General Surgery and Surgery of Esophagus and Stomach, Verona, Italy

**Francesco Falsetti** Division of General Surgery, Jesi Hospital, Jesi, Italy

**Emilio Feliciotti** Department of Surgery, "Ospedali Riuniti" University Hospital, Ancona, Italy

**Raffaella Ridolfo** Division of General Surgery, Senigallia General Hospital, Senigallia, Italy

**Walter Siquini** Division of General Surgery, "Madonna del Soccorso" Hospital, San Benedetto del Tronto, Italy

**Pierpaolo Stortoni** Division of General Surgery, "A. Murri" Hospital, Fermo, Italy

**Valerio Caracino** Division of General Surgery, Pescara Hospital, Pescara, Italy

# Position of the Patient

Raffaella Ridolfo, Pierpaolo Stortoni, Emilio Feliciotti, and Walter Siquini

This chapter illustrates patients' preparation and the correct positioning of patients and of the operating team. See illustrations following.

R. Ridolfo (✉)
Division of General Surgery, Senigallia General Hospital, Senigallia, Italy

Division of General Surgery
"A. Murri" Hospital, Fermo, Italy
e-mail: raffaella.ridolfo@email.it

P. Stortoni
Division of General Surgery,
"A. Murri" Hospital, Fermo, Italy
e-mail: pierpaolostortoni@libero.it

E. Feliciotti
Department of Surgery,
"Ospedali Riuniti" University Hospital,
Ancona, Italy
e-mail: feliciotti@live.it

W. Siquini
Division of General Surgery,
"Madonna del Soccorso" Hospital,
San Benedetto del Tronto, Italy
e-mail: walter.siquini@sanita.marche.it

W. Siquini (ed.), *Total, Subtotal and Proximal Gastrectomy in Cancer: A Color Atlas*,
DOI 10.1007/978-88-470-5749-4_1, © Springer-Verlag Italia 2015

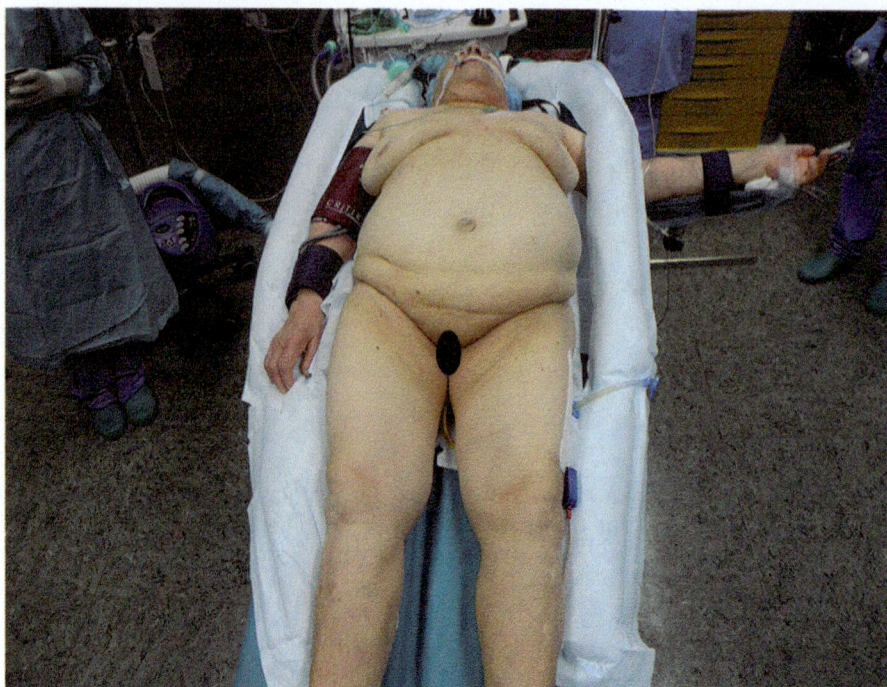

**Fig. 1.1** The patient is placed supine with the left arm abducted, as required by the anesthetist, and the right arm adducted to leave sufficient room for the surgeon and the assistant standing on the surgeon's left. A heating mat is placed between the patient and the surgical table.

A vesical catheter and a nasogastric tube are applied after induction of anesthesia.

Before taking the patient to the operating theater, body hair is removed with electric clippers from the intermammary line to the pubis vertically and between the midaxillary lines laterally

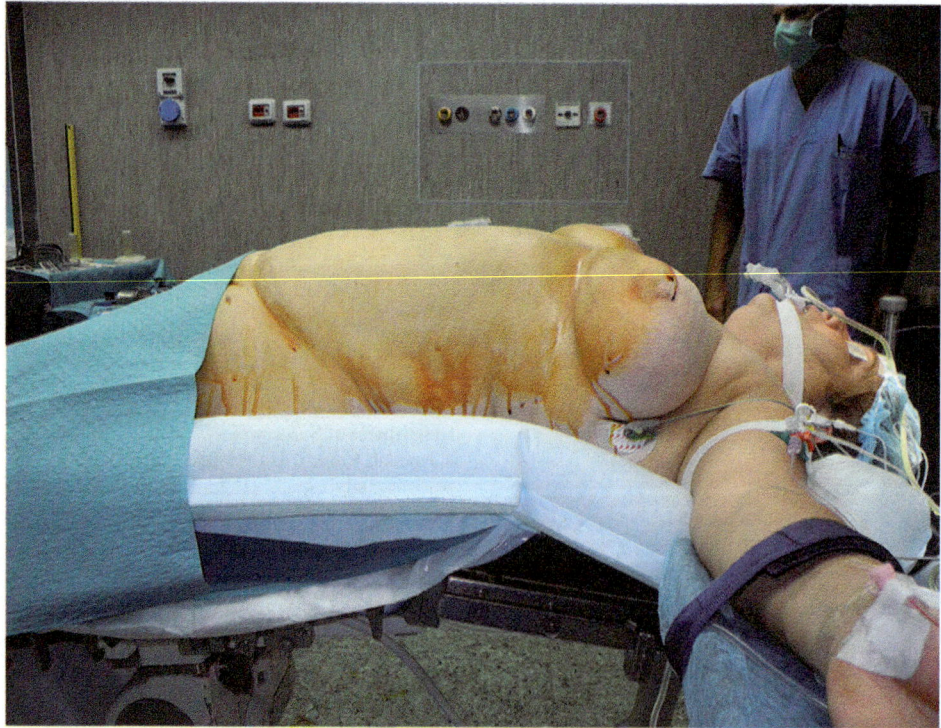

**Fig. 1.2** Optimal exposure of the operating field is obtained by breaking the operating table at the base of the patient's chest

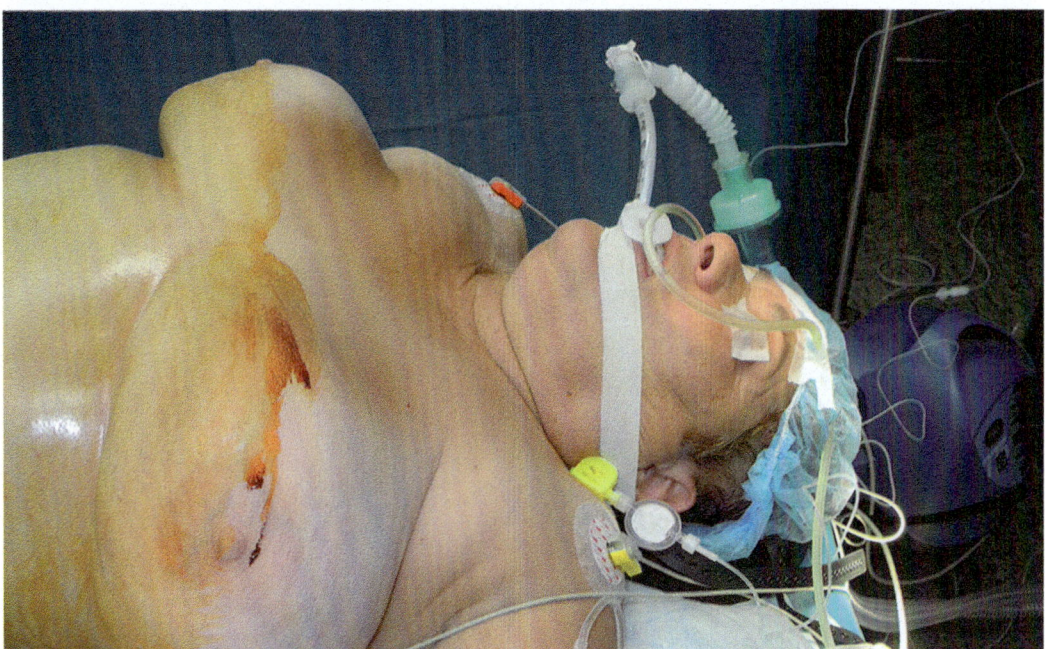

**Fig. 1.3** A peridural catheter for postoperative analgesia and a radial arterial line for arterial pressure evaluation are placed in the operating room

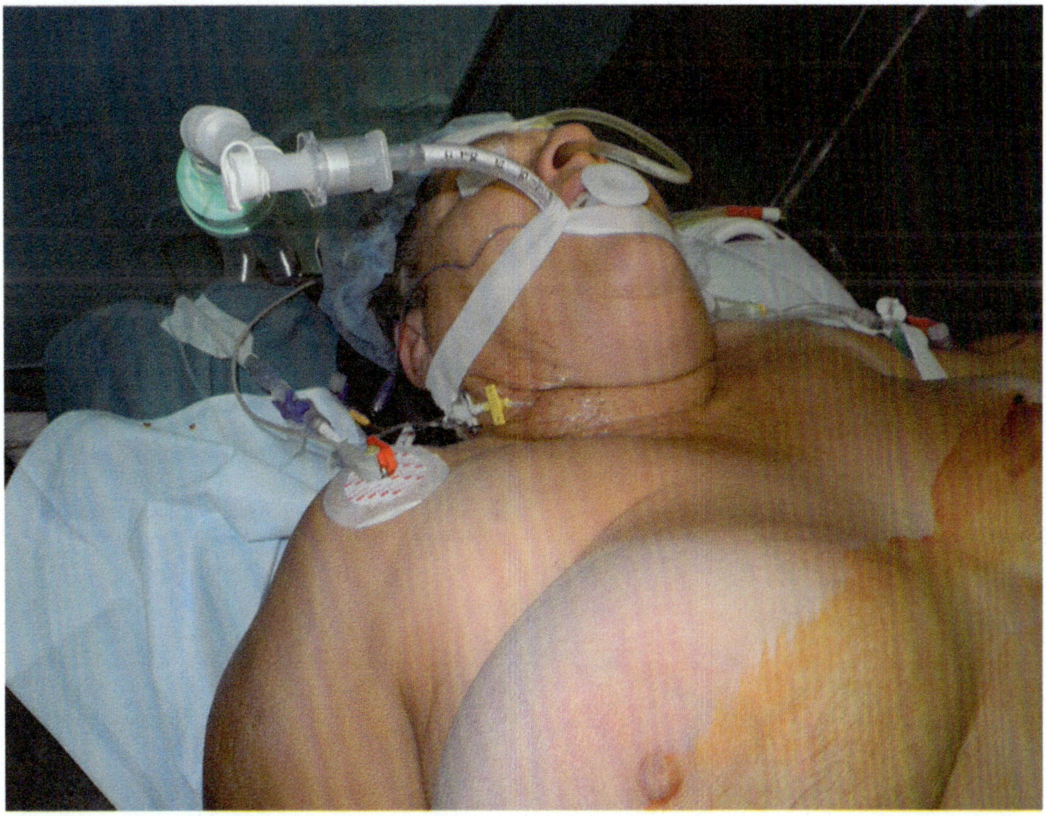

**Fig. 1.4** A central venous catheter (CVC) is placed in the operating room for postoperative parenteral nutritional support

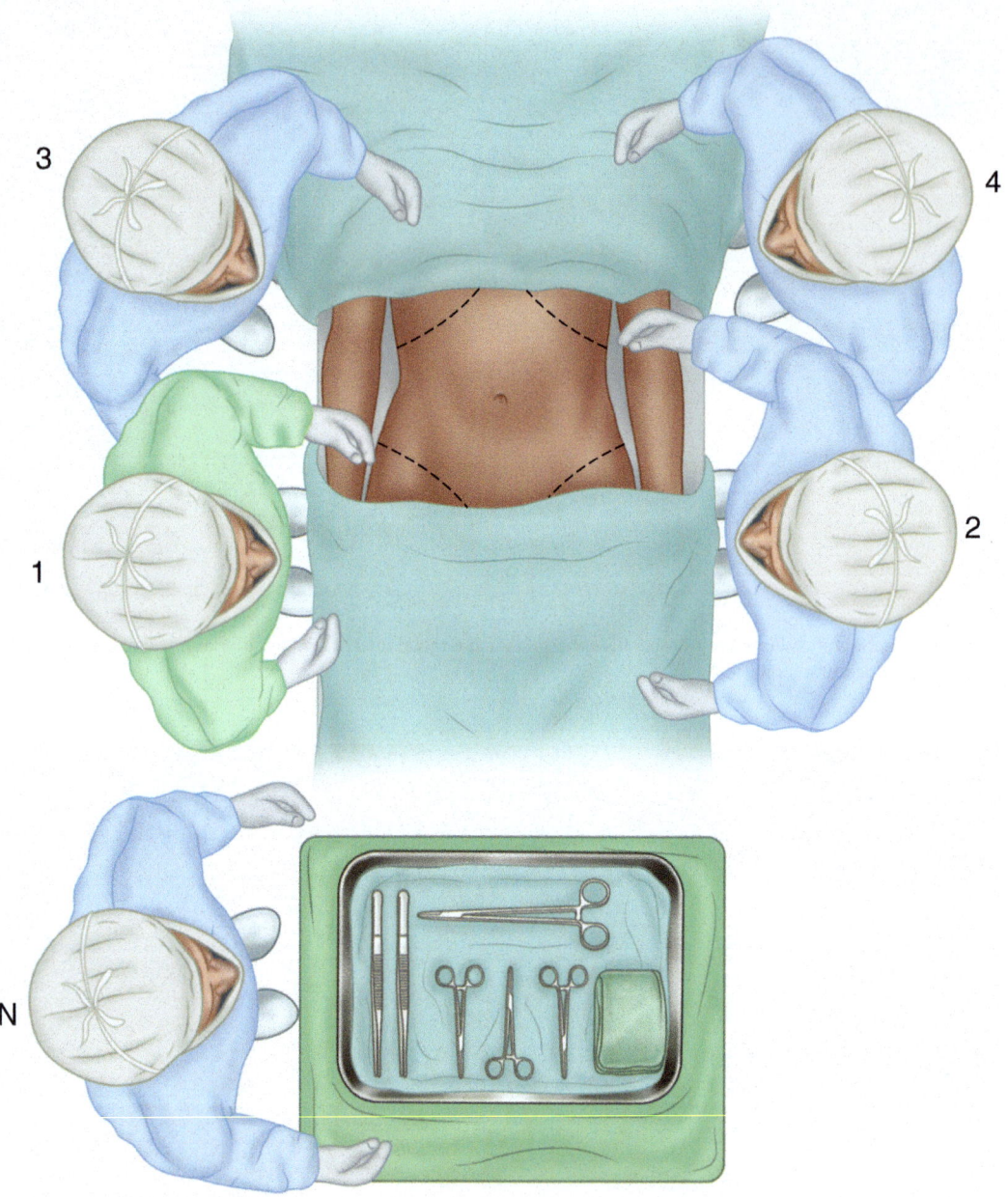

**Fig. 1.5** Position of the operating team: The surgeon (*1*) stands on the patient's right side, opposite the first assistant (*2*). Two further assistants stand, respectively, on the surgeon's left (*3*) and on the first assistant's right (*4*). The scrub nurse (*N*) stands on the surgeon's right

# Steps Shared by Total and Subtotal Gastrectomy

2

Pierpaolo Stortoni, Emilio Feliciotti, Raffaella Ridolfo, and Walter Siquini

There is no substitute for a well-planned and conducted operation on the stomach to provide the best possible surgical outcome. Correct and stable positioning of the patient is the first step for a successful operation, as well as a careful monitoring of the vital parameters by the anesthetist and a great attention on prevention and control of intraoperative hypothermia and of postoperative pain and malnutrition. Incision should be tailored on the surgical procedure and type of patient in order to provide the best exposure of the operating field, minimizing the risk of operation site infection. Exploration of the abdominal cavity and intraoperative cytology of peritoneal fluid or lavage are of paramount importance for tumor staging and prognosis. Then operation goes on through a gentle approach toward any anatomical structure and following precise steps of the surgical procedure. Detachment of the greater omentum from the transverse colon is followed by the division of the right gastroepiploic pedicle and of the pyloric vessels. The duodenum is then closed and resected. Finally, the left gastric vein and artery are divided.

P. Stortoni (✉)
Division of General Surgery,
"A. Murri" Hospital, Fermo, Italy
e-mail: pierpaolostortoni@libero.it

E. Feliciotti
Department of Surgery, "Ospedali Riuniti" University Hospital, Ancona, Italy
e-mail: feliciotti@live.it

R. Ridolfo
Division of General Surgery, Senigallia General Hospital, Senigallia, Italy
e-mail: raffaella.ridolfo@email.it

W. Siquini
Division of General Surgery,
"Madonna del Soccorso" Hospital,
San Benedetto del Tronto, Italy
e-mail: walter.siquini@sanita.marche.it

W. Siquini (ed.), *Total, Subtotal and Proximal Gastrectomy in Cancer: A Color Atlas*,
DOI 10.1007/978-88-470-5749-4_2, © Springer-Verlag Italia 2015

## 2.1 Incision

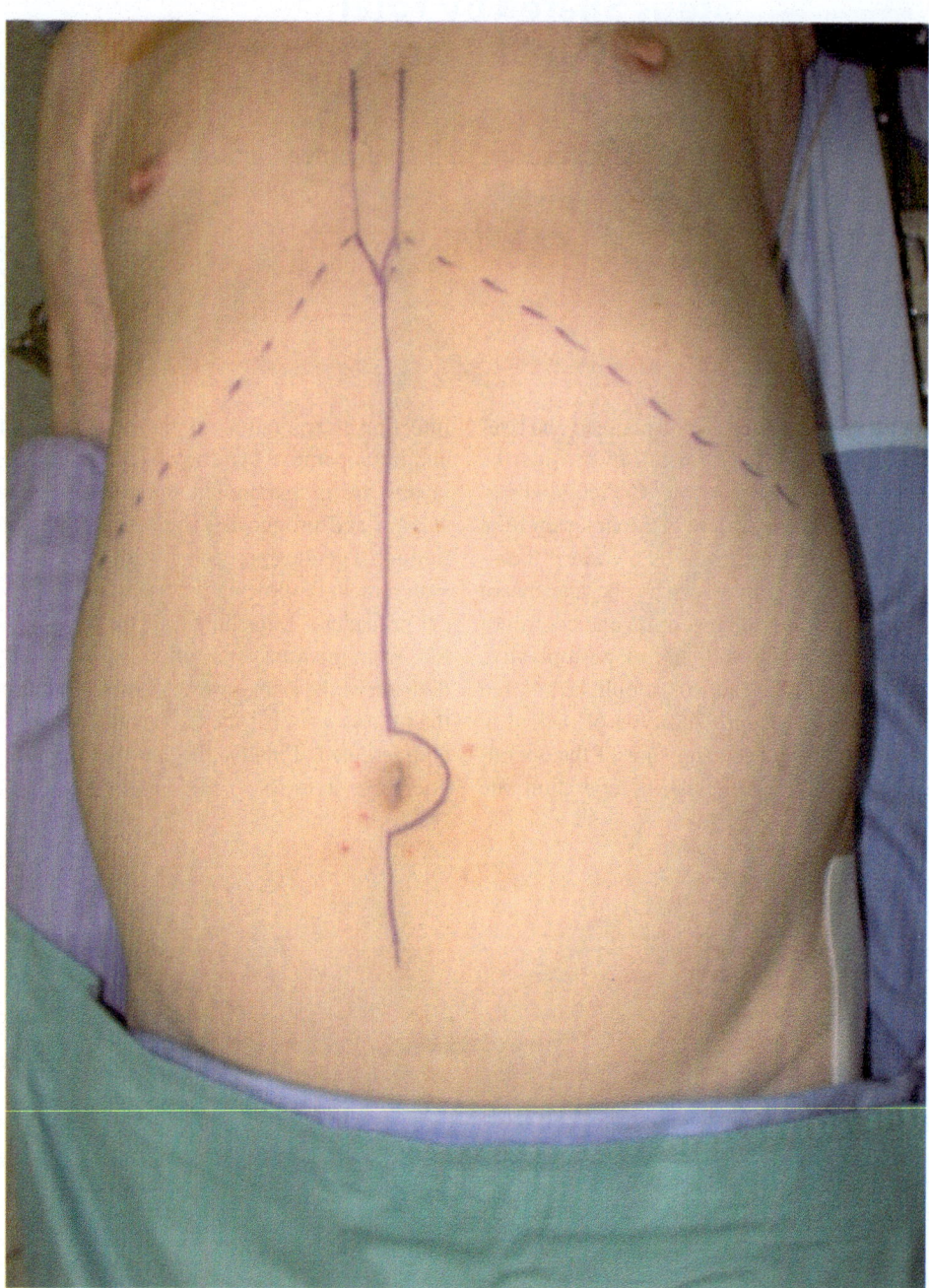

**Figs. 2.1, 2.2, and 2.3** After having disinfected the operating field by passing in succession two gauze pads soaked in povidone-iodine (or benzalkonium chloride if the patient is allergic to iodine), a midline incision from the xiphoid process to below the umbilicus is the most common approach for total and subtotal gastrectomy in patients with normal stature and weight. To minimize the risk of operation site infection, a gauze laparotomy pad soaked in povidone-iodine or benzalkonium chloride should be secured to either side of the incision with three full-thickness sutures, to protect the tissue layers in direct contact with the operating field. The operative field is exposed using Ulrich and Guarducci retractors

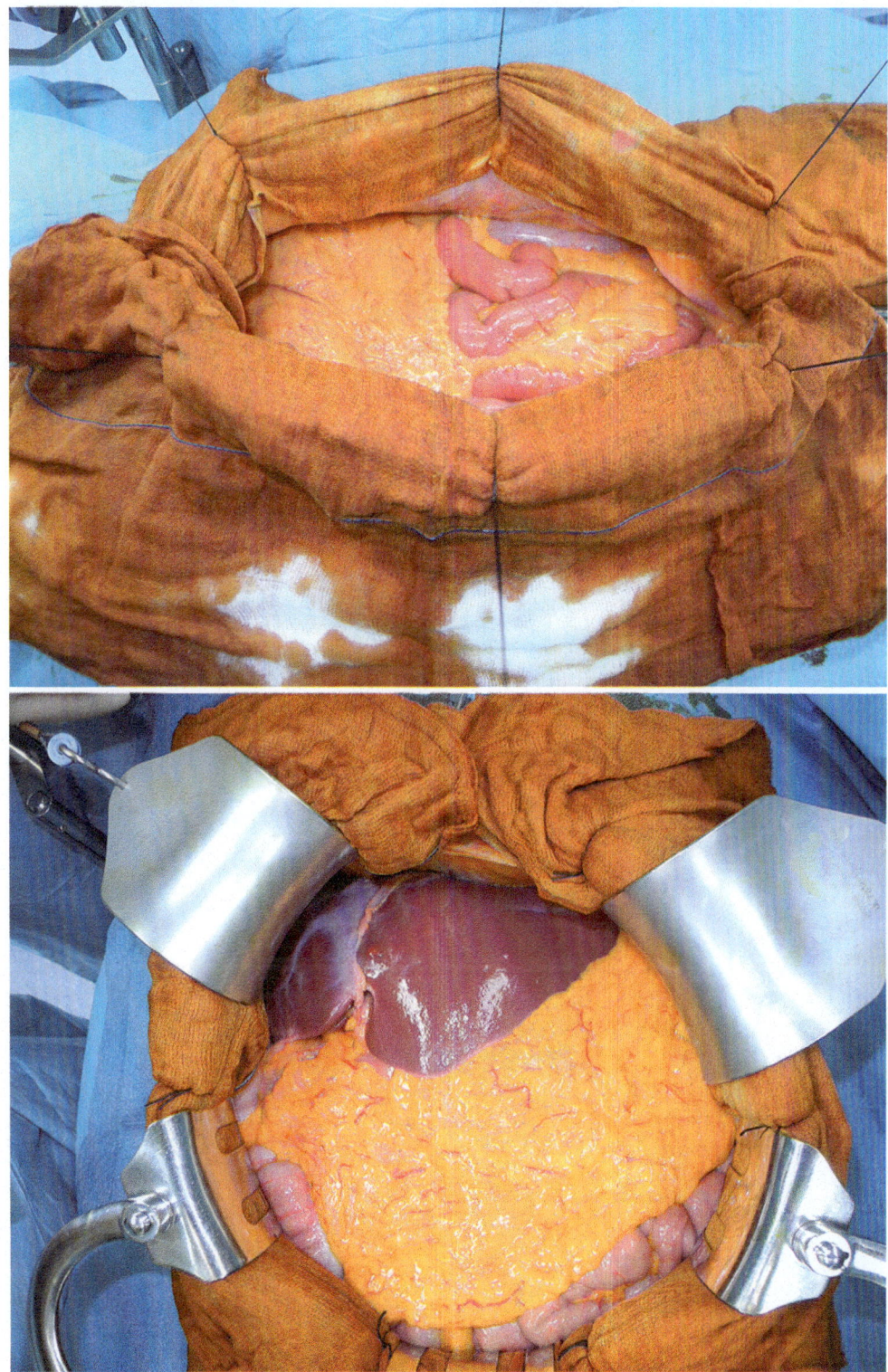

**Figs. 2.1, 2.2, and 2.3** (continued)

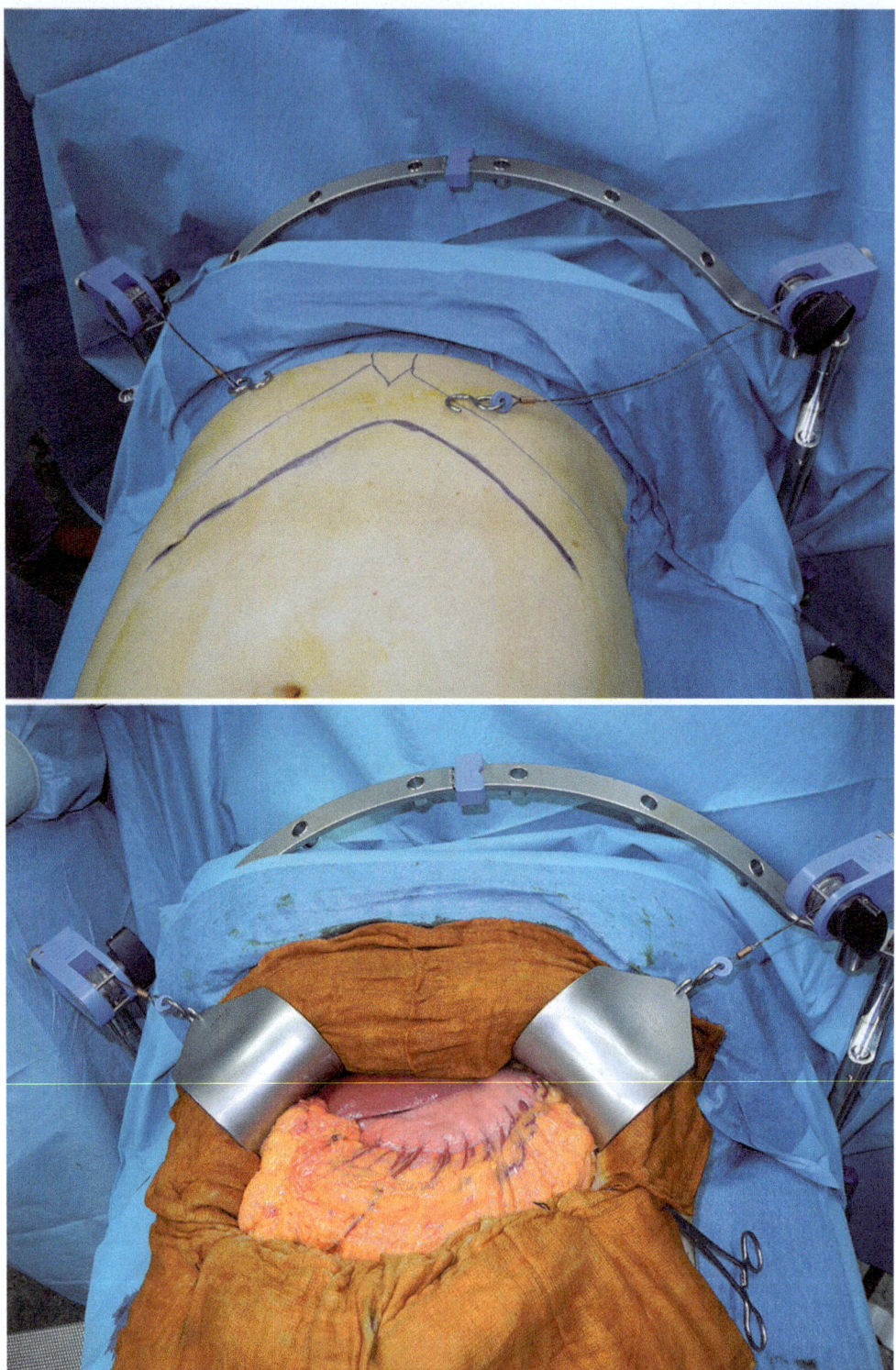

**Figs. 2.4 and 2.5** A bilateral subcostal incision provides better exposure in short and obese patients and in esophago-cardial tumors. The operative field is exposed using Ulrich or Kent or Rochard retractors

## 2.2   Exploration of the Abdominal Cavity and Lavage Cytology

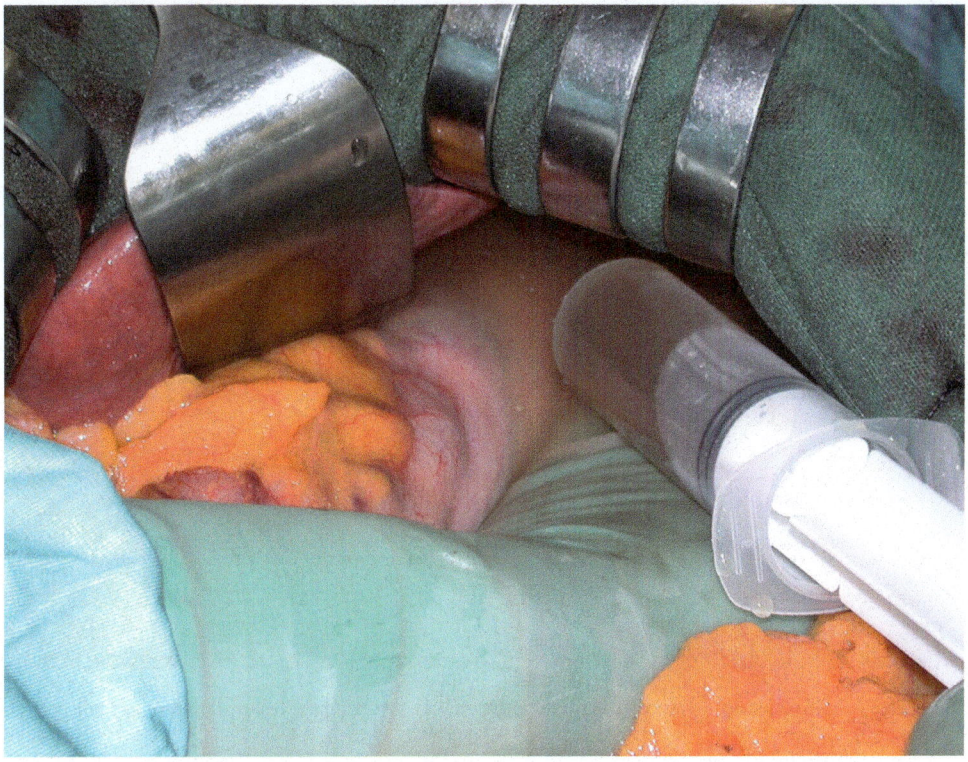

**Fig. 2.6** If no nodules of omental or peritoneal carcinosis are detected, but free fluid is found in the supramesocolic space, a sample of this is collected and submitted for intraoperative cytology. Otherwise, peritoneal lavage is performed with ca. 100 ml of saline poured upstream of the gastric wall involved by the neoplasm; the fluid is then recovered for intraoperative cytology

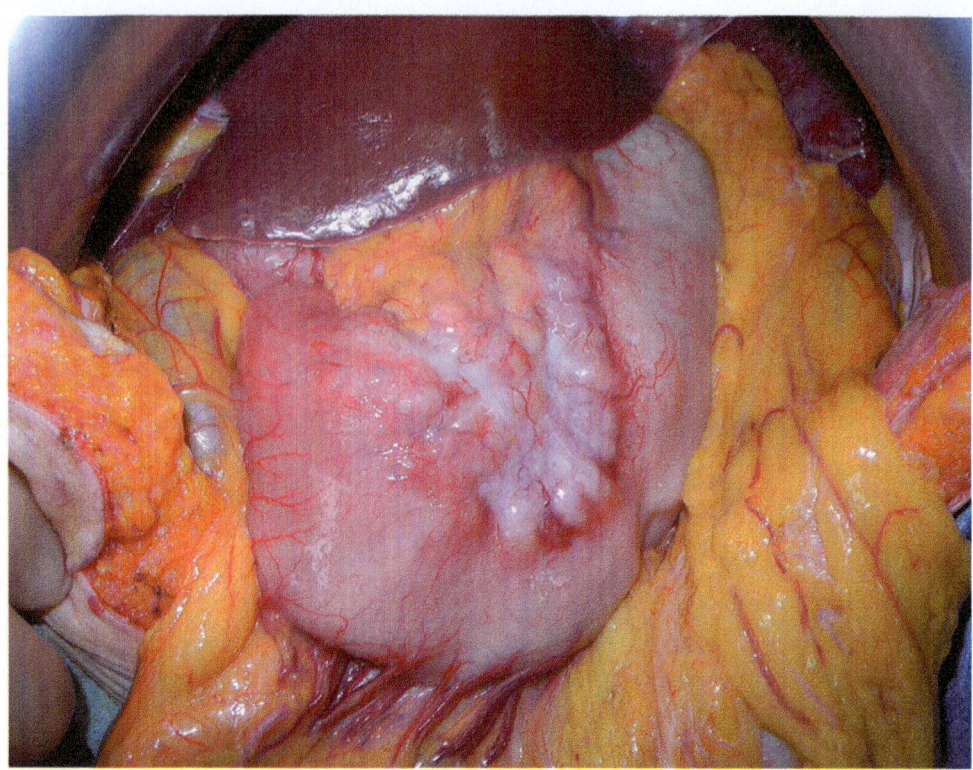

**Fig. 2.7** An example of locally advanced gastric tumor massively involving the lesser curvature and adjacent lymph nodes

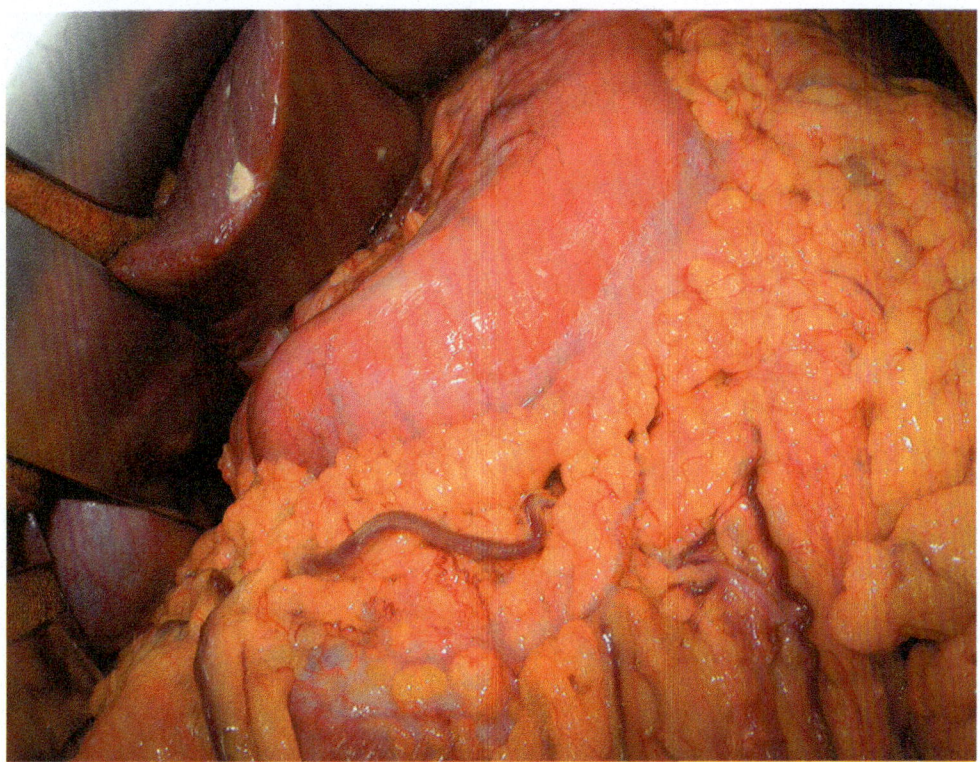

**Fig. 2.8** An example of gastric "linitis plastica," a diffuse intramurally infiltrating type of cancer in which the neoplastic cells invade throughout the stomach, resulting in the thickening and rigidity of the stomach wall. This stiff walled organ is also called "leather bottle stomach"

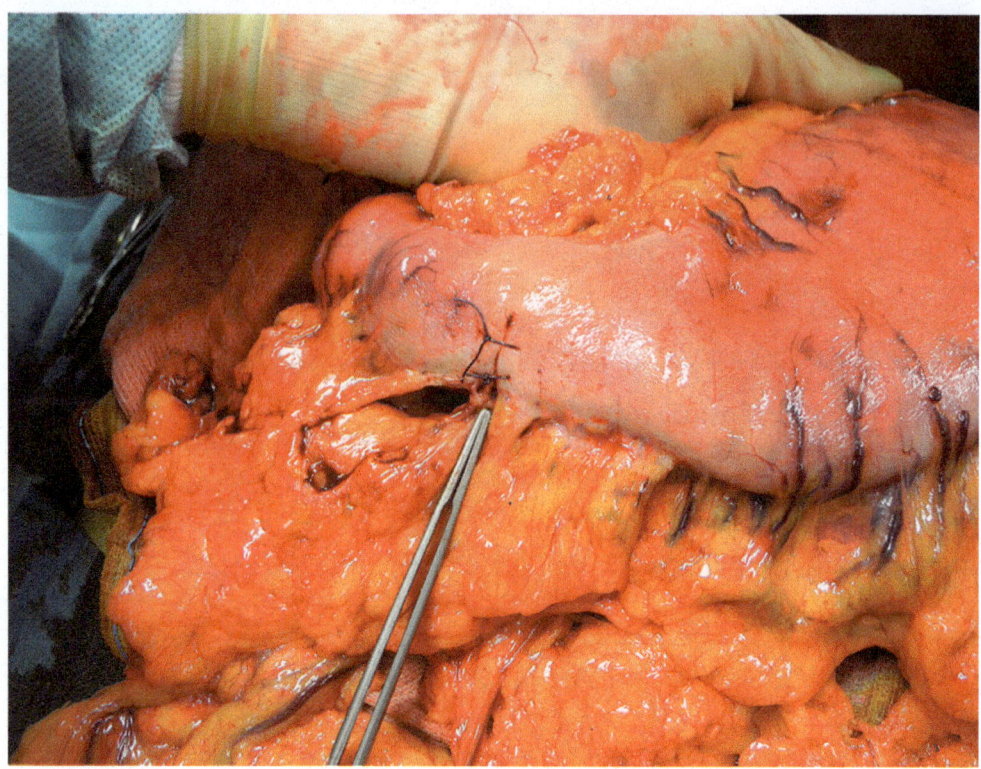

**Fig. 2.9** Since diagnosis of gastric "linitis plastica" through endoscopic biopsies is frequently difficult to obtain, an intraoperative full-thickness gastric wall biopsy is necessary to confirm the diagnosis of malignancy

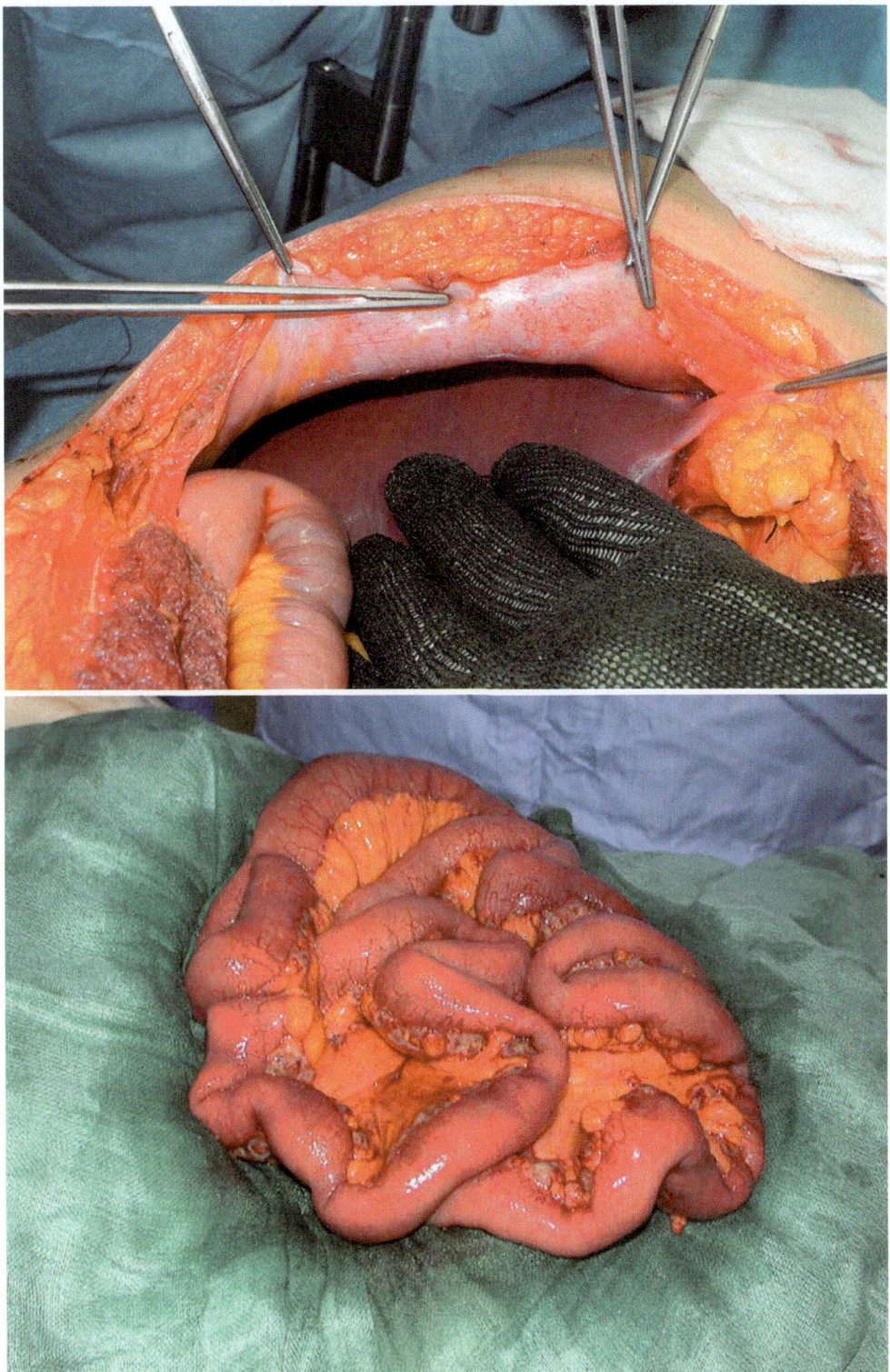

**Figs. 2.10, 2.11, and 2.12**  The supra- and inframesocolic spaces are explored for nodules of peritoneal, visceral, and omental carcinosis

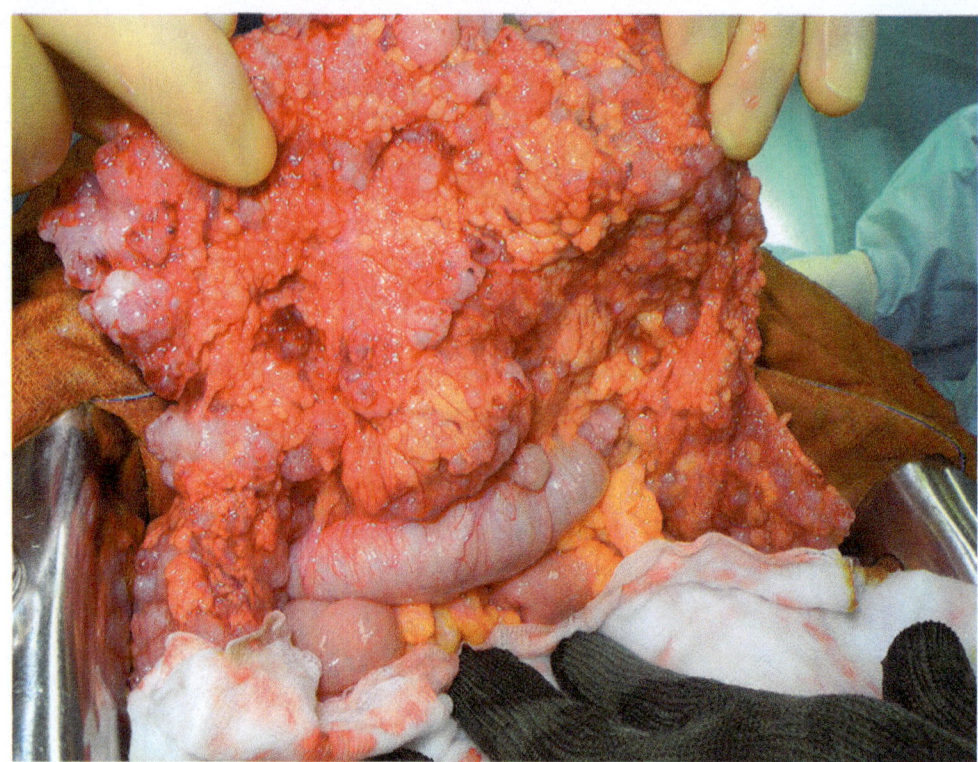

**Figs. 2.10, 2.11, and 2.12** (continued)

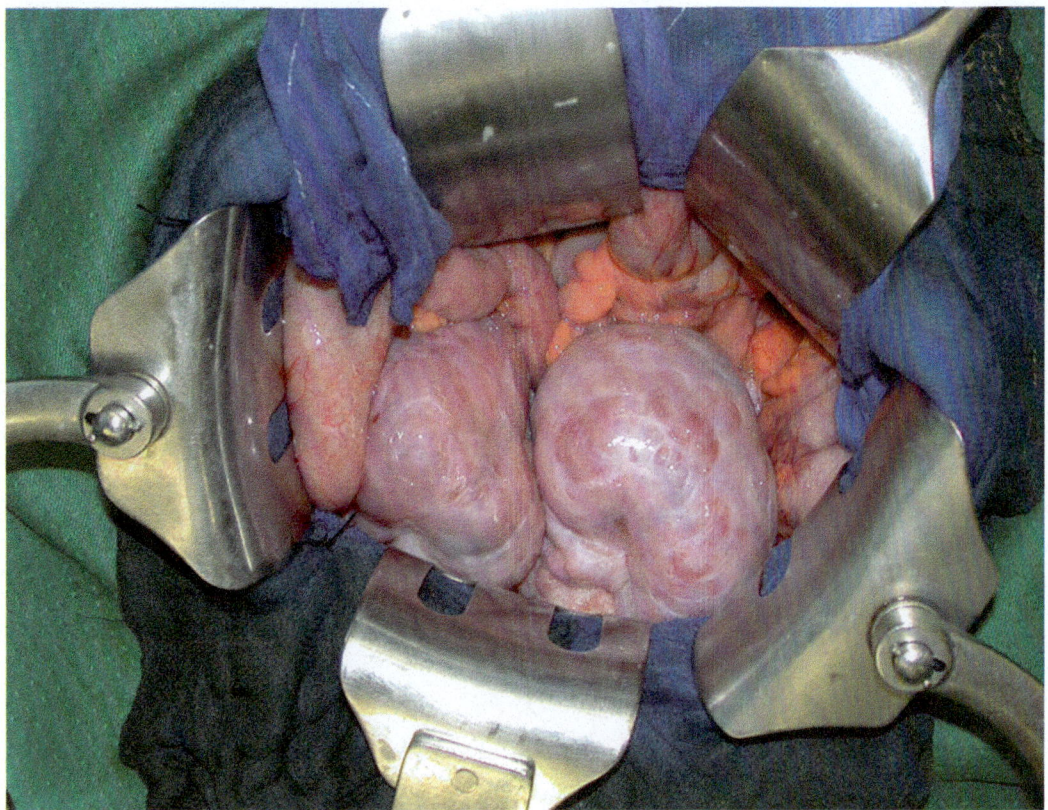

**Fig. 2.13** In female patients the ovaries are inspected to exclude metastatic disease (Krukenberg tumor)

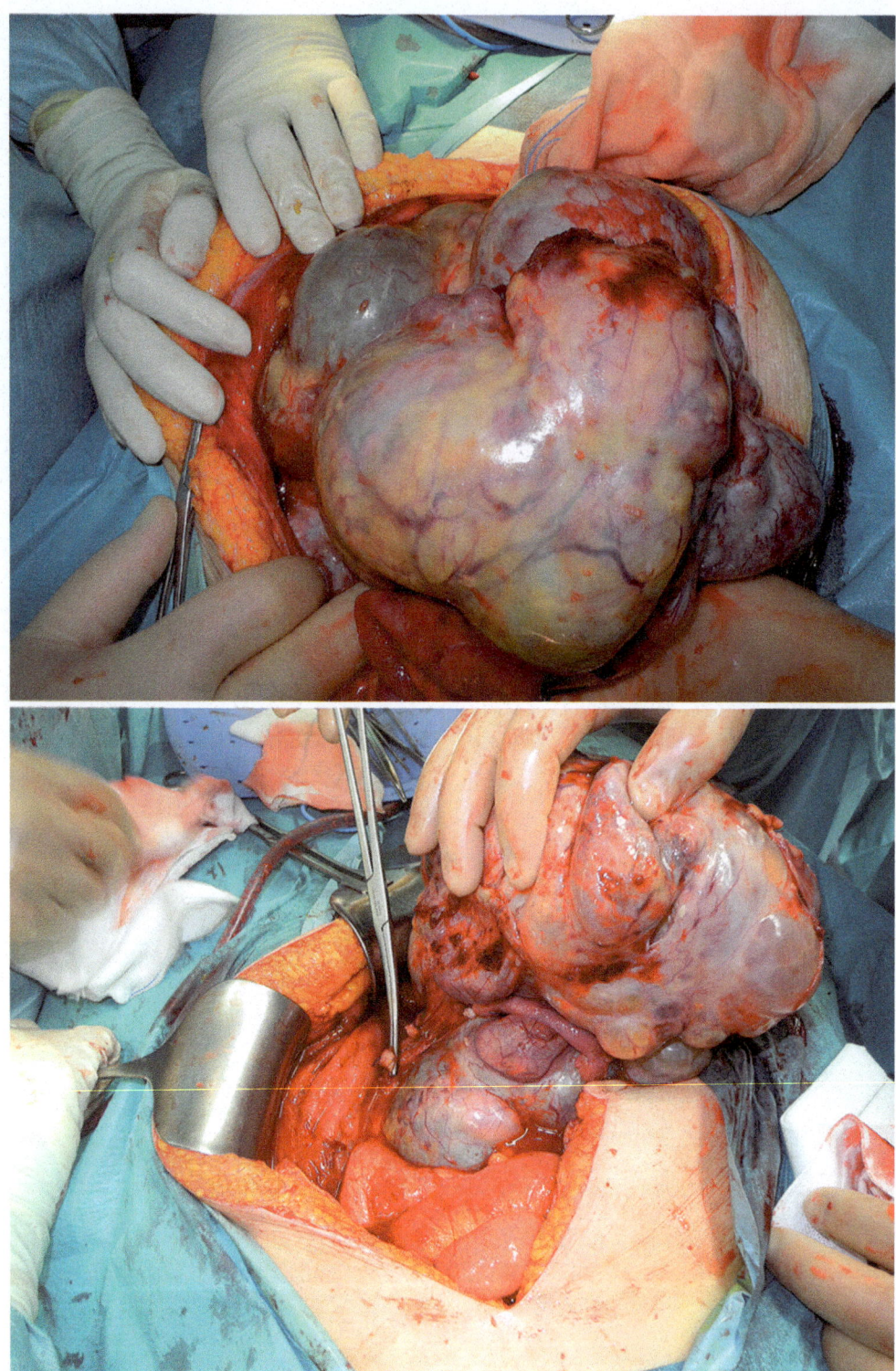

**Figs. 2.14 and 2.15** An extraordinary example of large bilateral Krukenberg tumor that causes an abdominal compartment syndrome by occupying more than half of the abdominal cavity volume

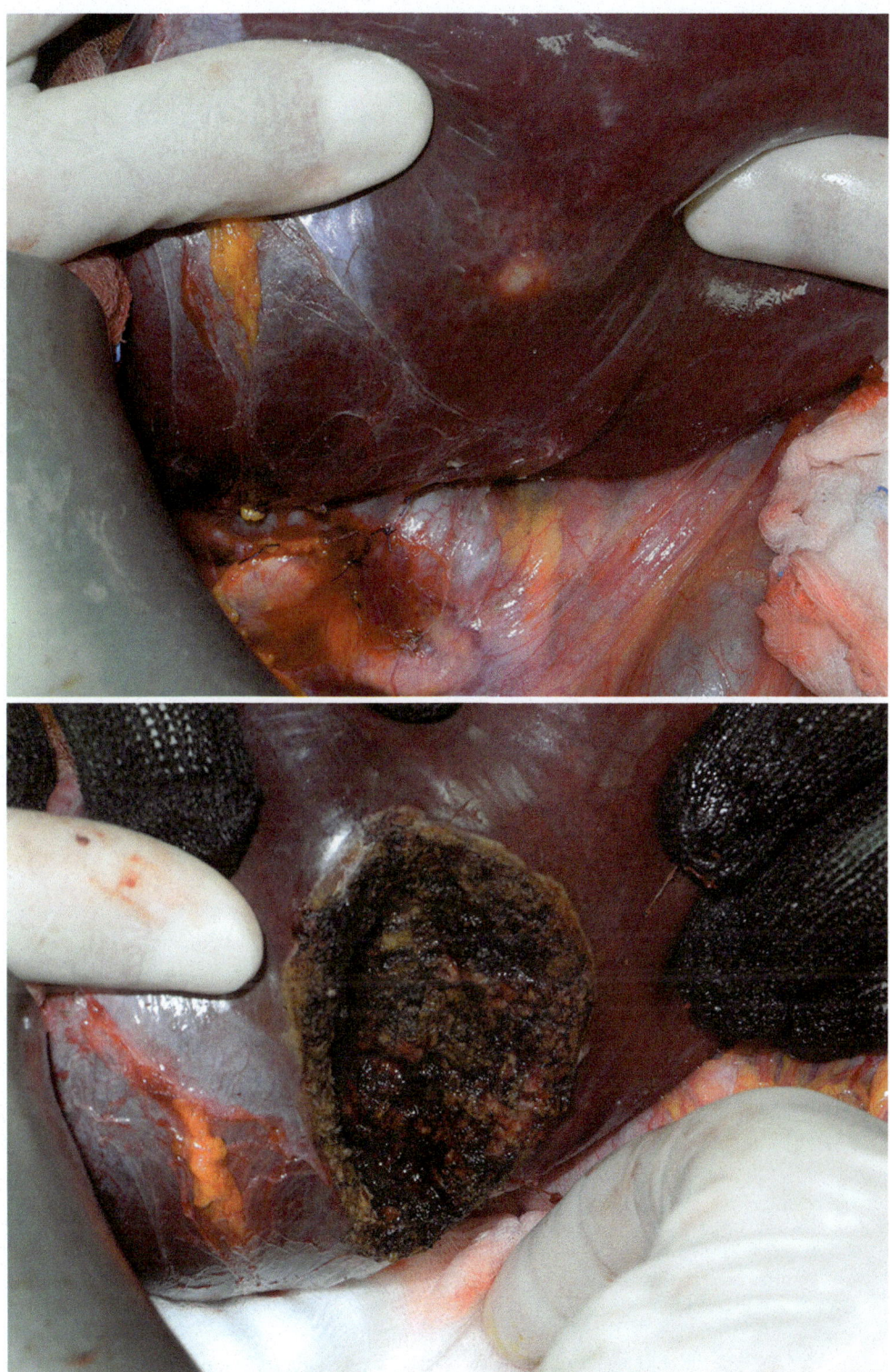

**Figs. 2.16 and 2.17** The liver is inspected, palpated, and subjected to ultrasound examination, to rule out any metastases not documented on preoperative CT or MR. The single and peripheral lesion is removed before gastrectomy

## 2.3 Detachment of the Greater Omentum from the Transverse Colon

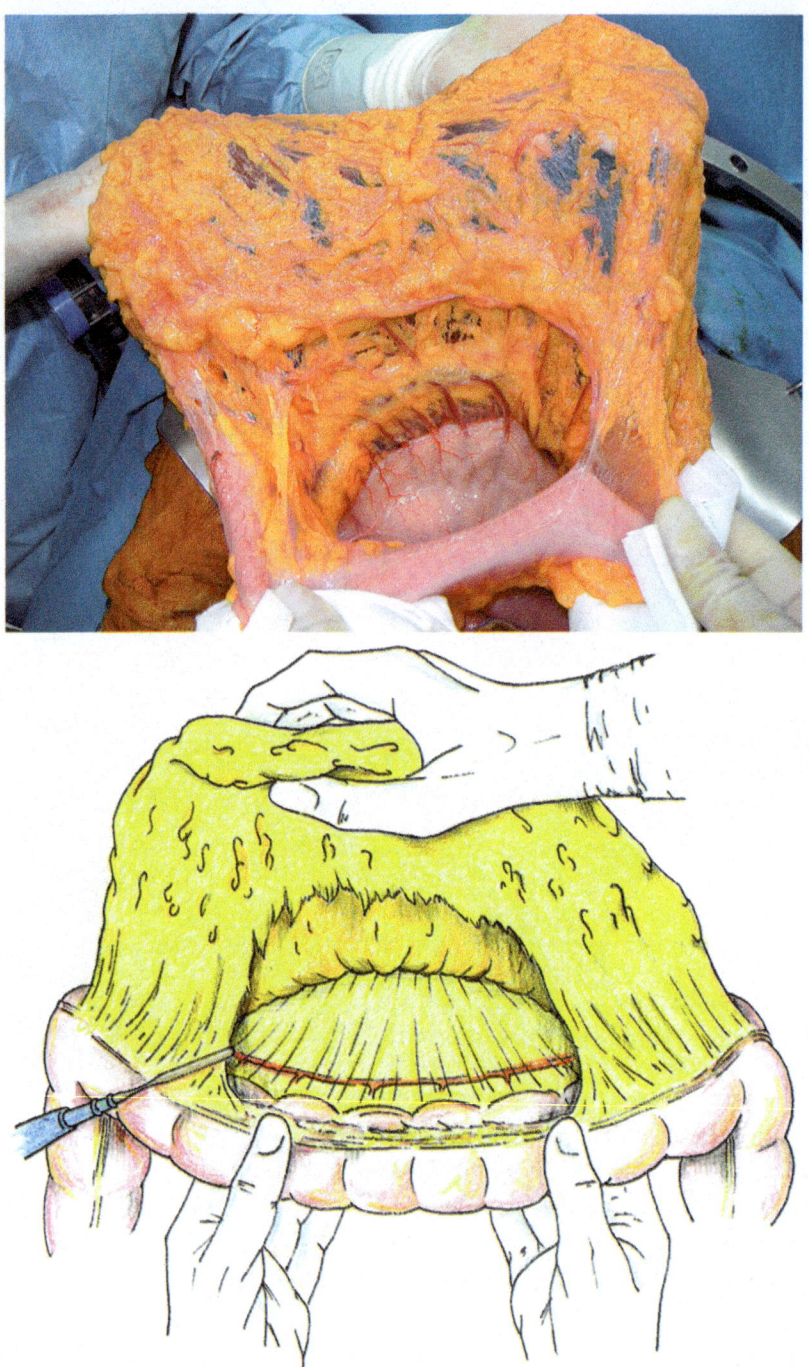

**Figs. 2.18 and 2.19** The surgeon identifies the avascular embryonic fusion plane between the greater omentum and the anterior layer of the transverse mesocolon and divides it from right to left. Complete detachment of the greater omentum from the transverse colon provides access to the lesser sac and exposure of the posterior wall of the stomach, anterior surface of the pancreas, right gastroepiploic vascular pedicle, and first and second portion of the duodenum. This leaves the right and left gastroepiploic arcade and the omentum attached to the stomach, allowing their en bloc removal

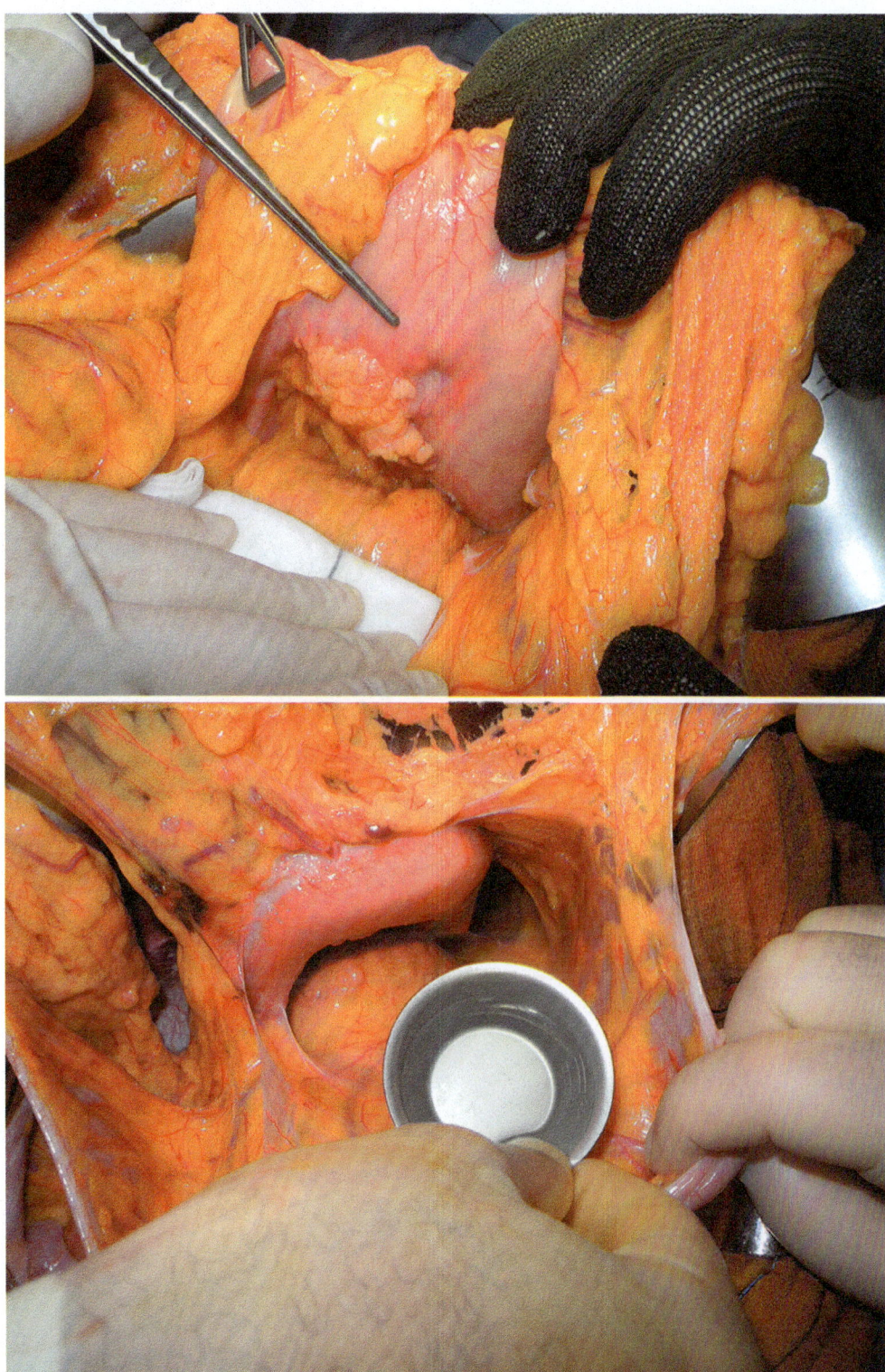

**Figs. 2.20 and 2.21** An example of tumor infiltrating the serosa of the posterior wall of the stomach. In this case, the exploration may show peritoneal carcinosis involving exclusively the lesser sac. In the absence of car-cinosis, more accurate staging is provided by sampling the fluid that may be found in the lesser sac. If no fluid is found, the neoplasm is flushed with saline, and the solution is recovered for intraoperative cytology

## 2.4    Division of the Gastroepiploic Pedicle

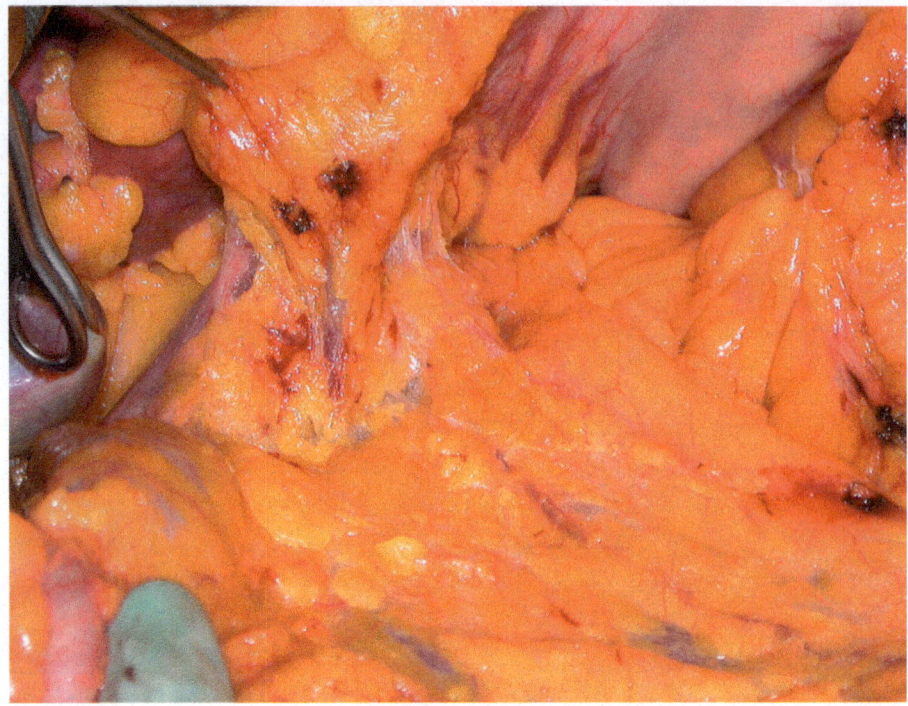

**Fig. 2.22** Detachment of the greater omentum from the transverse colon allows exposure of the right gastroepiploic pedicle

**Fig. 2.23** The right gastroepiploic vein and artery are isolated and divided at their origin between double ligatures

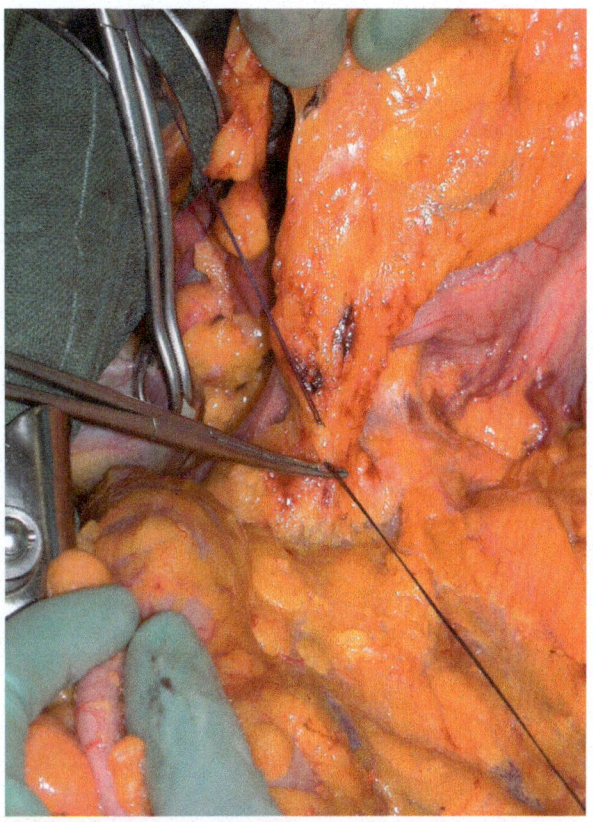

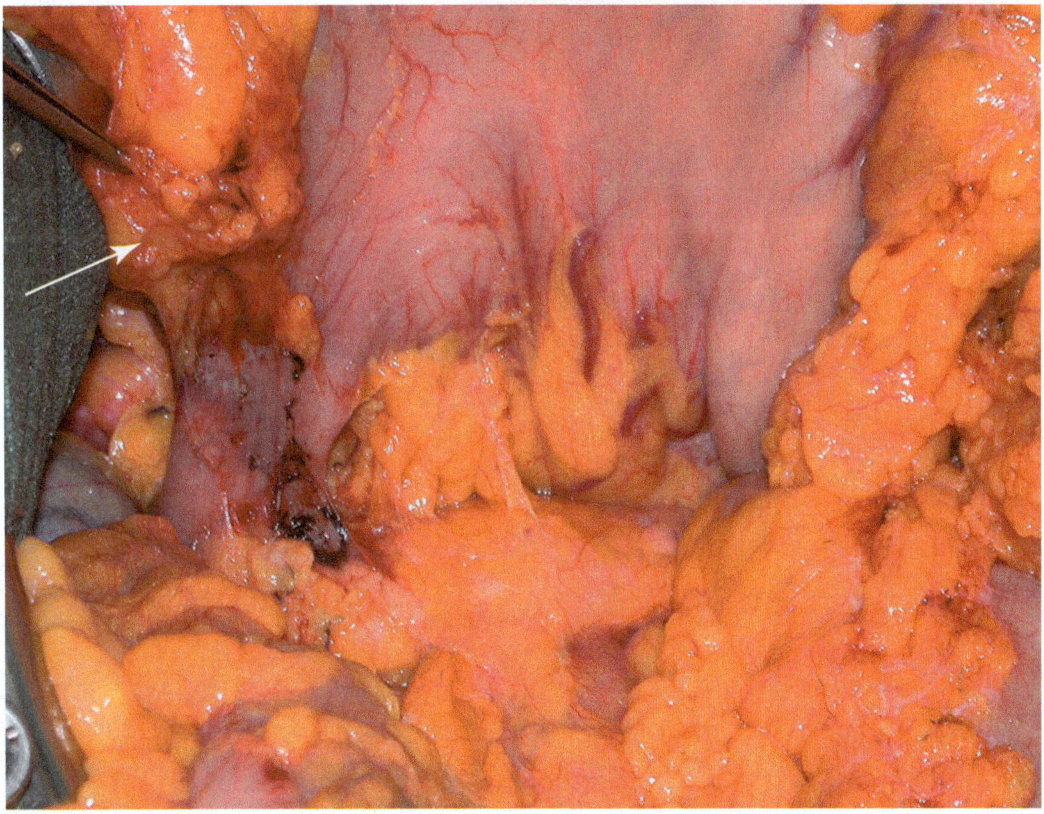

**Fig. 2.24** The infrapyloric lymph nodes (station 6, *arrow*) remain attached to the stomach

## 2.5    Division of Pyloric Vessels

**Figs. 2.25 and 2.26**
Isolation and division of the
right gastric vessels

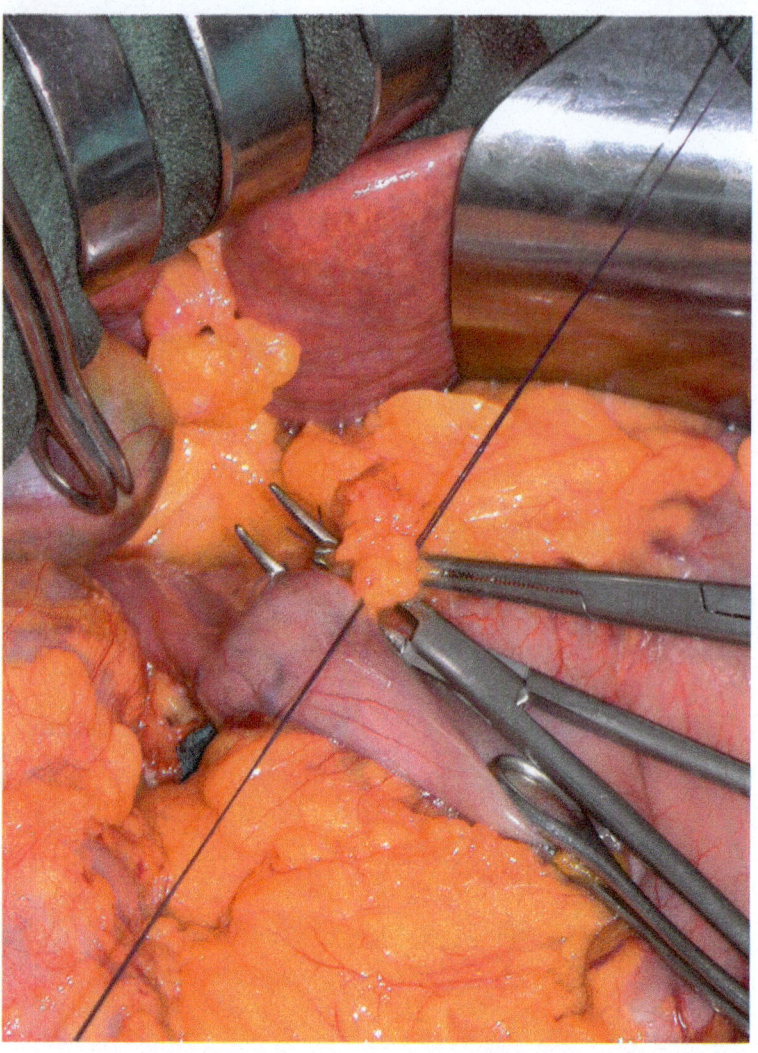

**Figs. 2.25 and
2.26**  (continued)

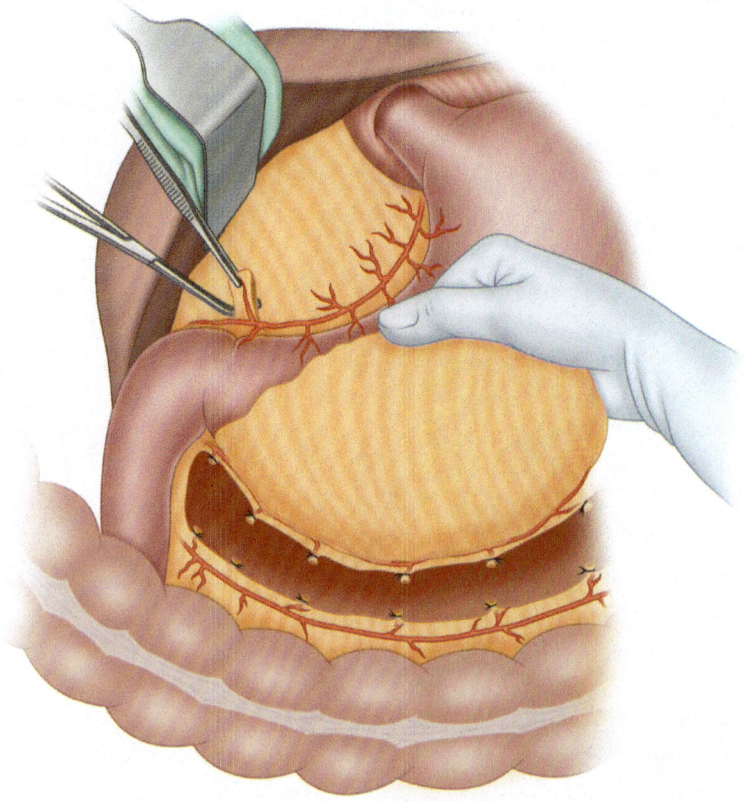

## 2.6    Duodenal Transection

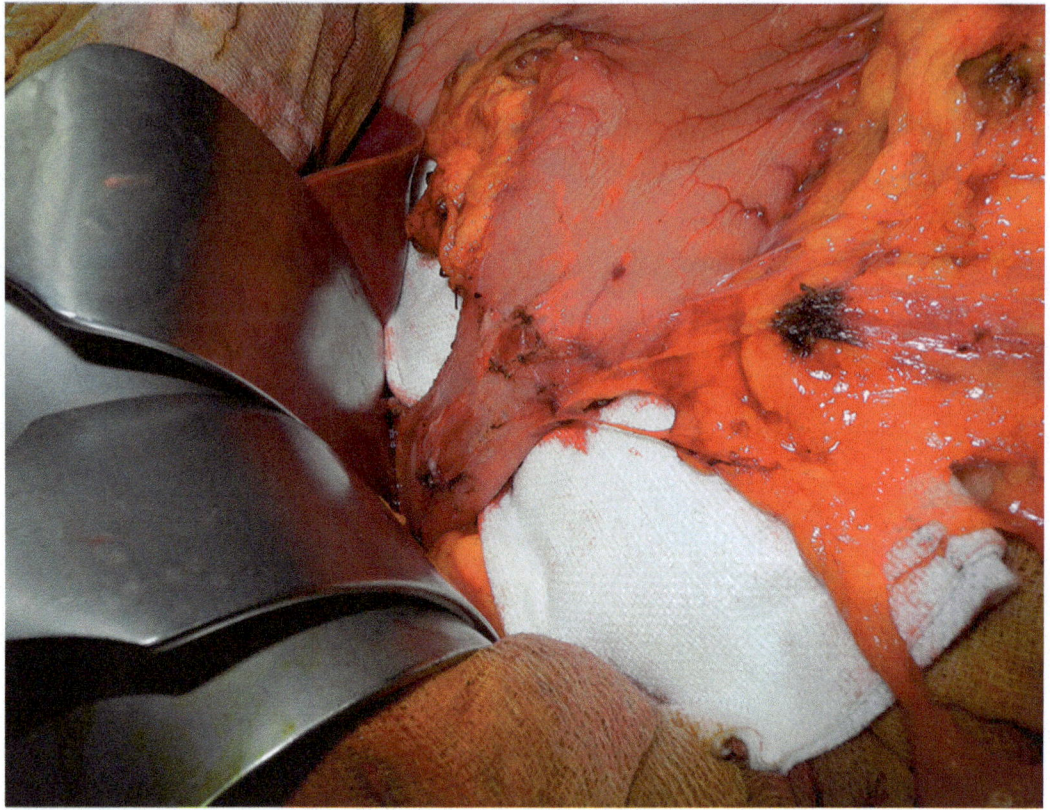

**Fig. 2.27** Anterior and posterior dissection of the pylorus and the duodenal bulb is performed for at least 3–4 cm

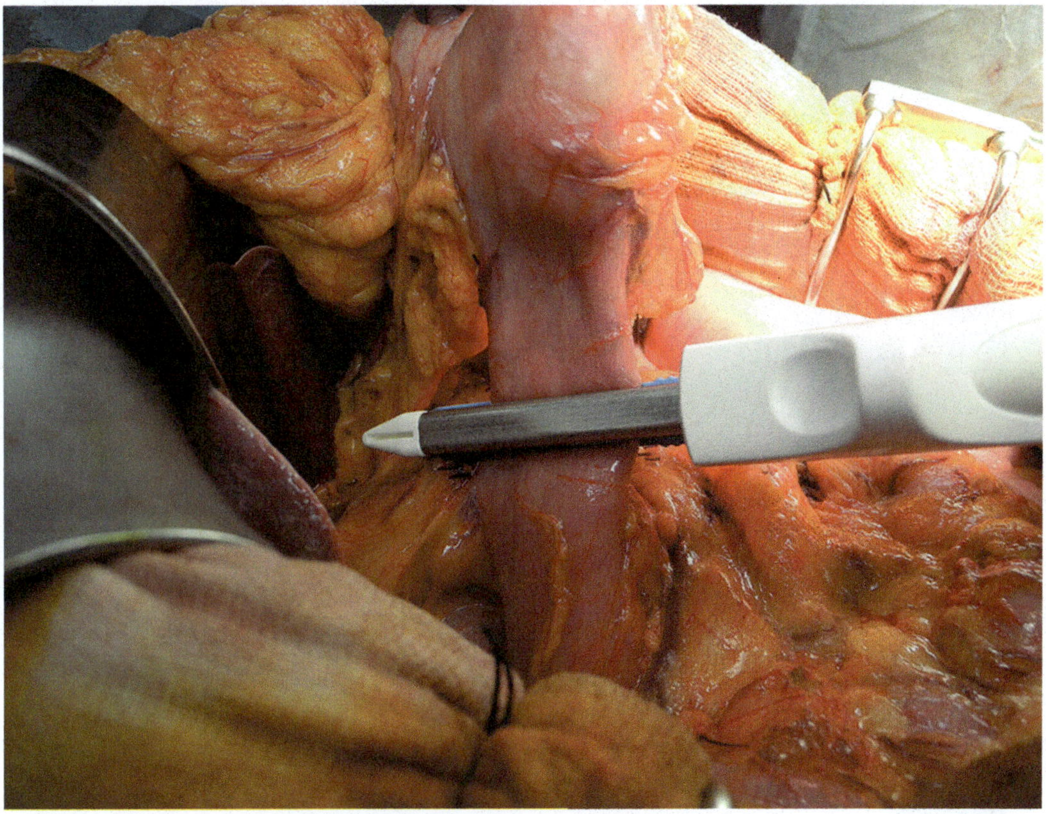

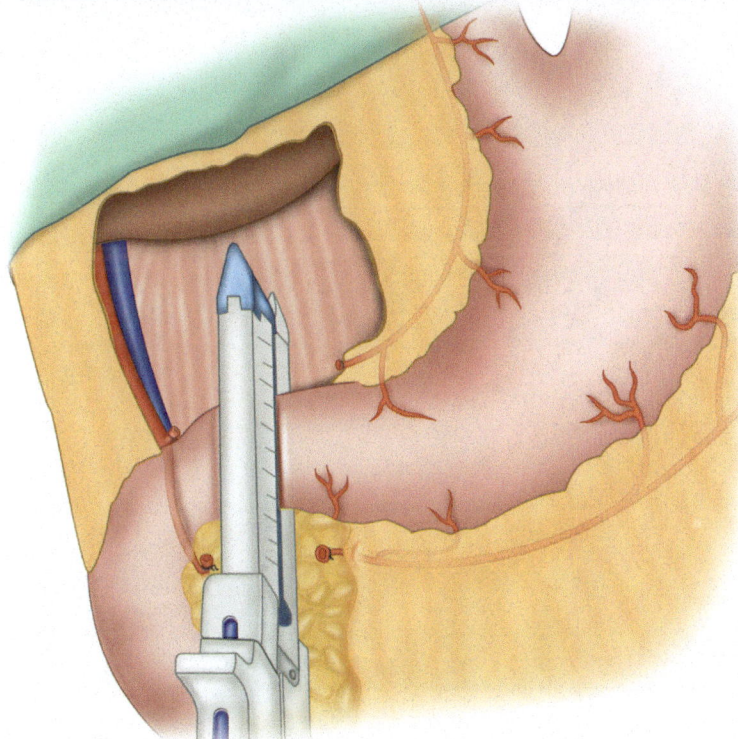

**Figs. 2.28 and 2.29** A mechanical linear stapler (GIA 55) is placed 2–3 cm below the pylorus leaving an inferior margin of duodenal wall of at least 1 cm to allow subsequent oversewing. After identification of the ideal resection level, the stapler's jaws are locked

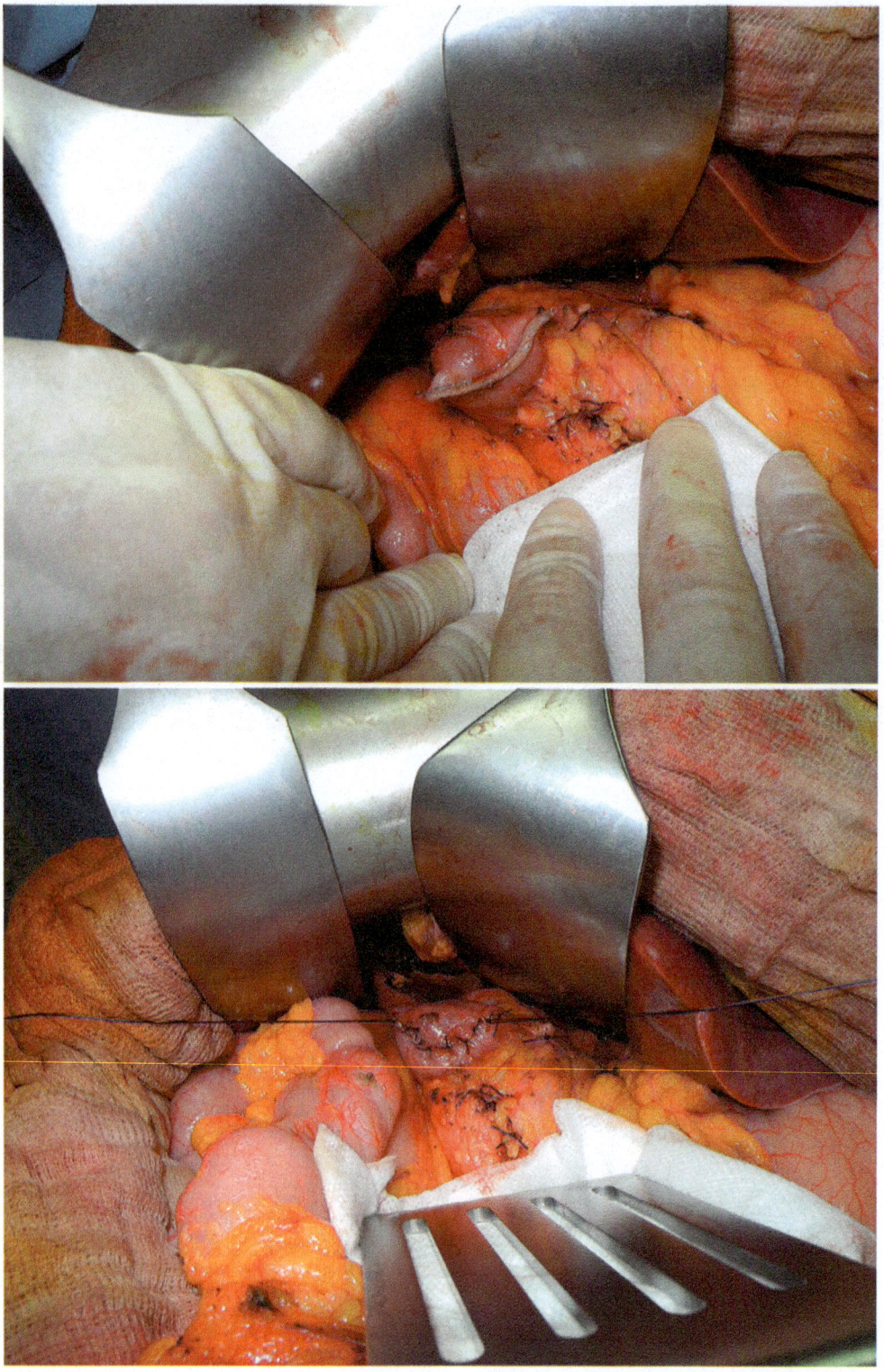

**Figs. 2.30, 2.31, and 2.32** The duodenum is closed and resected. A tampon soaked in povidone-iodine is passed on both stumps to minimize microcontamination. The sta- pler line of the duodenal stump is oversewn with inter- rupted seromuscular sutures using absorbable braided 3-0 thread, to reduce the risk of leakage

**Figs. 2.30, 2.31, and 2.32** (continued)

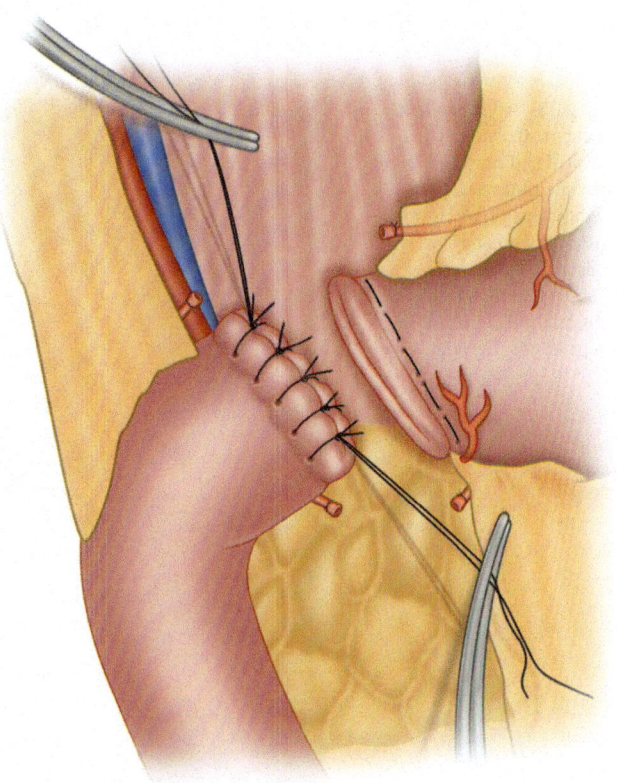

## 2.7    Division of the Left Gastric Pedicle

**Fig. 2.33** After duodenal resection, the stomach is elevated and retracted over the subcostal retractor, slightly tensioning its posterior wall and consequently the left gastric pedicle, which is thus easily identified and prepared for division

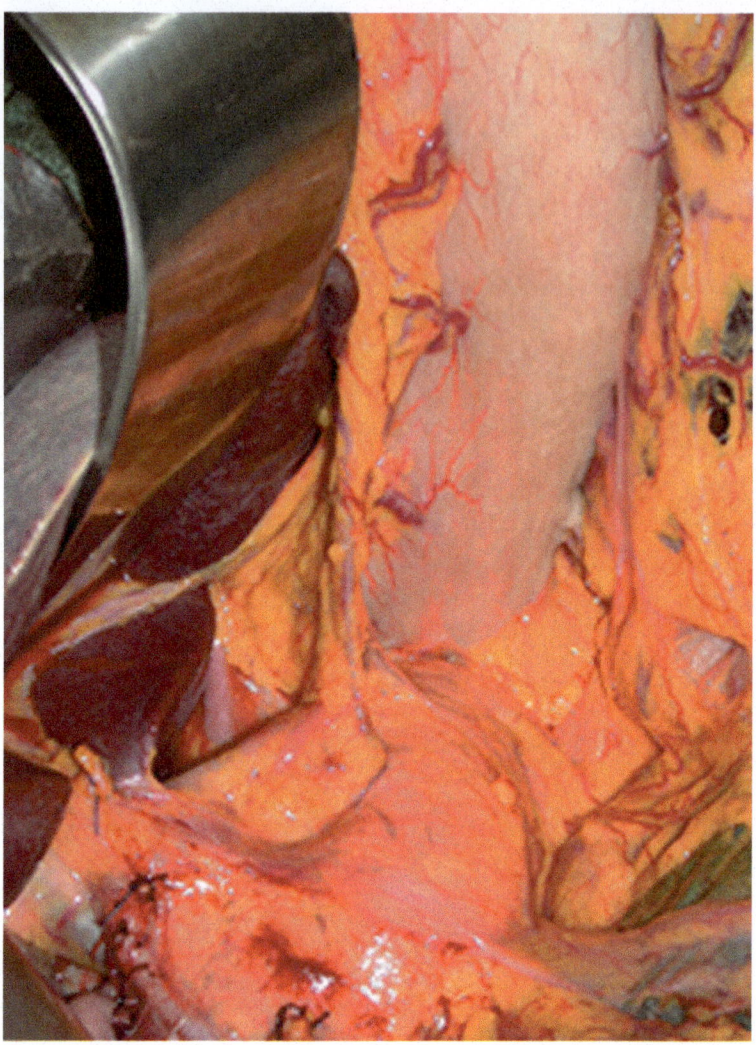

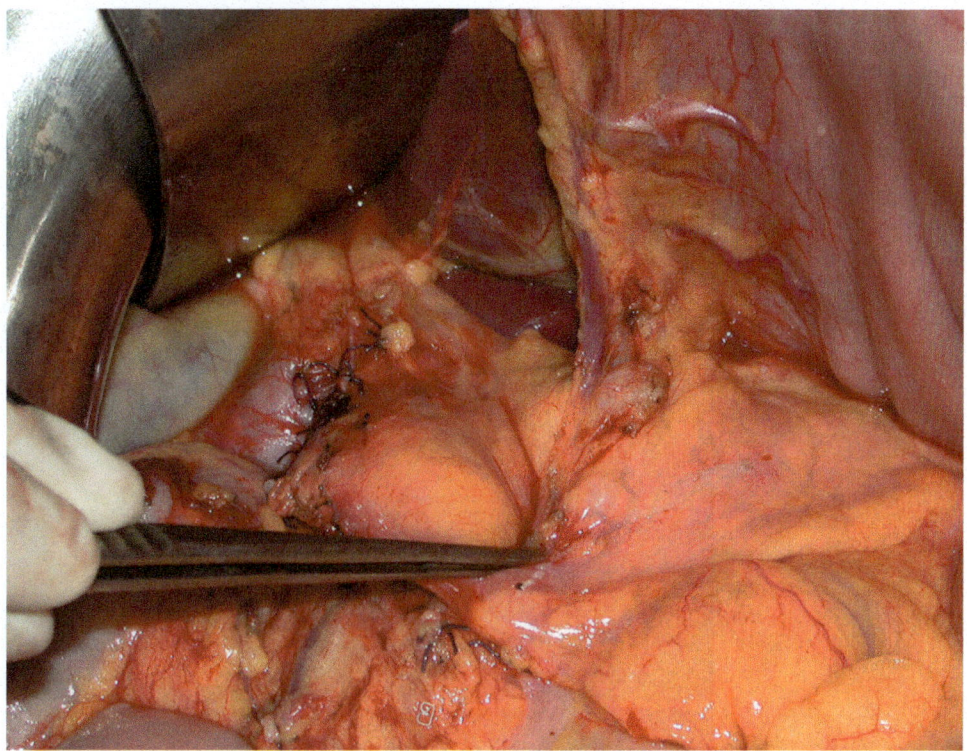

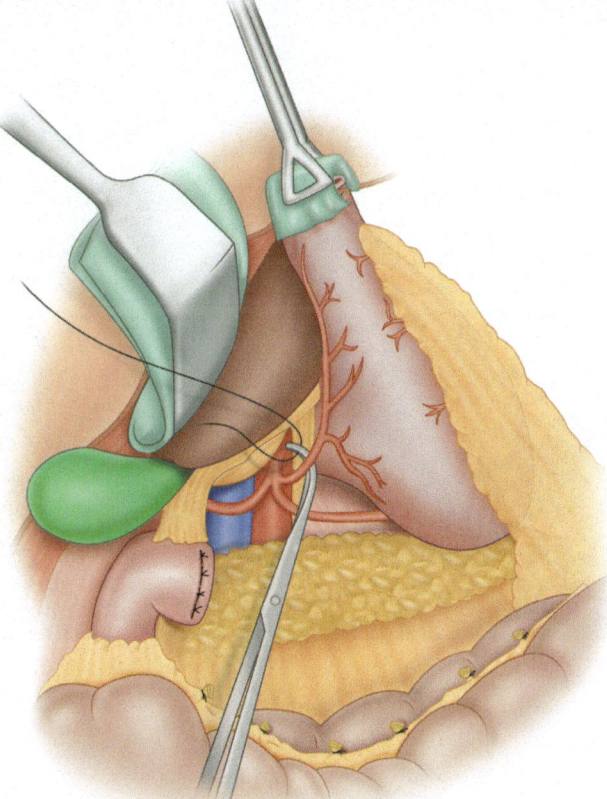

**Figs. 2.34 and 2.35** With the stomach elevated and retracted upward, the left gastric vein is usually seen anterior to the artery. The left gastric vein is dissected first and ligated at its origin, and then the artery, which is found immediately behind it, is resected at its origin with double ligature

**Figs. 2.36 and 2.37** Care must be taken during the dissection of the left gastric pedicle in order to detect a left hepatic artery originating from the left gastric artery (*red arrow*). It is a quite common vascular anomaly, since its incidence is reported to be 11.5 %. An accurate evaluation of the preoperative arterial phase CT scans enables to detect this anatomical variation prior to surgery

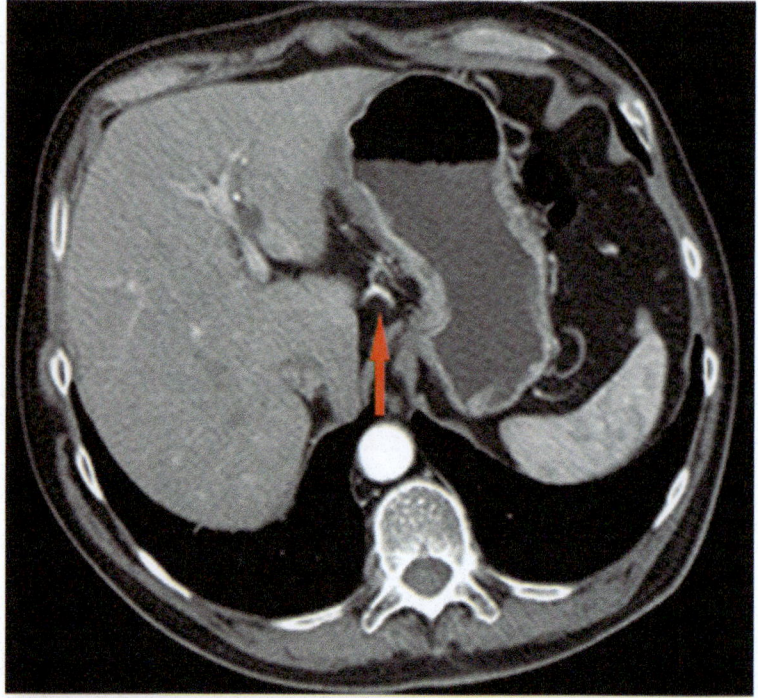

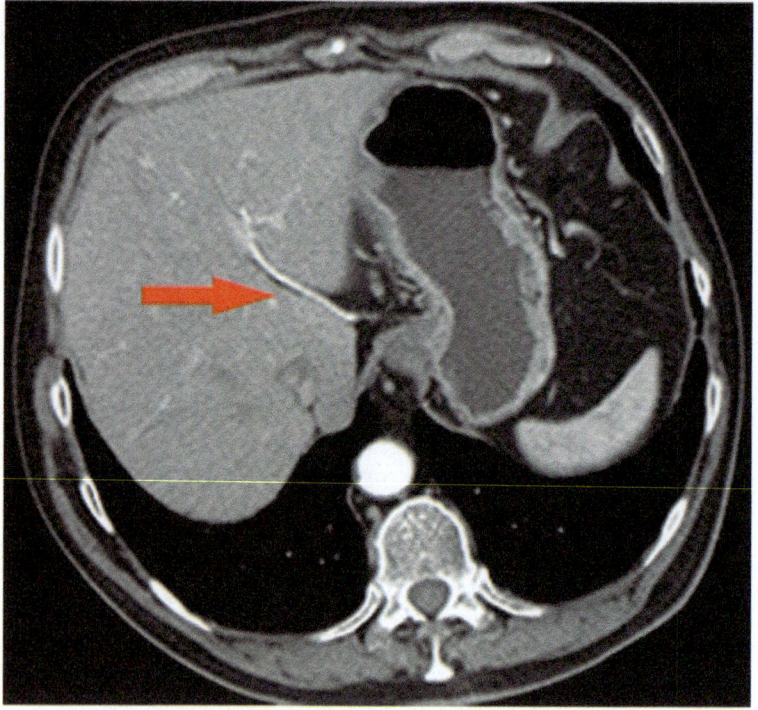

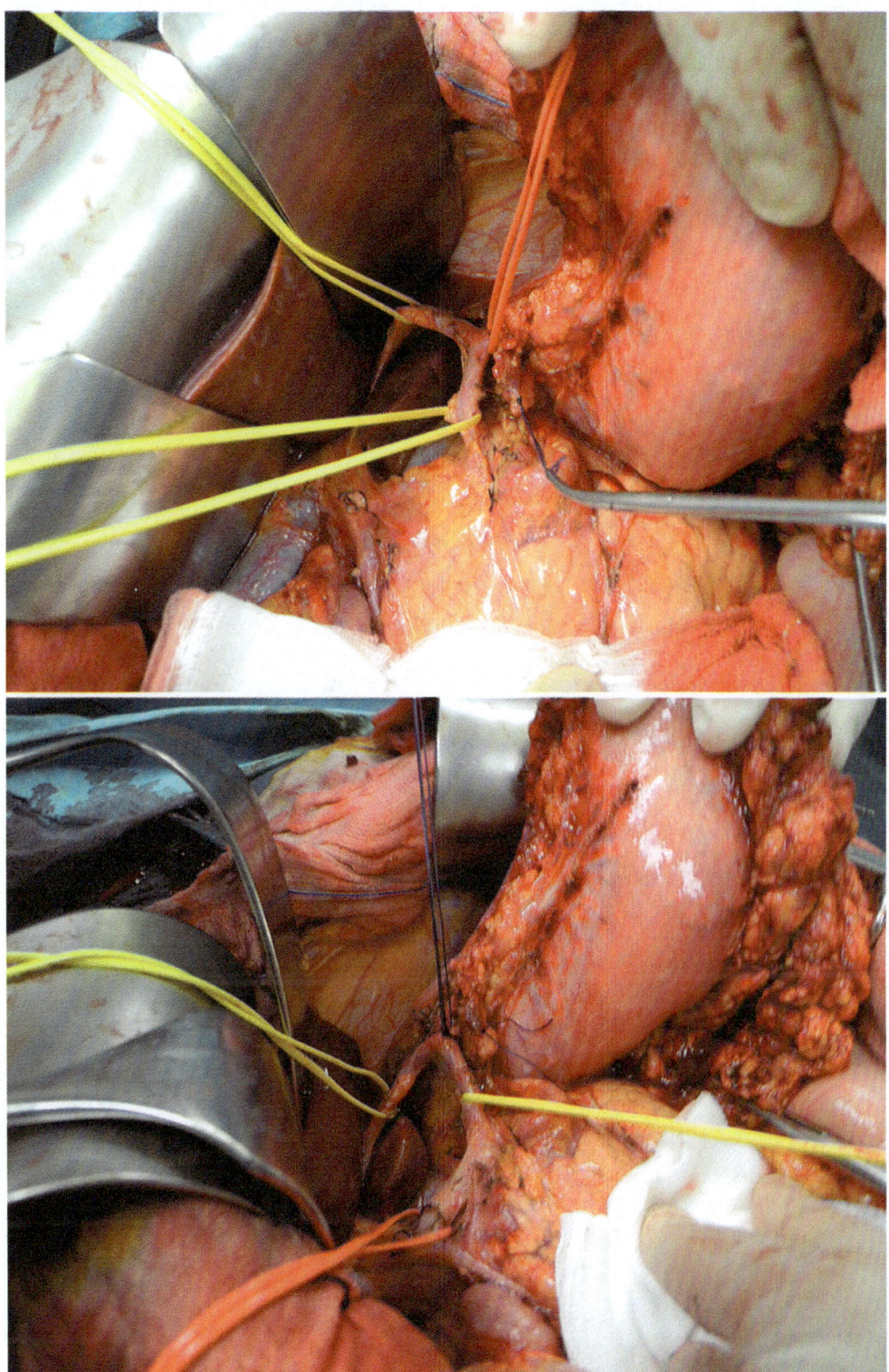

**Figs. 2.38 and 2.39** A left hepatic artery originating from the left gastric artery must be preserved, especially if it is relatively large in diameter, to avoid possible ischemia and dysfunction of the left lobe of the liver. This means that the left gastric artery must be selectively divided just below the origin of the anomalous left hepatic artery

# Total Gastrectomy

**3**

Emilio Feliciotti, Raffaella Ridolfo, Pierpaolo Stortoni, and Walter Siquini

The optimal surgical management of gastric cancer must be tailored to the extent and location of the disease. In the absence of distant metastatic spread, aggressive surgical resection of the gastric tumor is justified. In general, surgical resection of gastric cancer involves a wide enough resection to achieve negative margins as well as en bloc resection of lymph nodes and any adherent organ(s). The goal of curative surgical treatment is resection of all tumor (i.e., R0 resection). Thus all margins (proximal, distal, radial) should be negative and an adequate lymphadenectomy performed. Since gastric tumors are characterized by extensive intramural spread, the surgeon strives for a grossly negative proximal and distal margin of at least 4–6 cm, with intraoperative frozen section confirmation of histologically negative margins, to ensure a low rate of anastomotic recurrence. The appropriate surgical procedure should be determined by the location of the tumor and the known pattern of spread. Total gastrectomy generally is indicated for tumors of the body and fundus of the stomach.

In 1884 Connor attempted the first total gastrectomy in humans, but his patient did not survive the operation. In 1897 Schlatter carried out the first successful total gastrectomy. In 1892 Roux described a new procedure where the second jejunal loop was divided and the distal limb was joined to the esophagus. The proximal limb of the loop was anastomosed to the jejunum some 60 cm distal to the esophagus. Currently, Roux-en-Y reconstruction is still the most widely used procedure after total gastrectomy.

E. Feliciotti (✉)
Department of Surgery, "Ospedali Riuniti" University Hospital, Ancona, Italy
e-mail: feliciotti@live.it

R. Ridolfo
Division of General Surgery, Senigallia General Hospital, Senigallia, Italy
e-mail: raffaella.ridolfo@email.it

P. Stortoni
Division of General Surgery, "A. Murri" Hospital, Fermo, Italy
e-mail: pierpaolostortoni@libero.it

W. Siquini
Division of General Surgery, "Madonna del Soccorso" Hospital, San Benedetto del Tronto, Italy
e-mail: walter.siquini@sanita.marche.it

W. Siquini (ed.), *Total, Subtotal and Proximal Gastrectomy in Cancer: A Color Atlas*, DOI 10.1007/978-88-470-5749-4_3, © Springer-Verlag Italia 2015

## 3.1    Division of the Lesser Omentum

**Figs. 3.1 and 3.2** The inferior (pars flaccida) and superior (pars condensa) portions of the lesser omentum are resected close to the liver, so that they can be removed en bloc with the stomach. If the lesser omentum is divided up to the right crus of the diaphragm and the right esophageal wall, the lymphatic and adipose tissue of the lesser curvature and the right paracardial lymph nodes will remain attached to the stomach

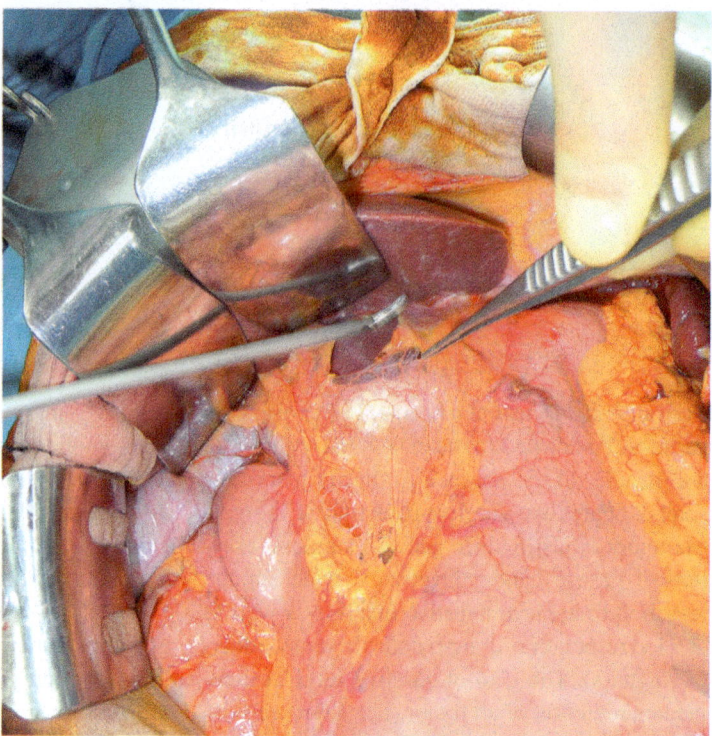

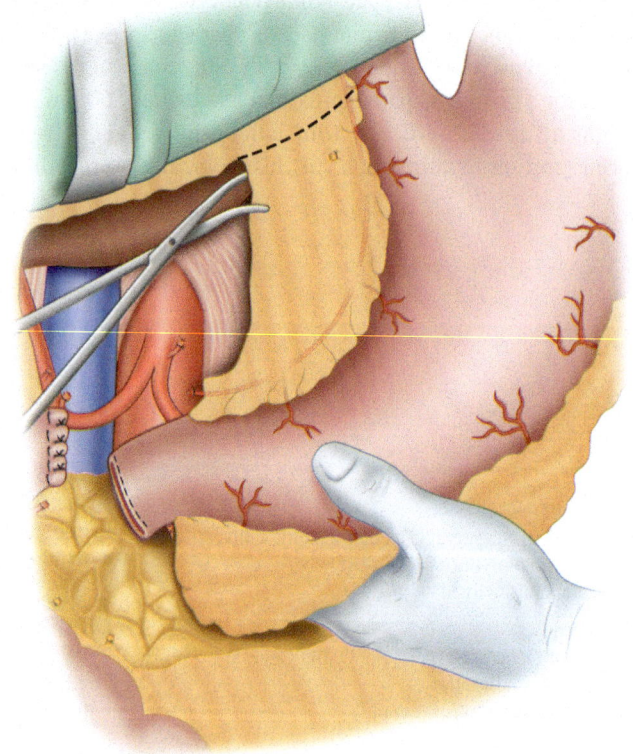

## 3.2    Resection of the Gastrosplenic Ligament

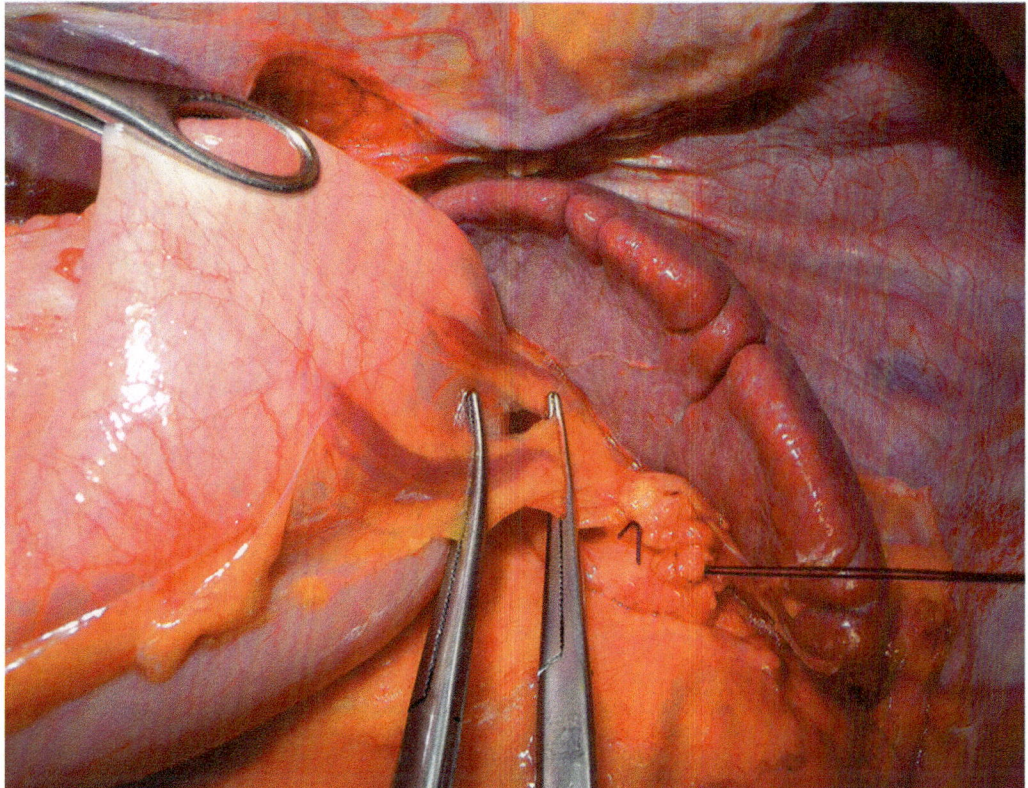

**Figs. 3.3 and 3.4**  On the side of the greater curvature, the gastrosplenic ligament is identified and resected, proceeding from low to high, carefully ligating its 4–6 short gastric vessels or dividing them with the ultrasonic or radiofrequency scalpel.

After ligation of the first and second short gastric vessels, the spleen is definitively freed from the stomach, and access is gained to the left paracardial region and crus of the diaphragm.

Only the tumor's close relationship to the spleen or the presence of multiple, macroscopically enlarged splenic hilar lymph nodes warrants splenectomy en bloc with the gastric specimen

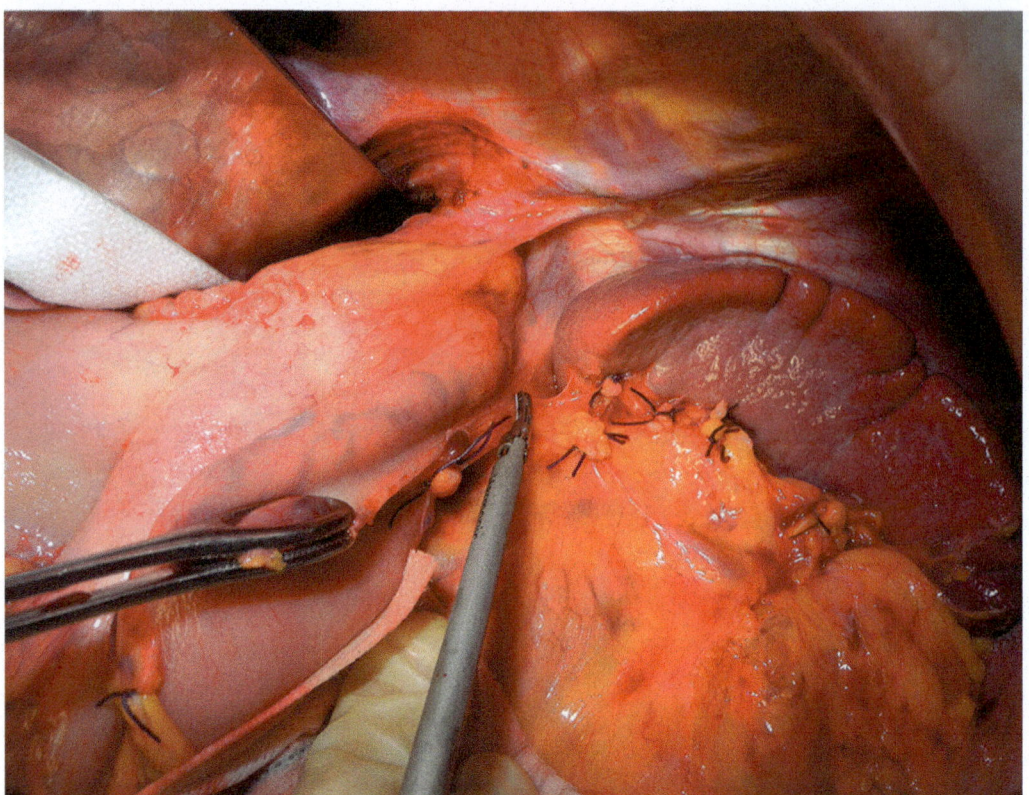

**Figs. 3.3 and 3.4** (continued)

## 3.3     Division of the Phrenoesophageal Membrane and Vagus Nerves

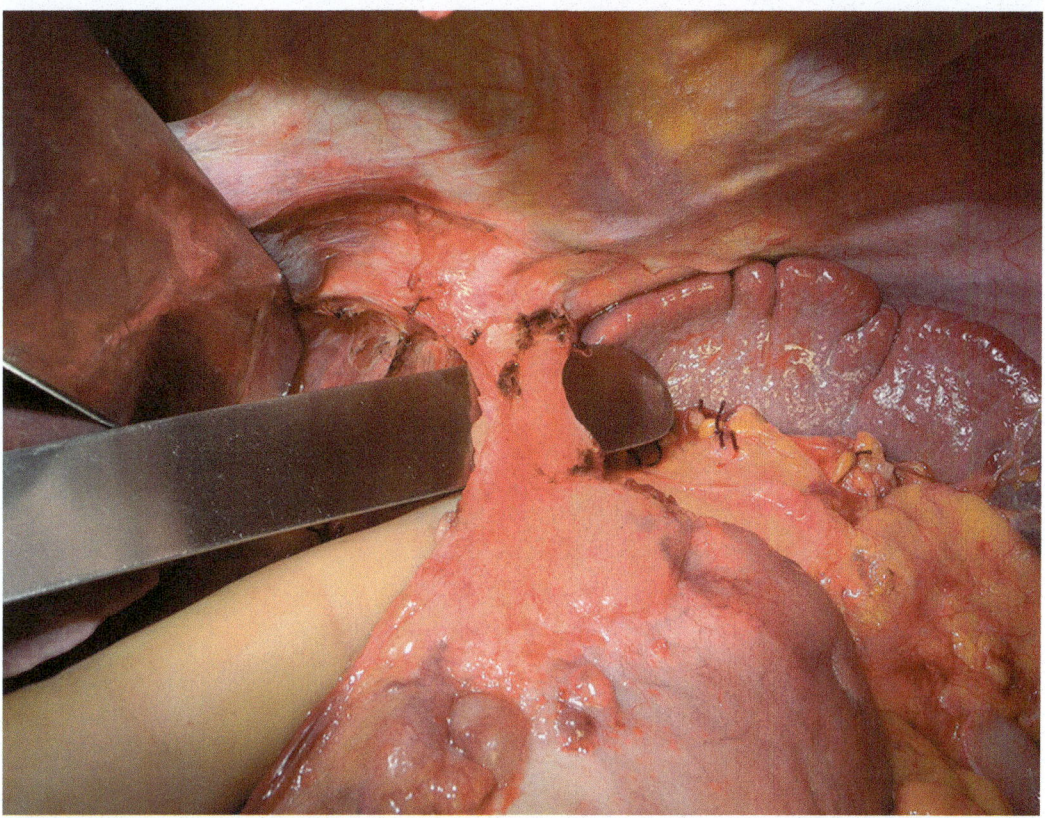

**Figs. 3.5, 3.6, and 3.7**  Section of the left triangular and coronary ligaments and right dislocation of the left leaver segments allow excellent exposure of the esophago-cardial region. Resection of the Lymer-Bertelli phreno-esophageal membrane releases the anterior esophageal wall and allows complete dissection of the intra-abdominal esophagus

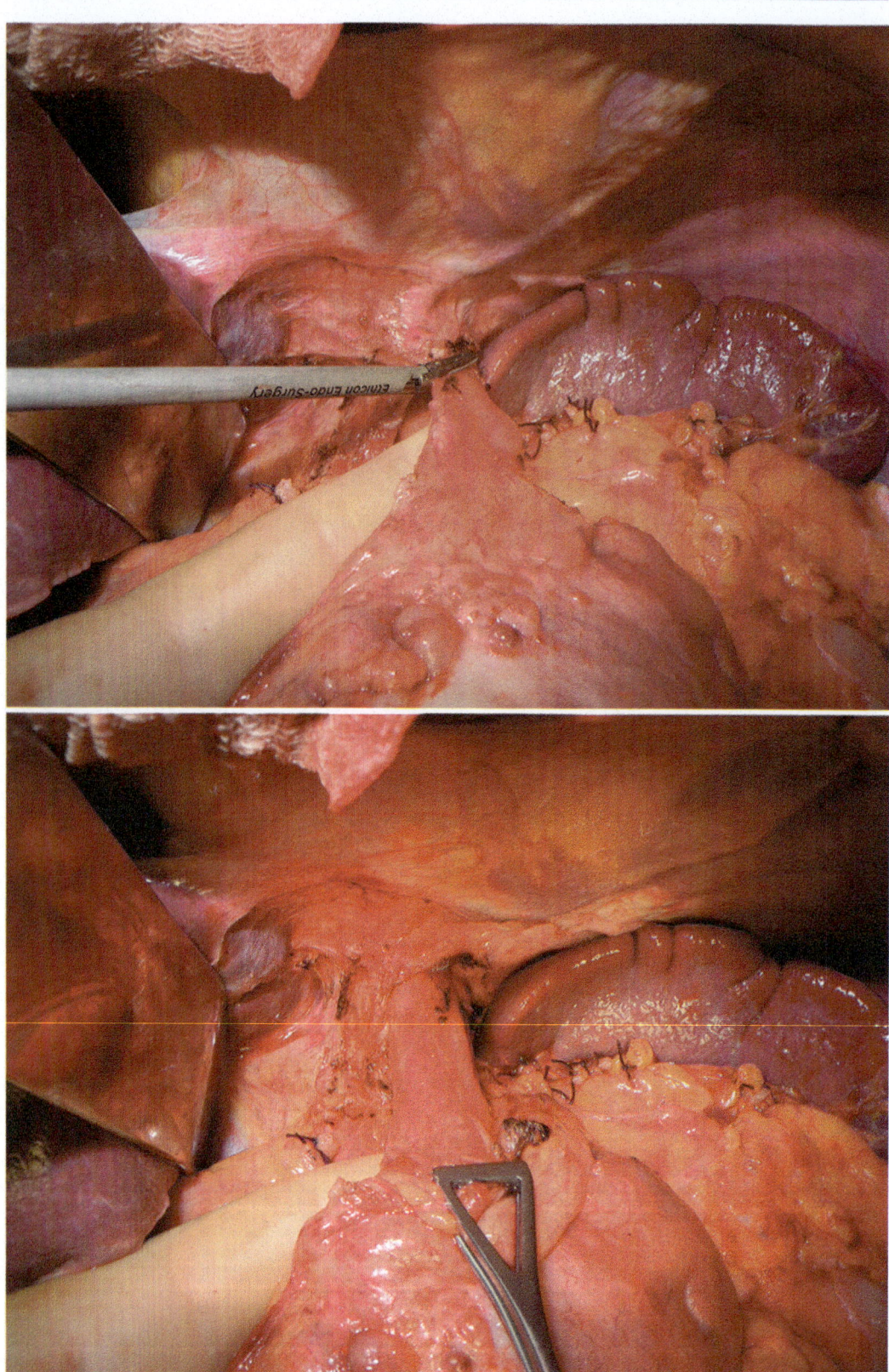

**Figs. 3.5, 3.6, and 3.7** (continued)

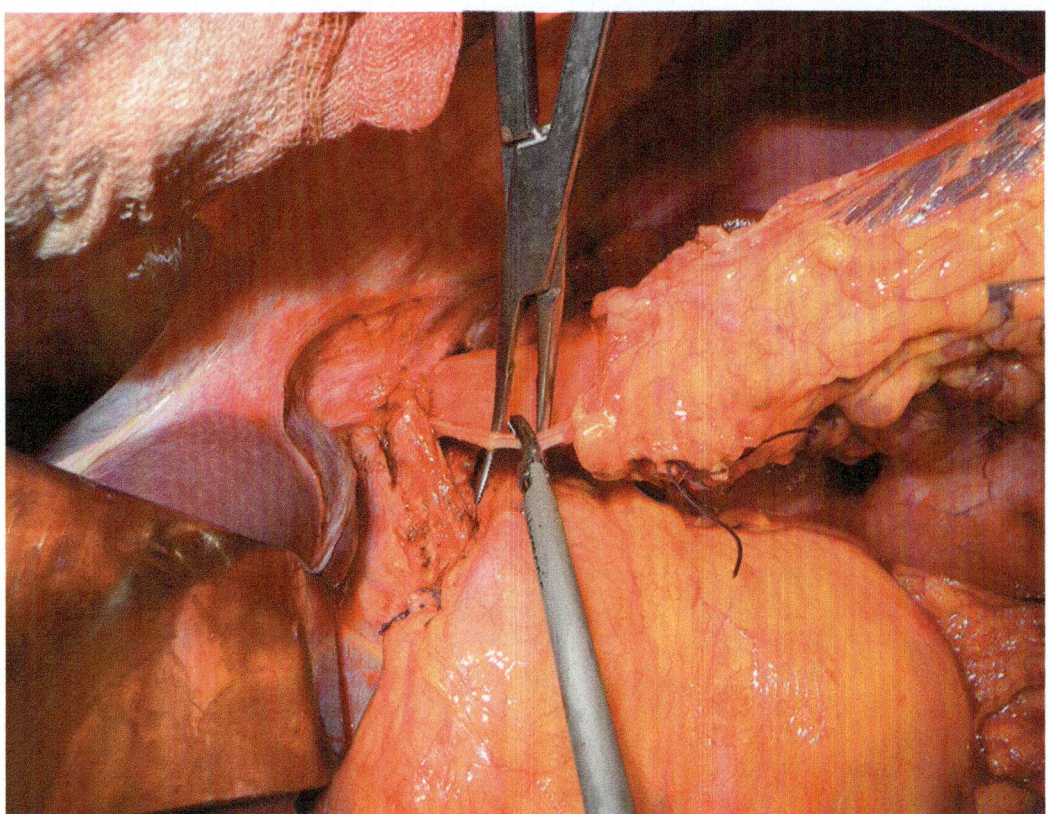

**Figs. 3.8 and 3.9** Division of the two vagus nerves, which are easily identified because they are strung longitudinally at the level of the external portion of the esophageal wall, allows further mobilization of the intra-abdominal esophagus. Their division after dissection results in immediate collapse or greater mobility of the intra-abdominal esophagus

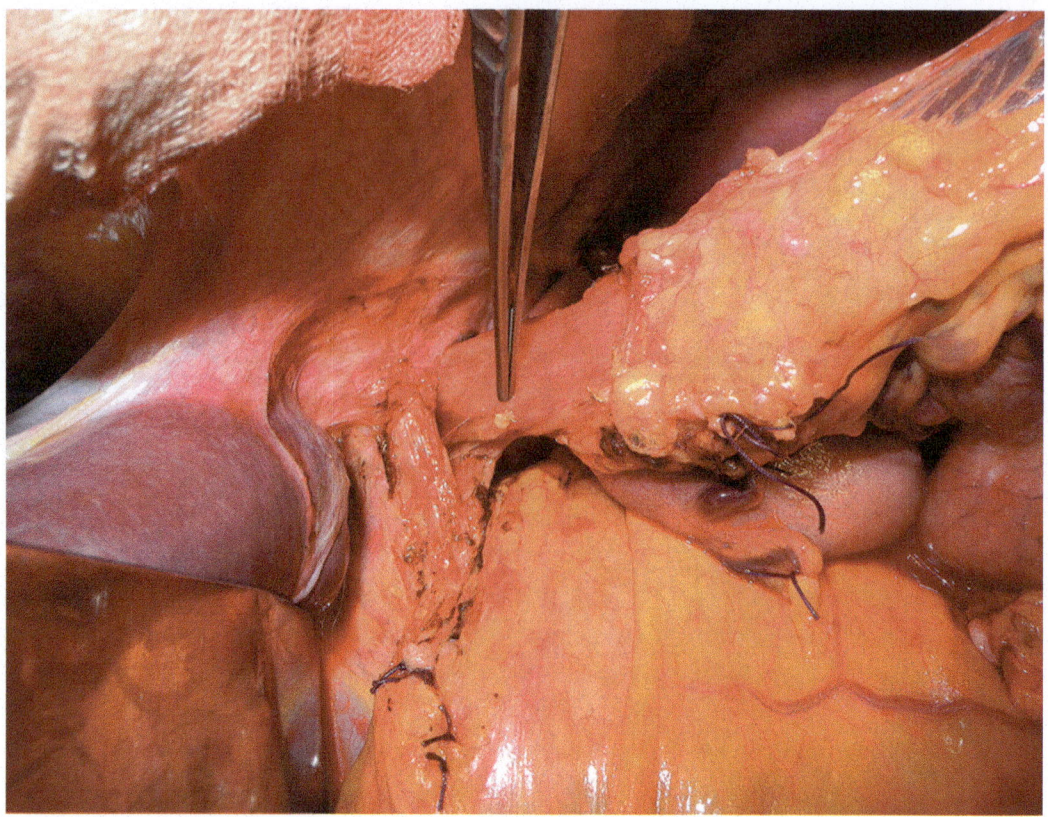

**Figs. 3.8 and 3.9** (continued)

## 3.4 Rake Clamp Positioning, Purse-String Suture, Esophageal Resection, and Stapler Anvil in the Distal Esophagus

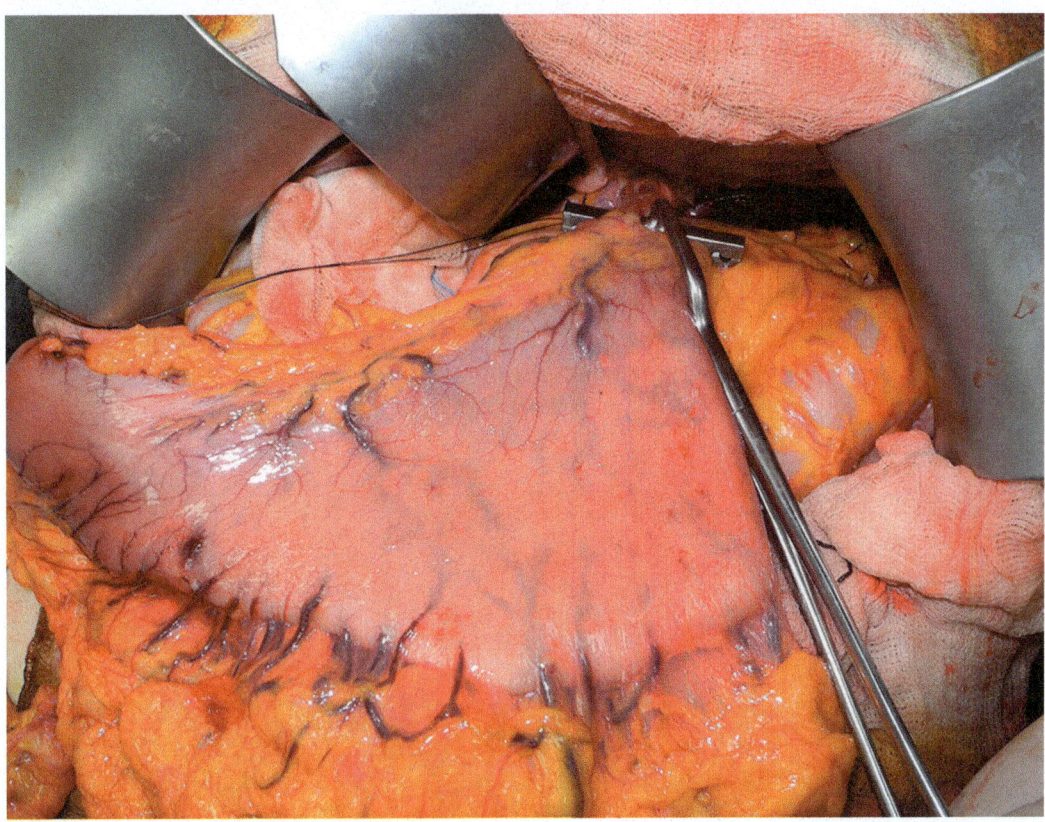

**Fig. 3.10** A rake clamp is positioned at the center of the intra-abdominal esophagus on macroscopically healthy tissue, 1–2 cm upstream of the cardia, carefully avoiding trapping the nasogastric tube. Two straight needles are inserted through the rake clamp jaws to execute a purse-string suture in the distal esophagus with nonabsorbable monofilament suture 2-0

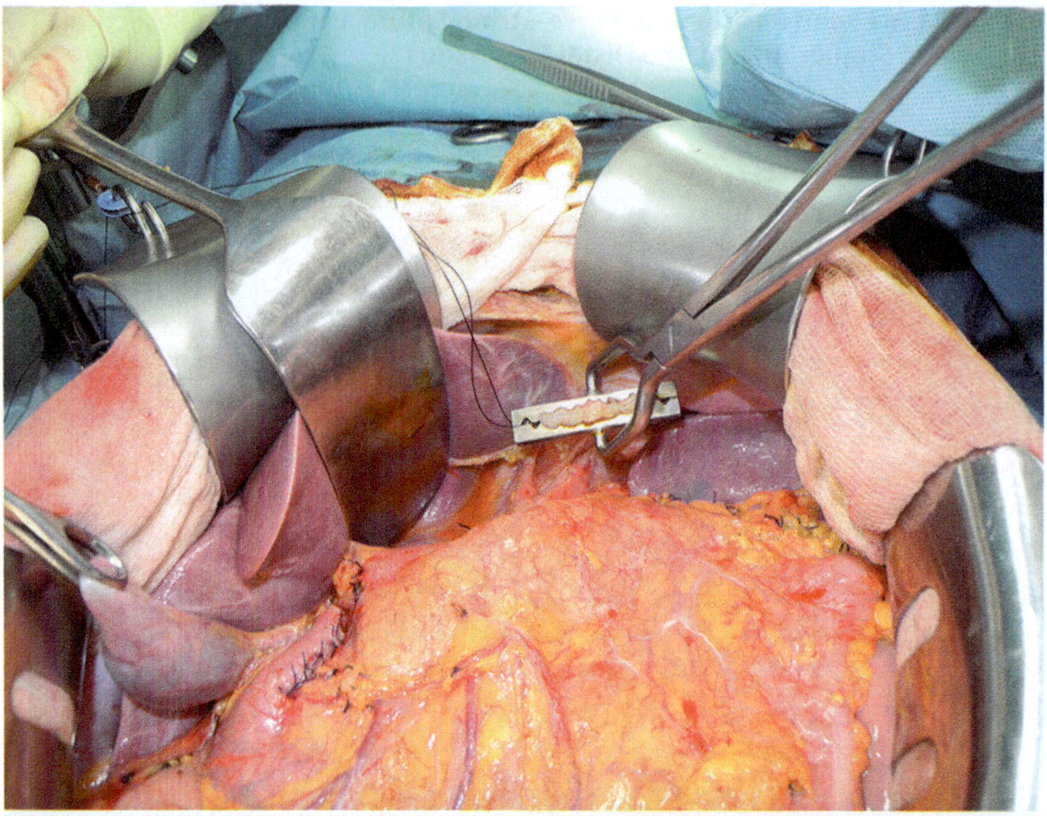

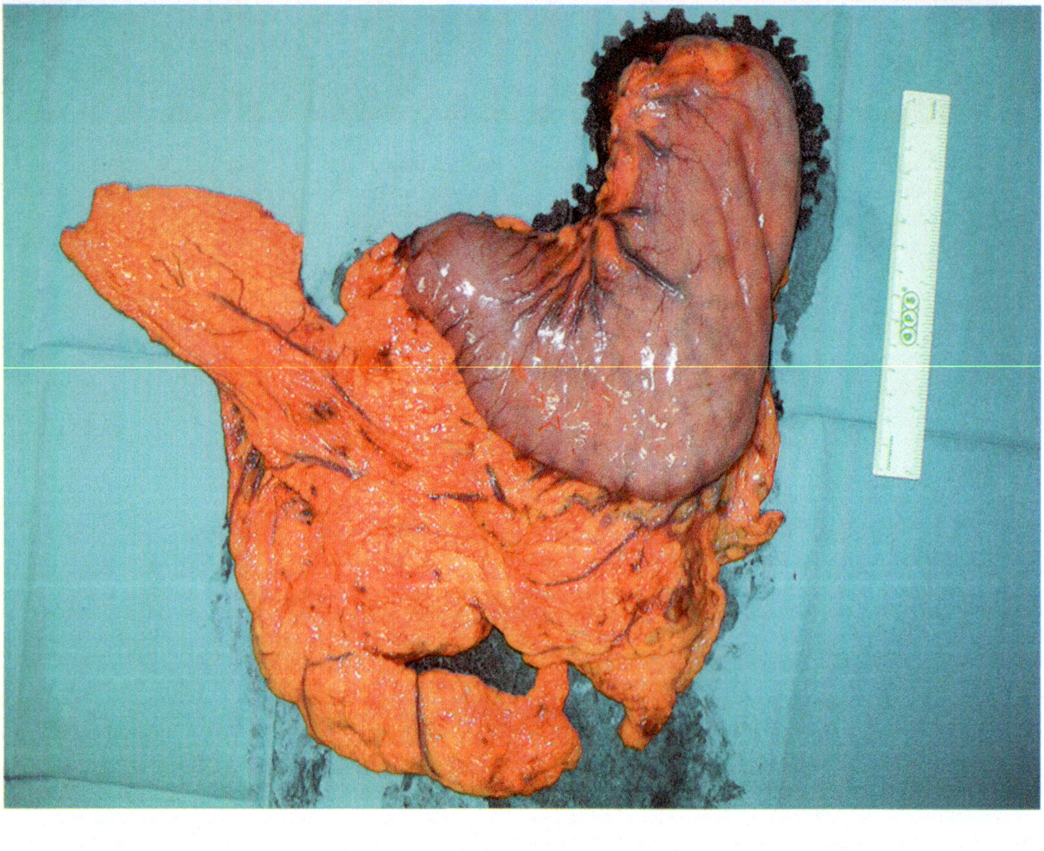

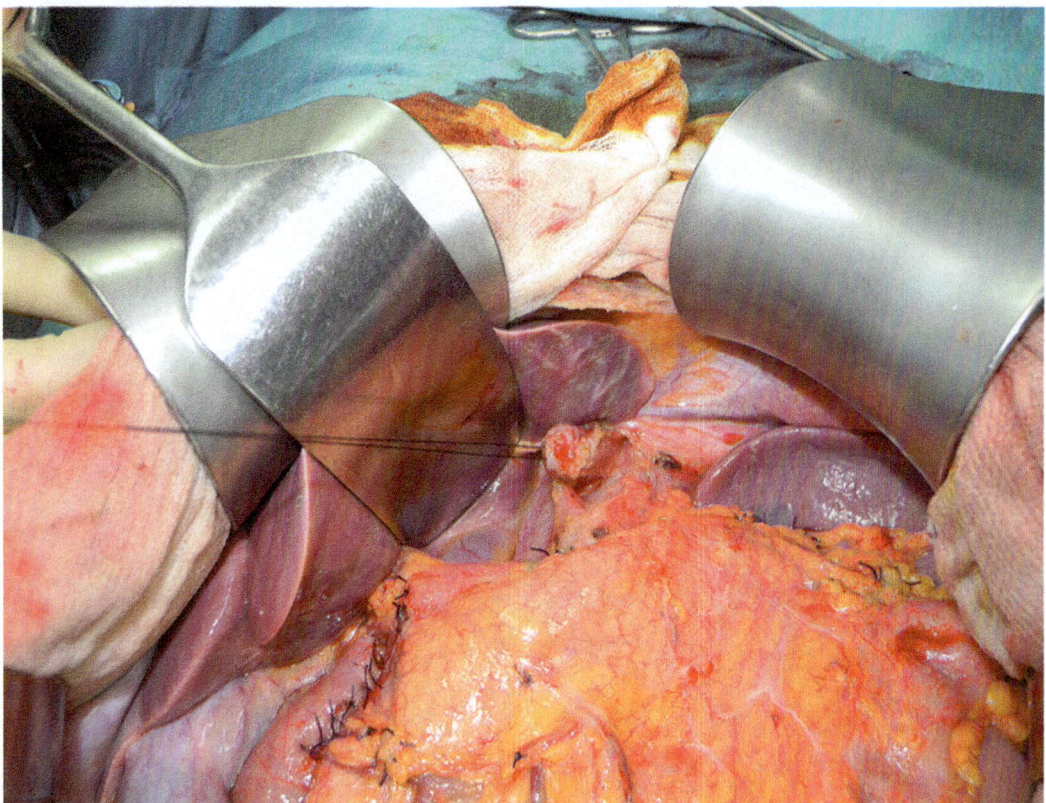

**Fig. 3.13** The surgeon opens the rake jaws with the right hand to remove it while tightening the purse-string suture with the left hand, to close the esophageal stump and avoid operative field contamination

**Figs. 3.11 and 3.12** The surgeon cuts the distal esophagus with curved scissors close to the rake clamp, thus freeing the specimen, which consists of the whole stomach, the omentum, and all first-level perigastric lymph nodes (stations 1–6). The specimen is submitted for intraoperative consultation to establish the tumor's distance from the proximal and distal margins and exclude microscopic positivity

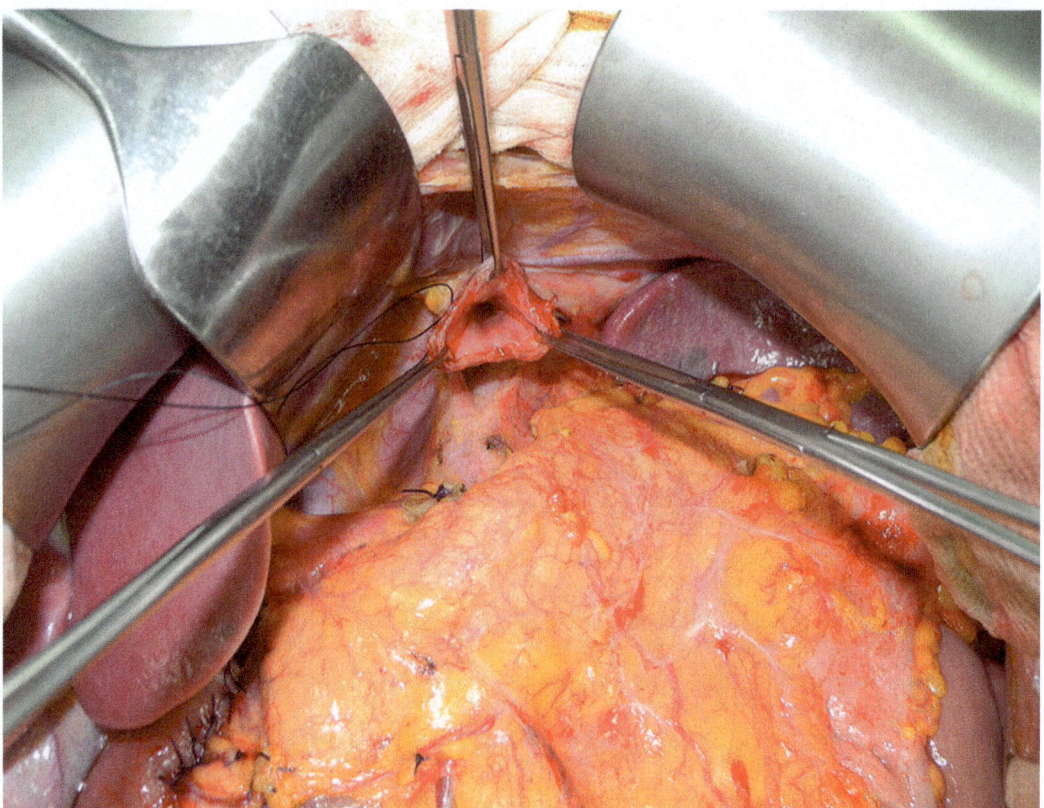

**Fig. 3.14** The purse-string suture is released and three Allis forceps are placed 120° apart along the esophageal stump, grasping the whole thickness of the wall. While the first and the second assistant open the esophageal stump by gently pulling the Allis clamps, the surgeon introduces a Carmalt clamp into the lumen, gently distending the wall to avoid mucosal tears, to establish the caliber of the circular mechanical stapler required for the esophagojejunal anastomosis

**Figs. 3.15 and 3.16** The surgeon introduces the oiled anvil of the stapler into the esophagus with the right hand, tightening the pouch strings with the left hand as the first and the second assistant remove the Allis clamps. The purse-string suture is then tied at the base of the anvil's shaft, and the esophageal stump is ready for the anastomosis. A 25 mm stapler (Premium Plus CEEA) or, less commonly, a 21 mm stapler is used in most cases. The two ends of the purse-string suture on the anvil are held together by a Pean clamp, and at the time of the anastomosis, gentle pulling of the strings will allow safe and easy recovery

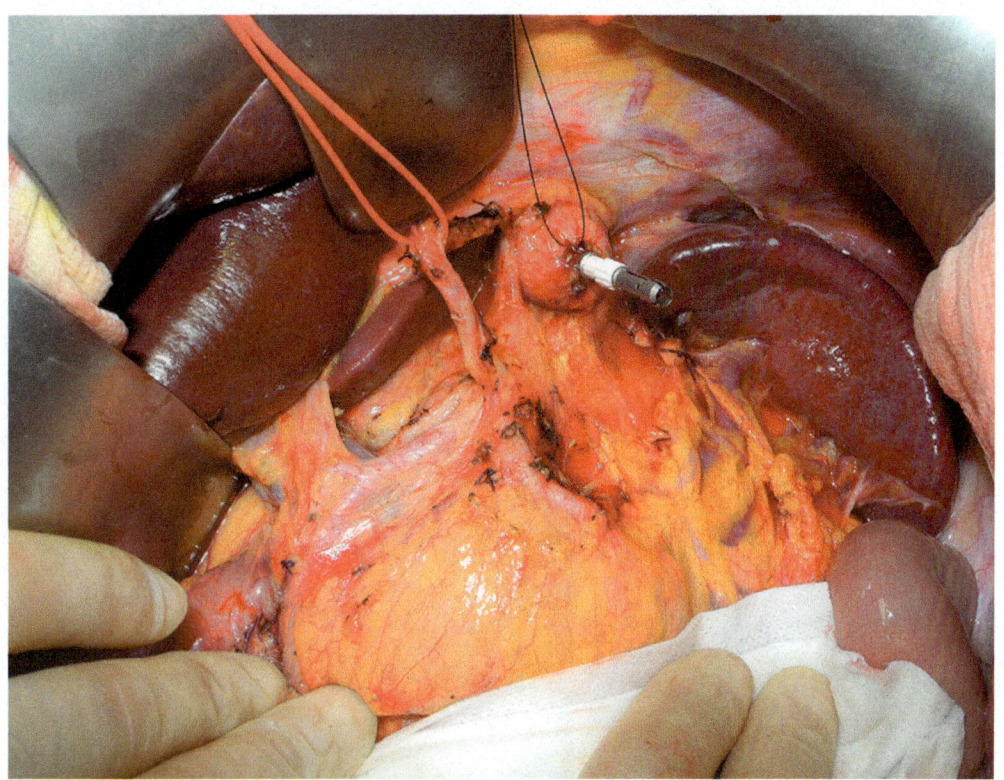

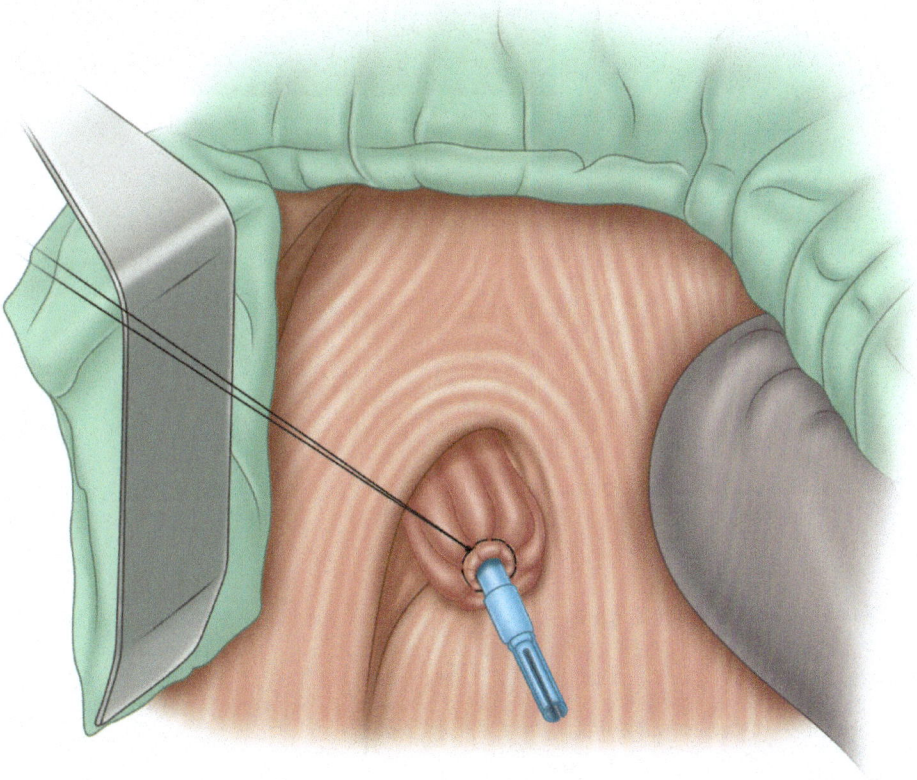

## 3.5     Preparation of the Jejunal Loop and Roux Limb Transposition to the Supramesocolic Compartment

**Fig. 3.17** With the transverse colon gently retracted, the second jejunal loop is spread to examine the anatomy of the arterial arcades by transillumination

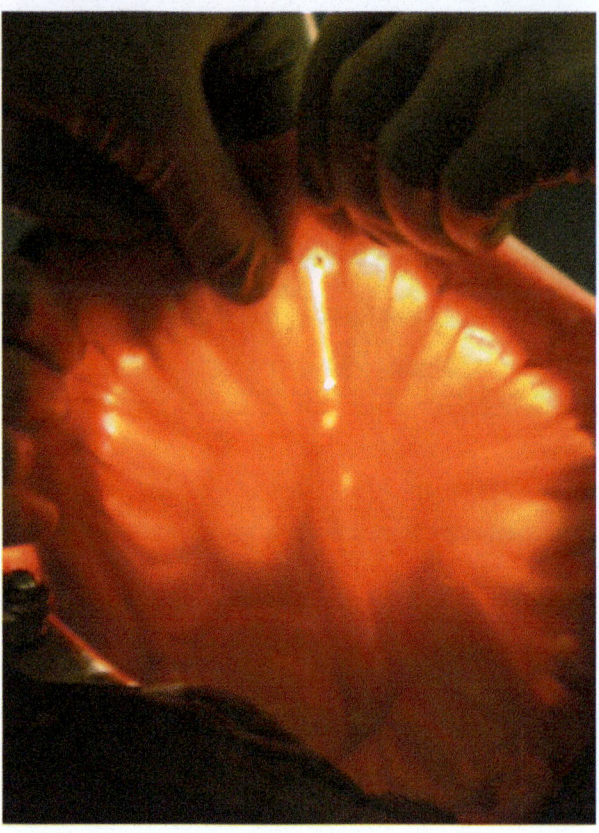

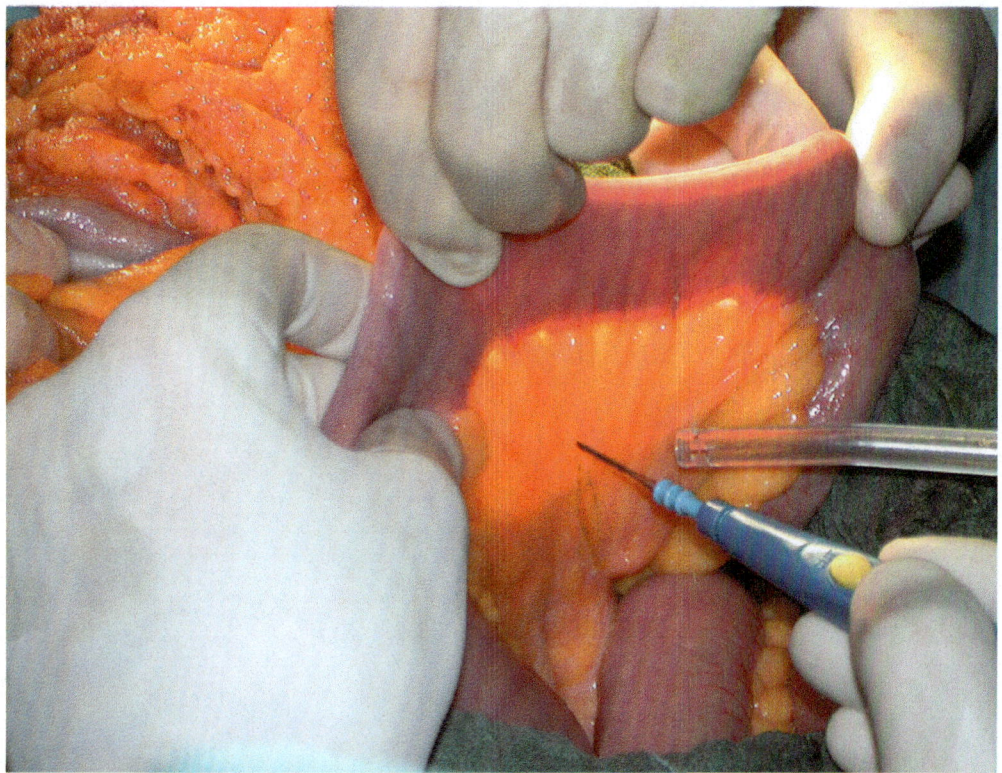

**Fig. 3.18** The arcades are divided nearly up to the base of the mesentery, to mobilize the jejunum and gain tension-free access to the cardial region

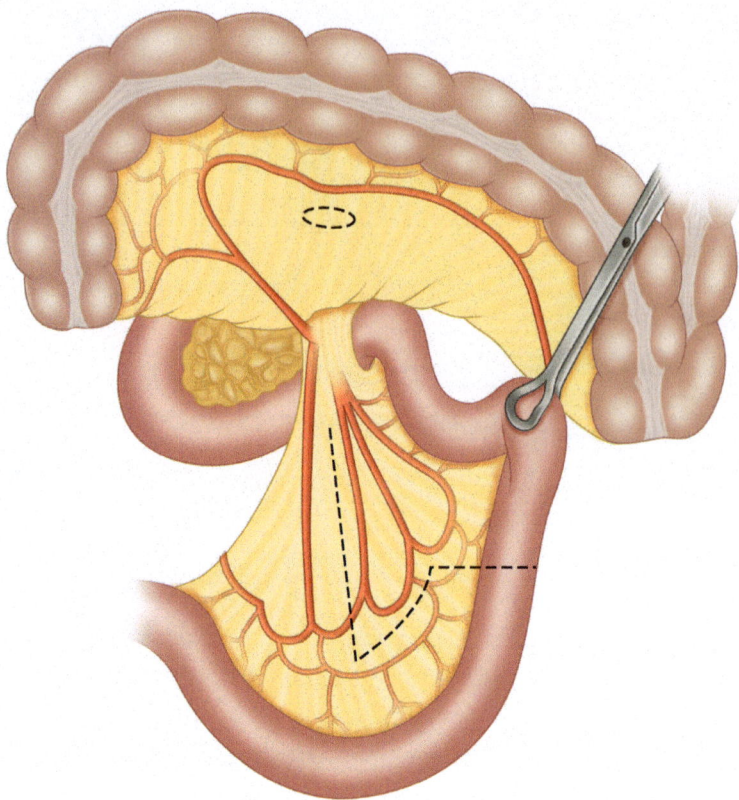

**Fig. 3.19** After two non-crushing intestinal clamps have been placed upstream and downstream of the resection site, the jejunal loop is resected and the two stumps are disinfected. The afferent loop, closed with a non-crushing intestinal clamp and covered with gauze, is abandoned in the abdomen. With the transverse mesocolon still gently retracted, an avascular area in its left inferior paramedian portion is identified by transillumination and excised, to allow transposition of the efferent jejunal limb to the supramesocolic compartment through the transverse mesocolon

## 3.6    Stapled End-to-Side Esophagojejunostomy

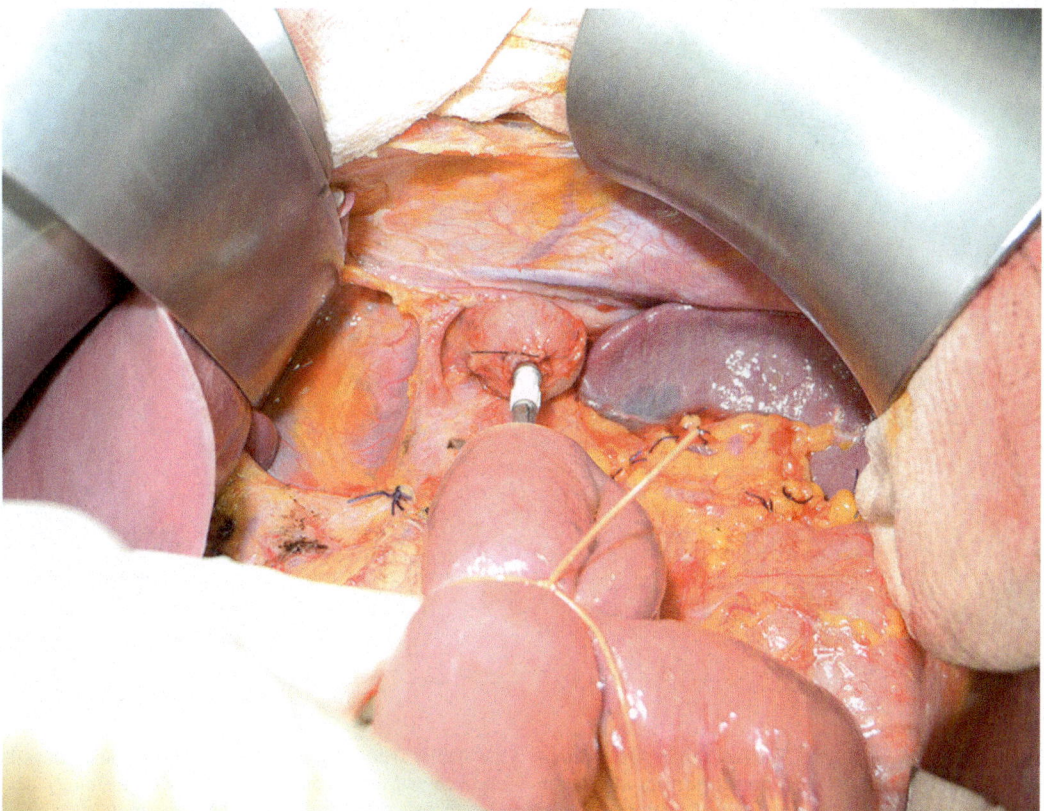

**Fig. 3.20** The surgeon inserts the oiled circular stapler 10–15 cm into the Roux limb. The site of the jejunal limb to be perforated with the spike is identified. There must be no mechanical tension between the esophageal stump and the jejunal limb itself. The jejunal wall is perforated, and the anvil is joined to the stapler

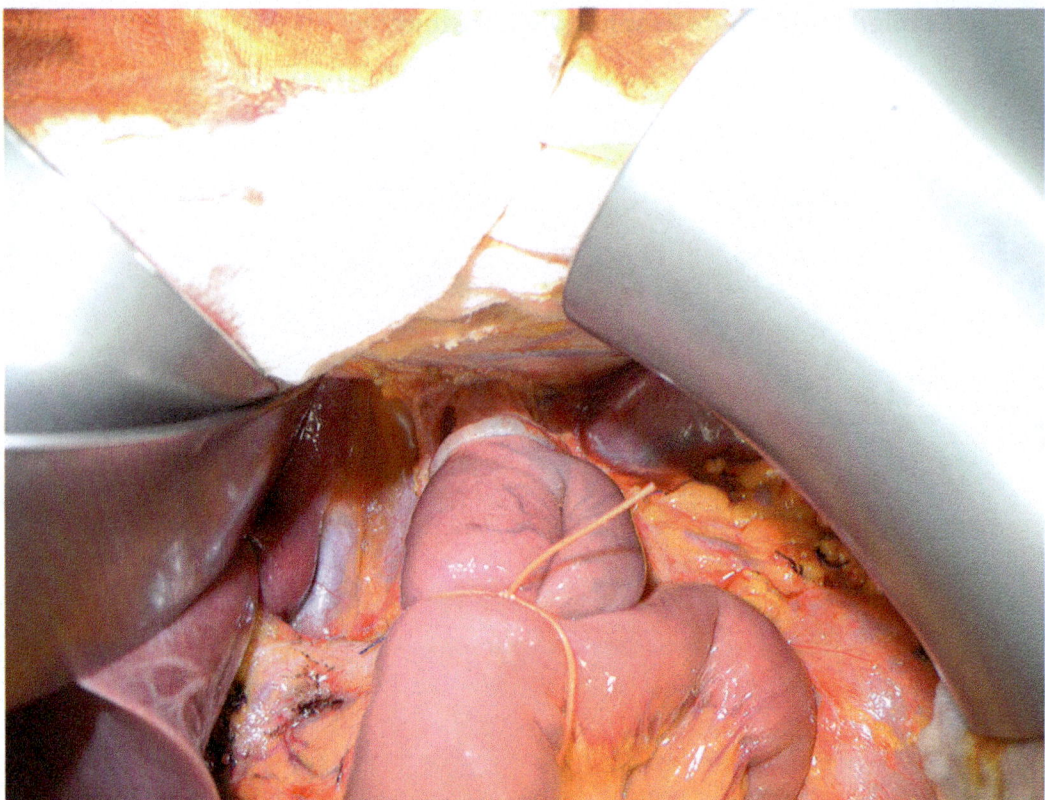

**Figs. 3.21, 3.22, and 3.23** The two stumps are approximated by screwing the stapler shut; correct approximation of the margins is signaled by a green light, authorizing firing. Two full turns tilt the anvil, allowing extraction of the stapler. The integrity of the two anastomotic rings is checked and the esophageal ring sent for histology. The anastomosis must be supple and tension-free

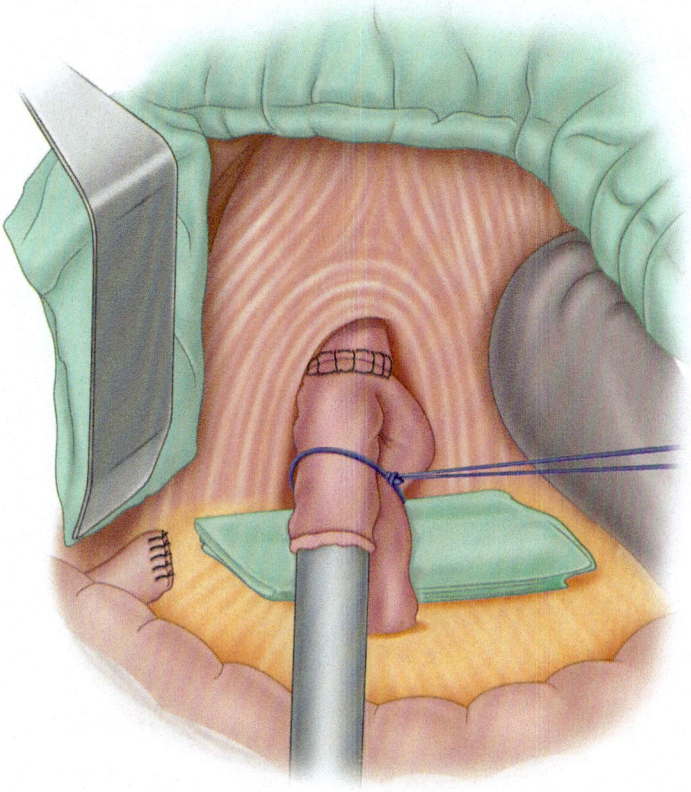

**Figs. 3.21, 3.22, and 3.23** (continued)

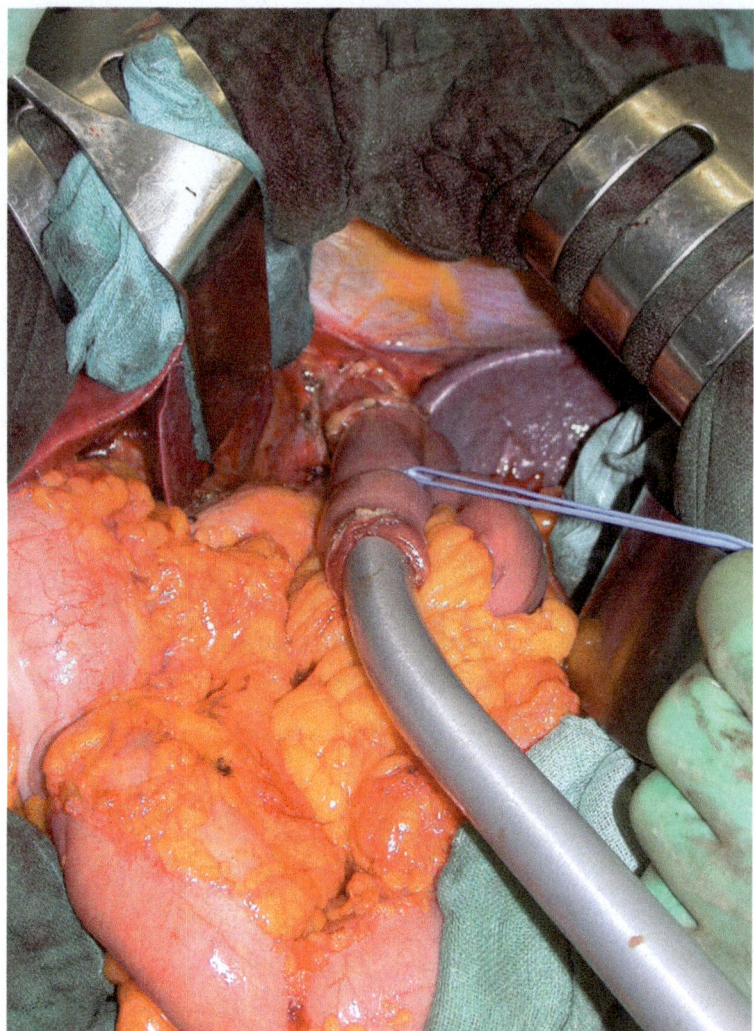

**Figs. 3.21, 3.22, and 3.23** (continued)

**Figs. 3.24, 3.25, 3.26, and 3.27** The gentle traction exerted on the edge of the jejunal loop allows its spread and identification of the ideal site for closing the jejunal stump. The mesentery is resected and then the jejunal loop is closed and transected with a mechanical linear stapler (GIA or TA) 2–3 cm lateral to the esophagojejunal anastomosis

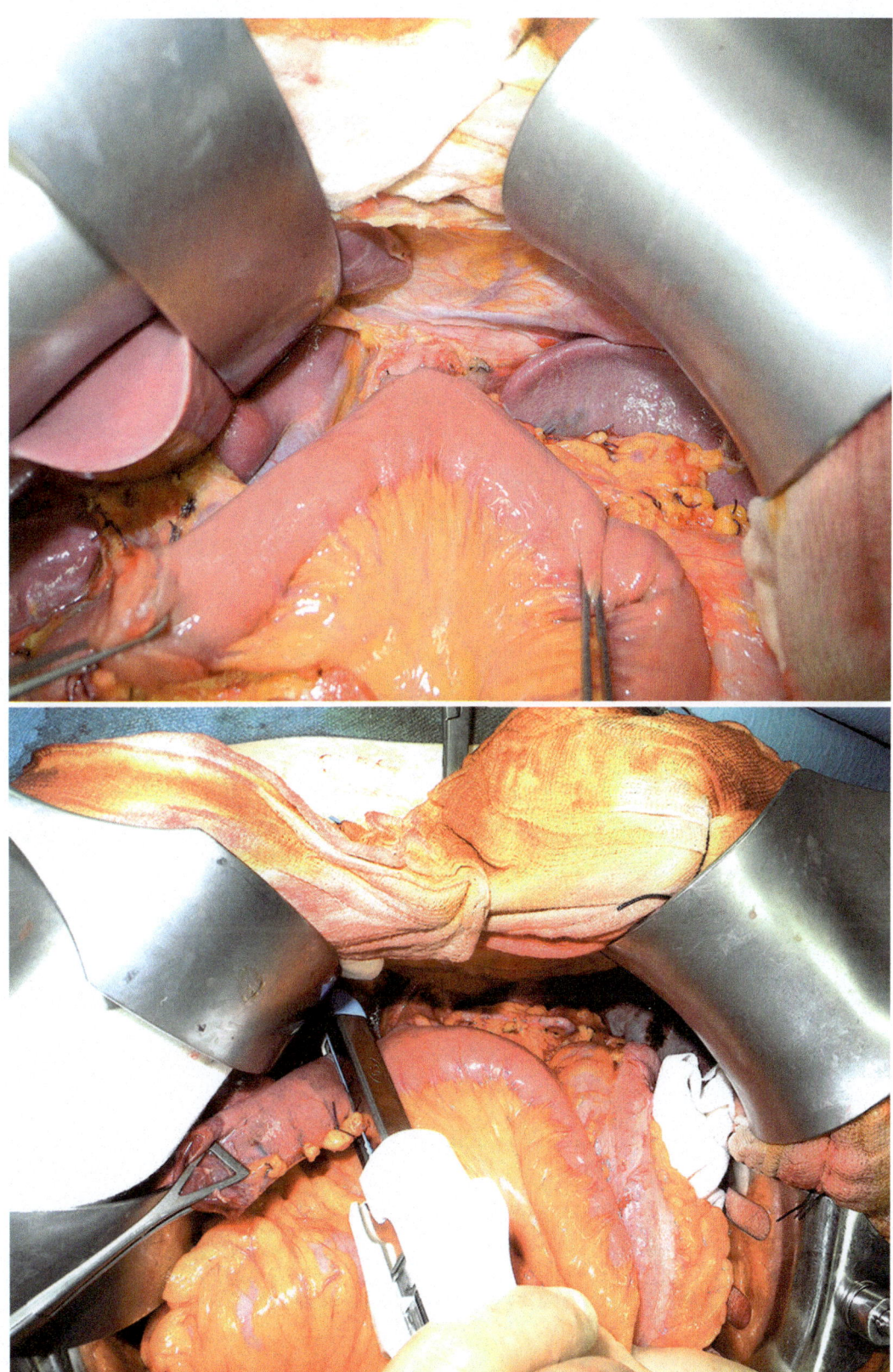

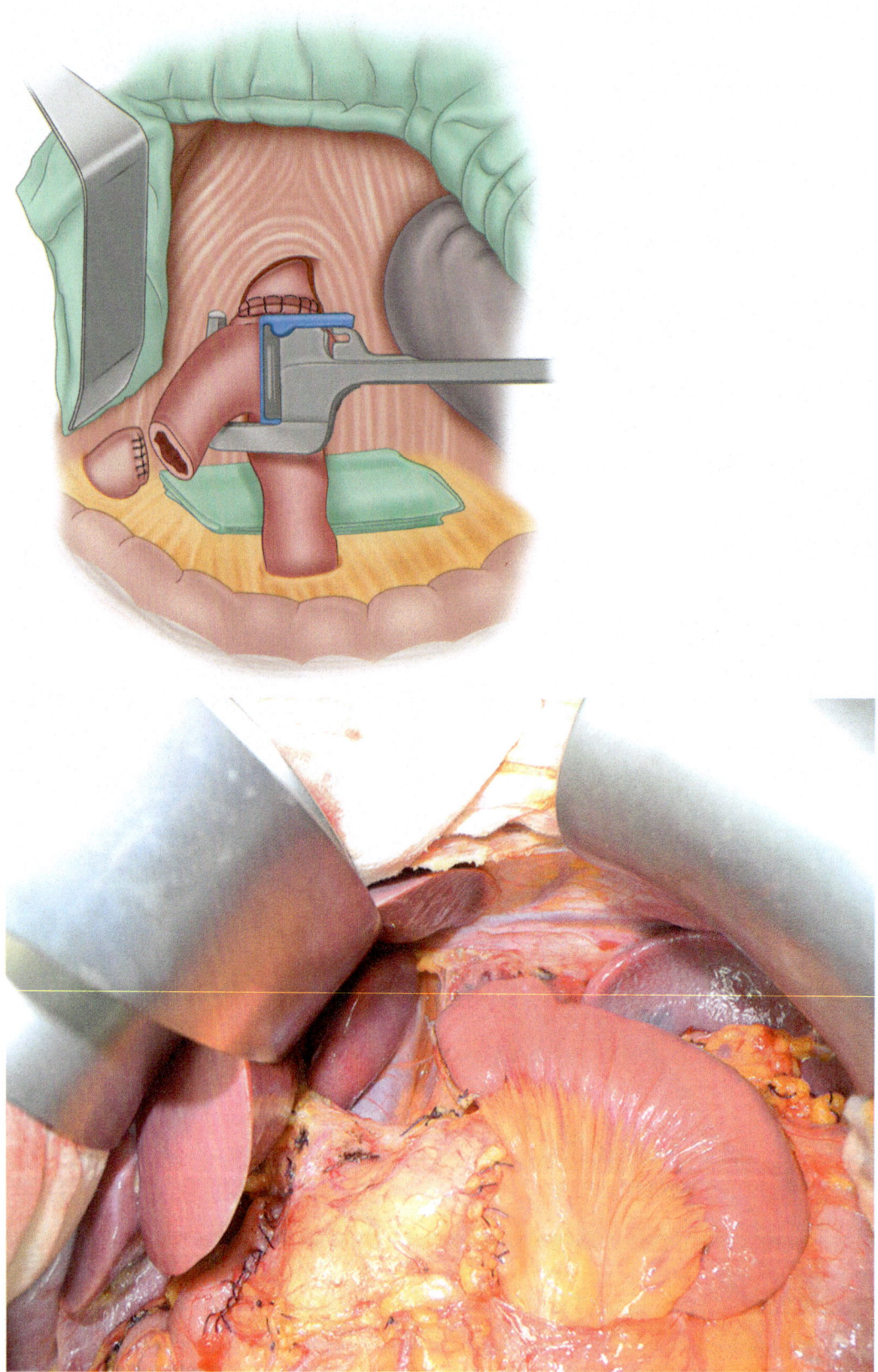

**Figs. 3.24, 3.25, 3.26, and 3.27** (continued)

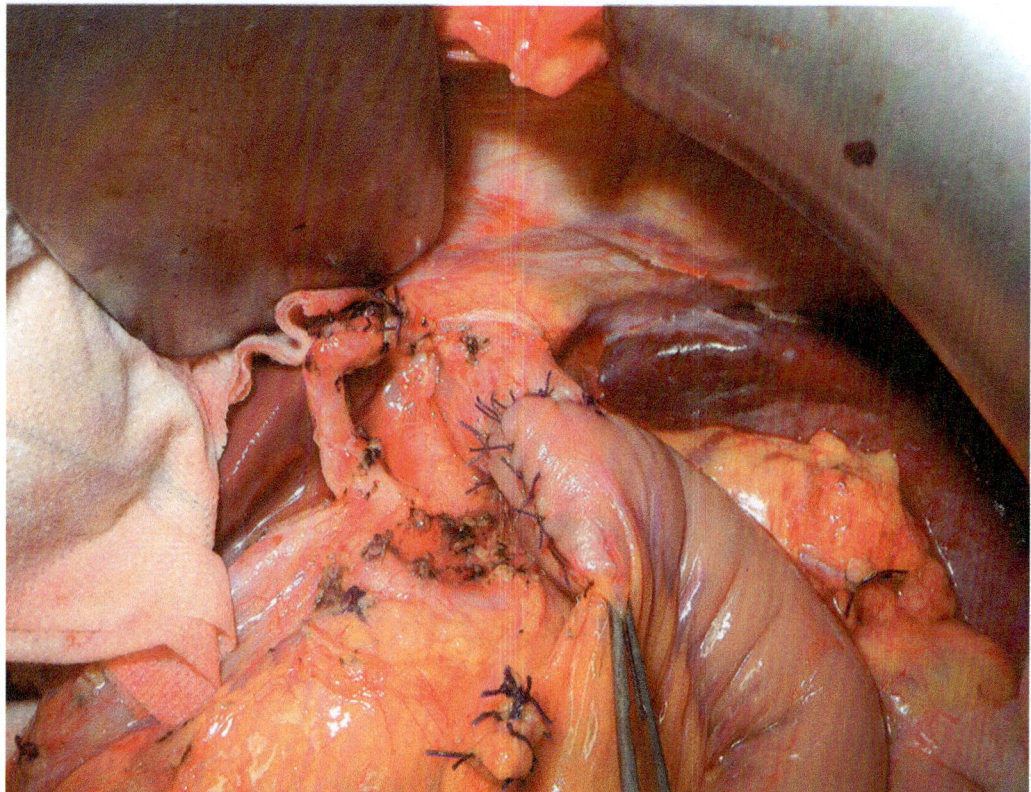

**Figs. 3.28 and 3.29**  The closed jejunal stump is disinfected and oversewn using interrupted slowly absorbable braided 3-0 sutures to obtain a short jejunal stump that does not disturb the esophagojejunal transit. To minimize the risk of leakage of the esophagojejunal anastomosis, absorbable interrupted seromuscular 3-0 sutures are applied all around the anastomosis (360°) to avoid staple line tension and reinforce the anastomosis

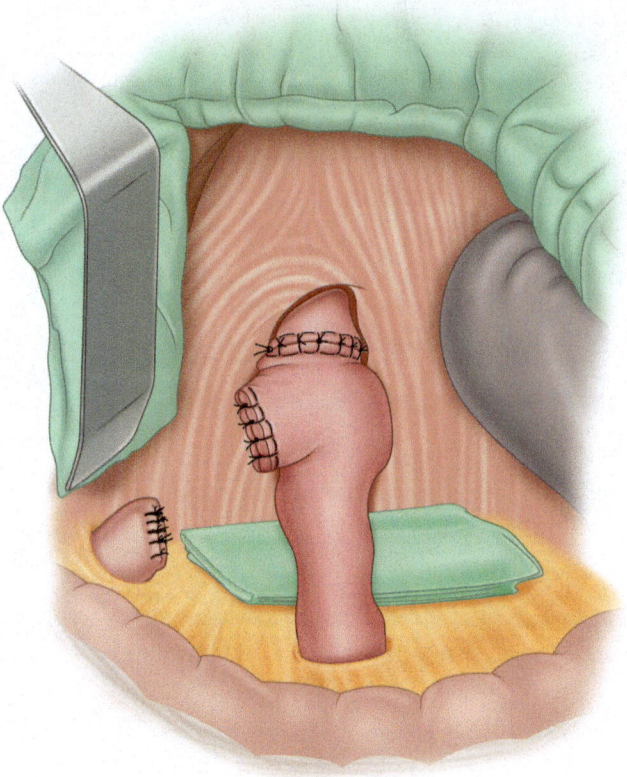

**Figs. 3.28 and 3.29** (continued)

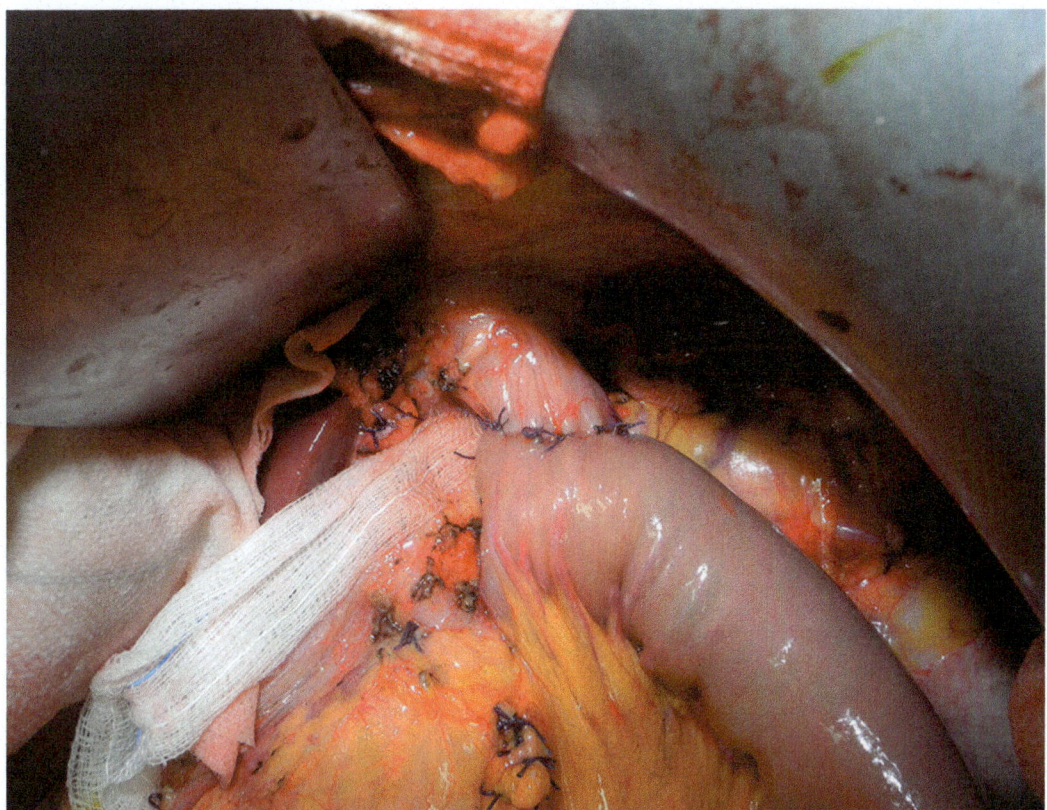

**Figs. 3.30, 3.31, and 3.32** A non-crushing intestinal clamp is placed on the jejunal loop 10 cm downstream of the anastomosis; the nasogastric tube is then gently advanced ca. 5 cm past the suture and injected with 40–60 ml of saline added with methylene blue for anasto-motic leak testing. The solution is then pumped out through the nasogastric tube, the clamp is removed, and the nasogastric tube is removed. Water-soluble contrast swallow is performed 7 days after total gastrectomy to assess anastomotic integrity before restoring oral intake

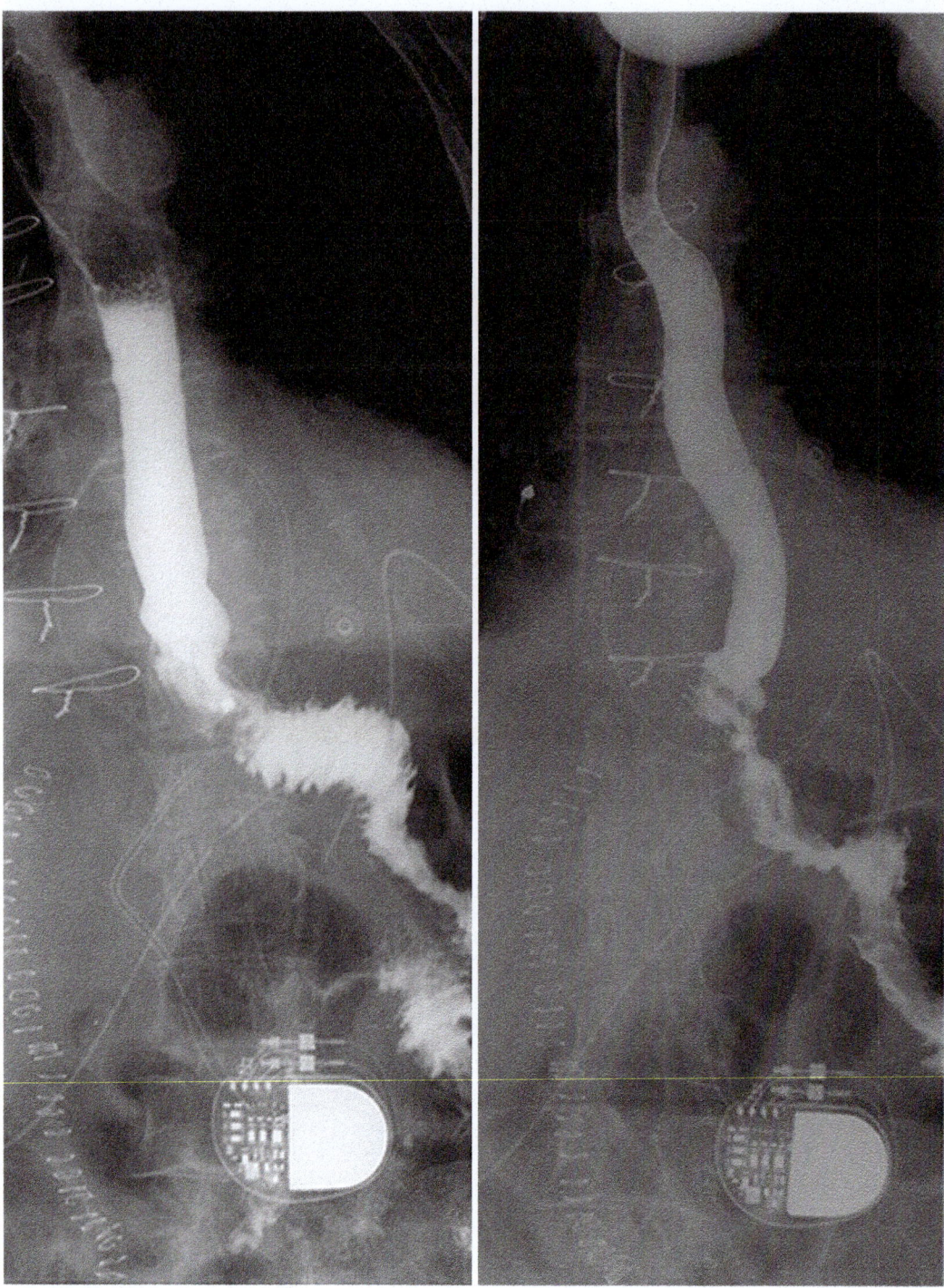

**Figs. 3.30, 3.31, and 3.32** (continued)

## 3.7    Enteroenterostomy and Drains

**Fig. 3.33** To reestablish intestinal continuity
the afferent jejunal stump is recovered, and a
two-layer, end-to-side jejunojejunal anastomosis is performed on the efferent jejunal loop
60 cm from the esophagojejunal anastomosis
using interrupted slowly absorbable 3-0
sutures. The mesenteries are closed with
interrupted slowly absorbable 3-0 sutures to
minimize the risk of internal herniation.
Finally, two abdominal drains are placed, the
right one coursing posterior to the esophagojejunal anastomosis below the hepatoduodenal
ligament, also draining the duodenal stump,
and the left one running anterior to the
esophagojejunal anastomosis, also draining the
left hypochondrium

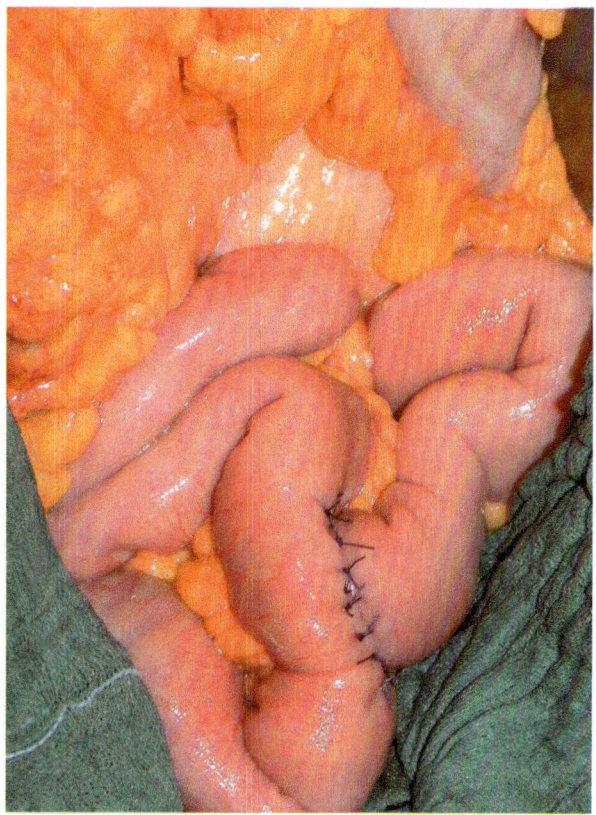

# Manual Subtotal Gastrectomy

**4**

Raffaella Ridolfo, Pierpaolo Stortoni, Emilio Feliciotti, and Walter Siquini

## 4.1 Introduction

Distal and antral tumors account for about 35 % of all gastric cancers.

A complete margin-negative resection (R0) remains the only potentially curative treatment for gastric adenocarcinoma.

In an effort to lower the positive margin rate, in the past years it has been proposed that total gastrectomy should be considered the only operation of choice for all operable gastric cancers.

Prospective trials have indicated no difference in 5-year survival between patients undergoing potentially curative subtotal and total gastrectomy.

Subtotal gastrectomy is appropriate for patients in whom a negative margin resection can be performed with less morbidity and a better quality of life than does a total gastrectomy.

According to the Japanese gastric cancer treatment guidelines 2010 (ver. 3) [1] of the Japanese Gastric Cancer Association, a proximal margin of at least 3 cm is recommended for T2 or deeper tumors with an expansive growth pattern (Types 1 and 2), and 5 cm is recommended for those with infiltrative growth pattern (Types 3 and 4).

When these rules cannot be observed, it is advisable to examine the proximal resection margin by frozen section.

When the tumor border is unclear, preoperative endoscopic marking of the tumor border will be helpful for decision-making regarding the resection line.

Although there are several options for reconstruction, including various types of interposition loops and pouches, we will discuss the type of reconstruction we usually perform: the Roux-en-Y retrocolic, isoperistaltic, end-to-side, and oralis partialis gastrojejunostomy.

We prefer this technique in order to minimize the incidence of bile reflux gastritis and esophagitis, avoid the afferent limb syndrome described in the Billroth II patients, reduce the risk of anastomotic leakage and reduce gastric stump cancerization.

R. Ridolfo (✉)
Division of General Surgery, Senigallia General Hospital, Senigallia, Italy
e-mail: raffaella.ridolfo@email.it

P. Stortoni
Division of General Surgery, "A. Murri" Hospital, Fermo, Italy
e-mail: pierpaolostortoni@libero.it

E. Feliciotti
Department of Surgery, "Ospedali Riuniti" University Hospital, Ancona, Italy
e-mail: feliciotti@live.it

W. Siquini
Division of General Surgery,
"Madonna del Soccorso" Hospital,
San Benedetto del Tronto, Italy
e-mail: walter.siquini@sanita.marche.it

W. Siquini (ed.), *Total, Subtotal and Proximal Gastrectomy in Cancer: A Color Atlas*,
DOI 10.1007/978-88-470-5749-4_4, © Springer-Verlag Italia 2015

## 4.2    Dissection of the Upper Portion of the Lesser Curvature

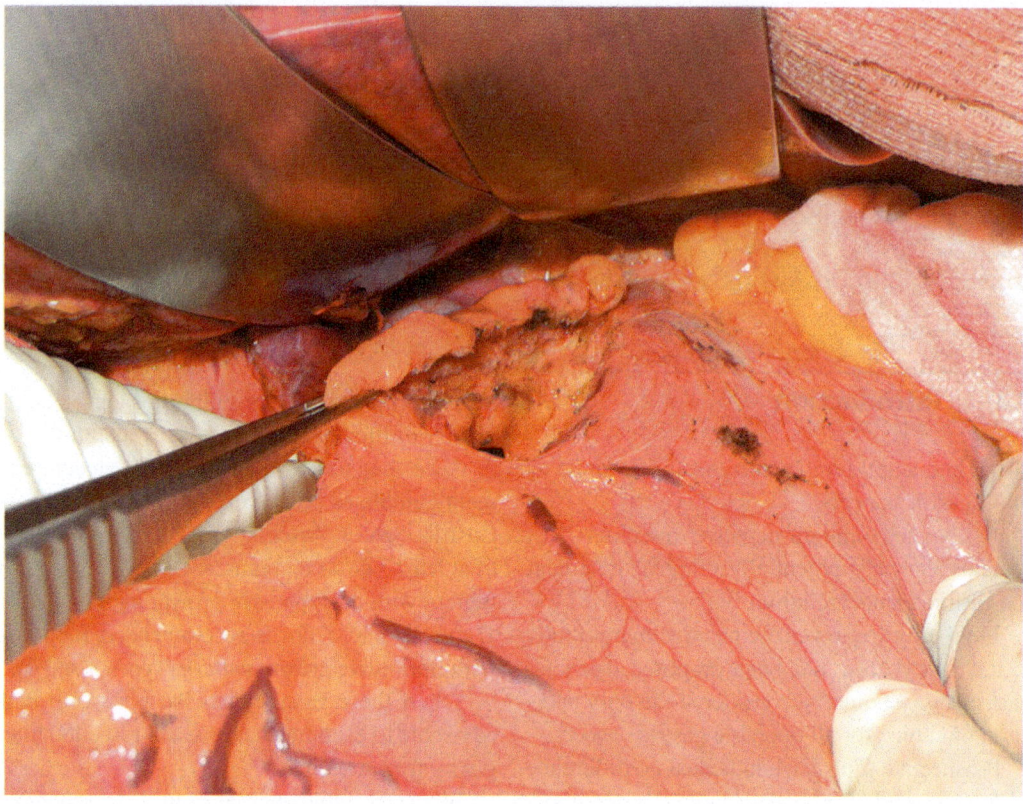

**Fig. 4.1** Complete removal of lymphatic and adipose tissue of the proximal portion of the lesser curvature up to the right wall of the cardia exposes the medial wall of the stomach and the esophagogastric junction, ensuring optimal exposure and safe closure of the medial portion of the gastric stump

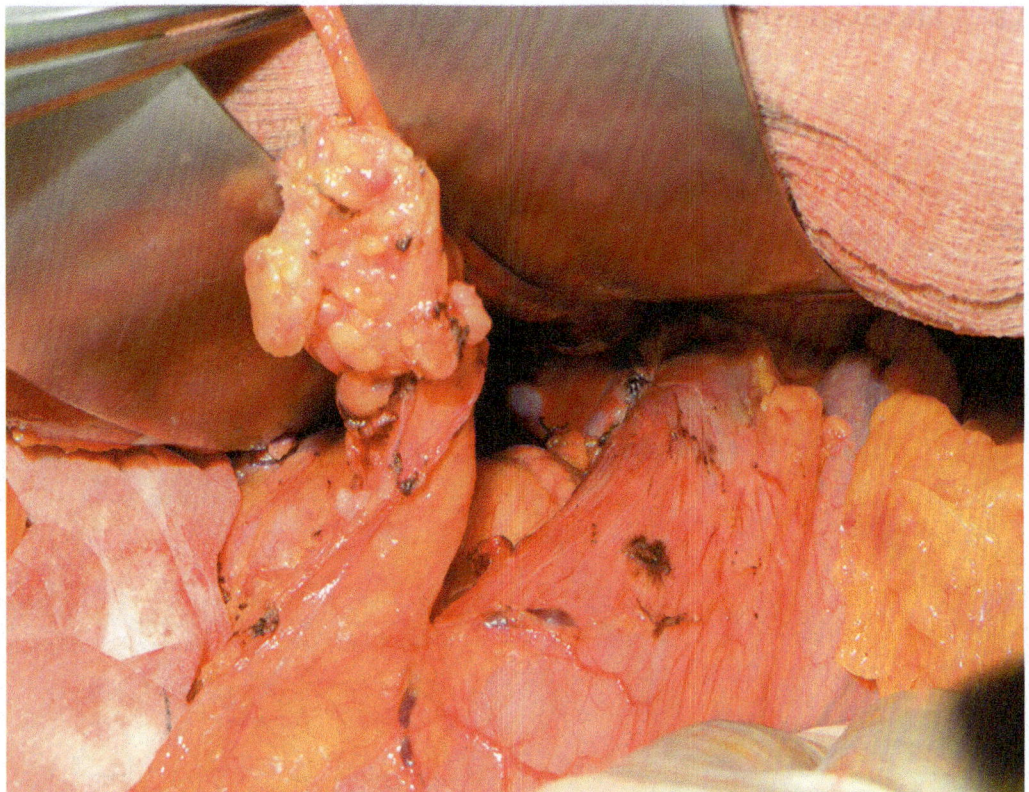

**Fig. 4.2** The right paracardial (station 1) and proximal lymphatic and adipose tissue of the lesser curvature (station 3) is thus removed, dissected, and sent for definitive histology. The arteriovenous branches of the left gastric pedicle, which penetrate the gastric wall, also need to be ligated close to the gastric wall

## 4.3 Preservation of Gastric Stump Vascularity

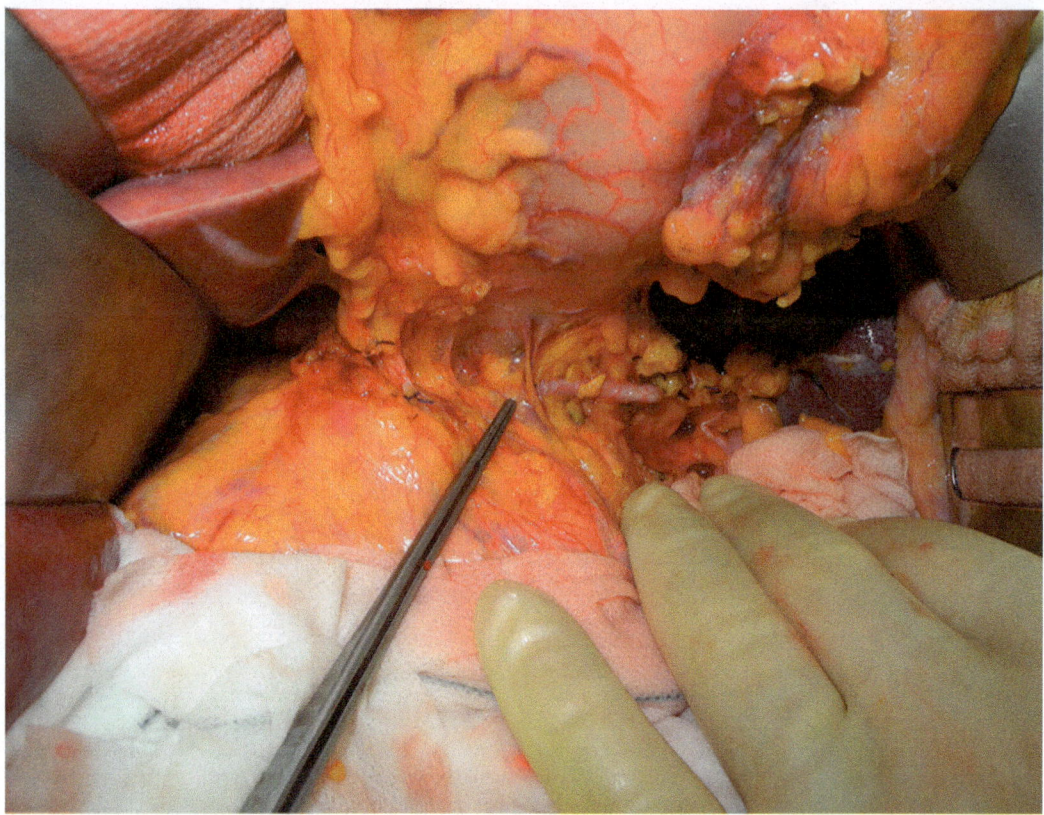

**Fig. 4.3** After identification of the transection point on the greater curvature, the gastric wall is dissected at this level, carefully preserving two or more short gastric vessels and the posterior gastric artery to ensure viability and trophism of the gastric stump

## 4.4    Preparation of the Jejunal Loop and Roux Limb Transposition to the Supramesocolic Compartment

**Fig. 4.4** With the transverse colon gently retracted, the second jejunal loop and the associated mesentery are spread to examine the anatomy of its arterial arcades by transillumination

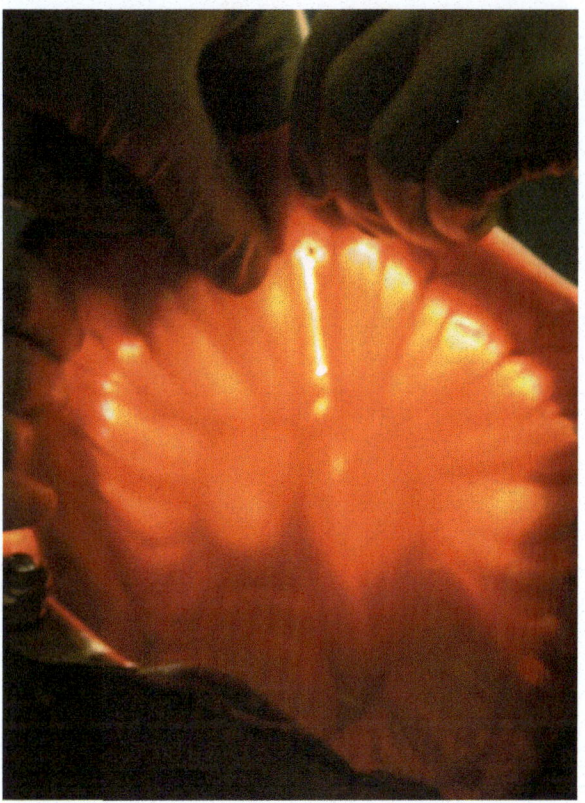

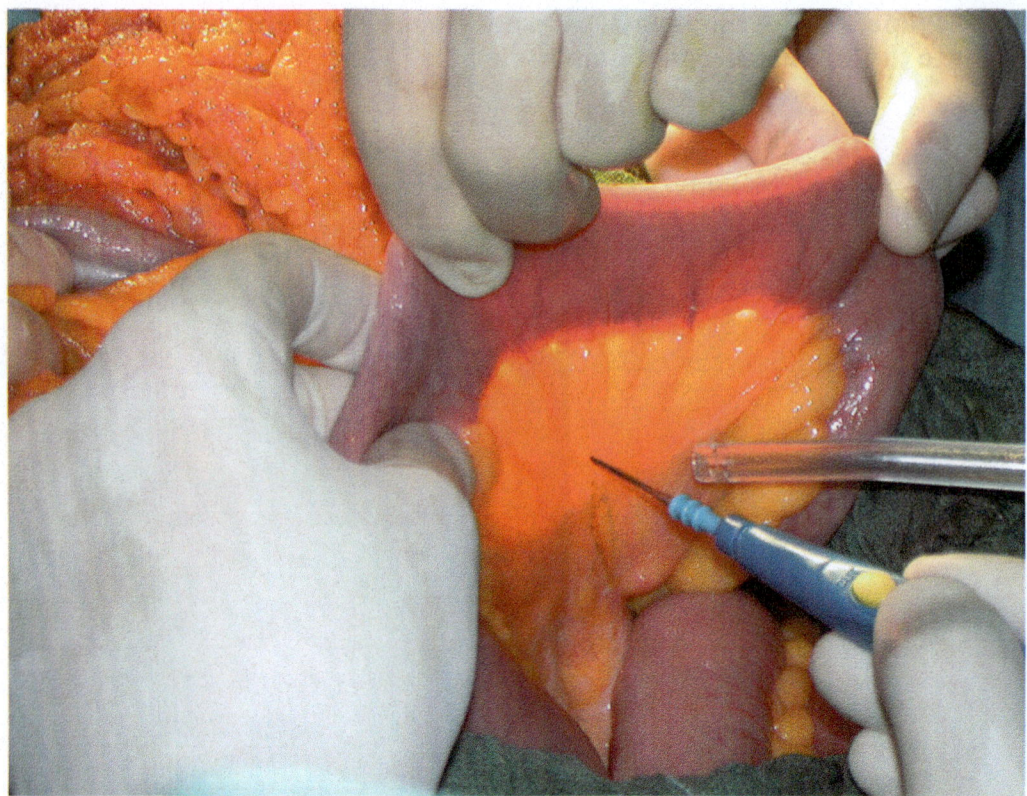

**Fig. 4.5** The arcades are then divided nearly up to the base of the mesentery, to mobilize the jejunum and gain tension-free access to the gastric stump

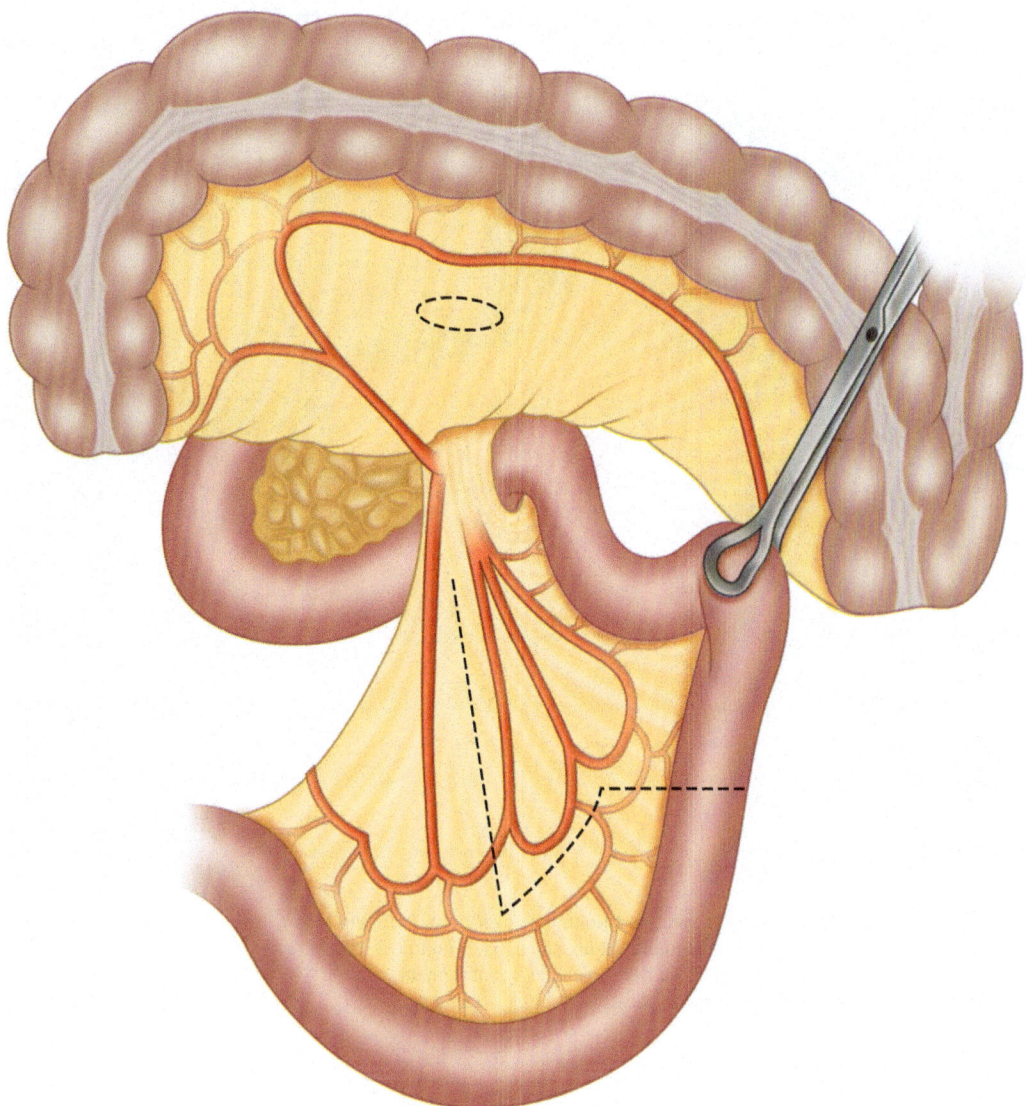

**Fig. 4.6** The resection site on the jejunum is then identified, and the jejunum is closed with a TA 30 linear stapler; after placement of a non-crushing intestinal clamp, the afferent portion is also resected with a traditional blade and remains open. The stapled efferent portion is oversewn with interrupted slowly absorbable 3-0 sutures. With the transverse colon still gently retracted, an avascular area in its left inferior paramedian portion is identified by transillumination and incised to allow transposition of the efferent jejunal limb to the supramesocolic compartment through the transverse mesocolon

## 4.5    Placement of the Haberer Intestinal and Stomach Clamp

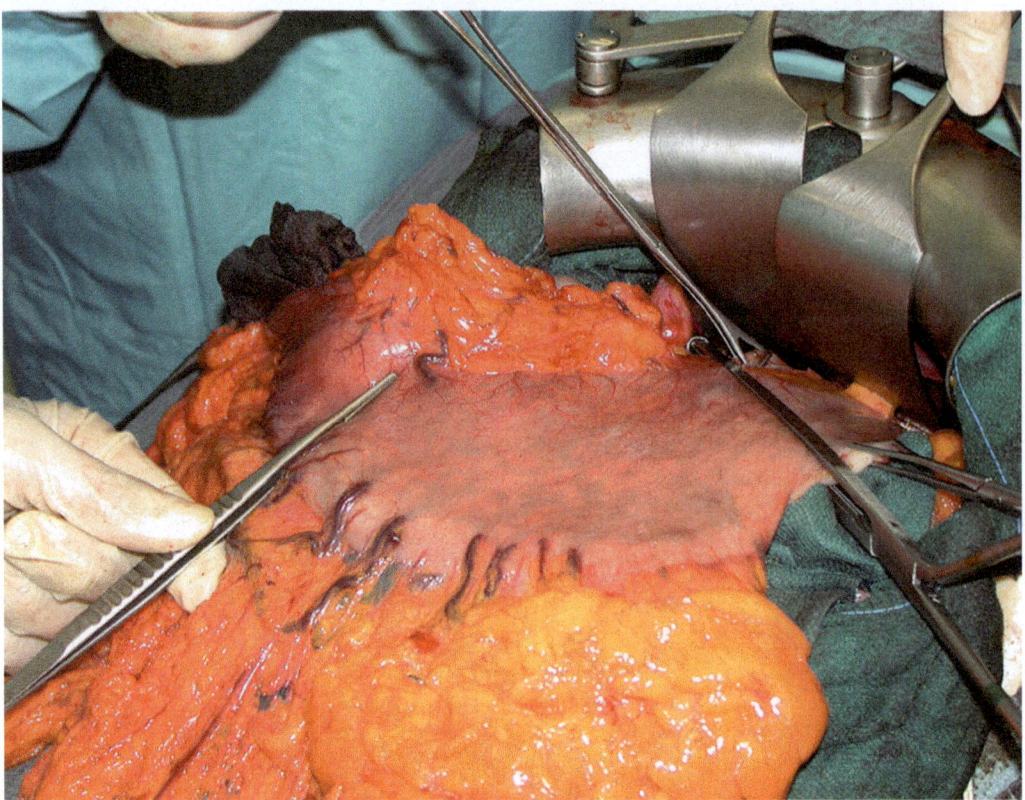

**Fig. 4.7** The gastric tool of the Haberer intestinal and stomach clamp is applied to the gastric fundus at an adequate distance between the proximal tumor pole and resection line, considering that the anastomosis will be executed ca. 2 cm below the clamp. The nasogastric tube is withdrawn before closing the clamp, to avoid its entrapment

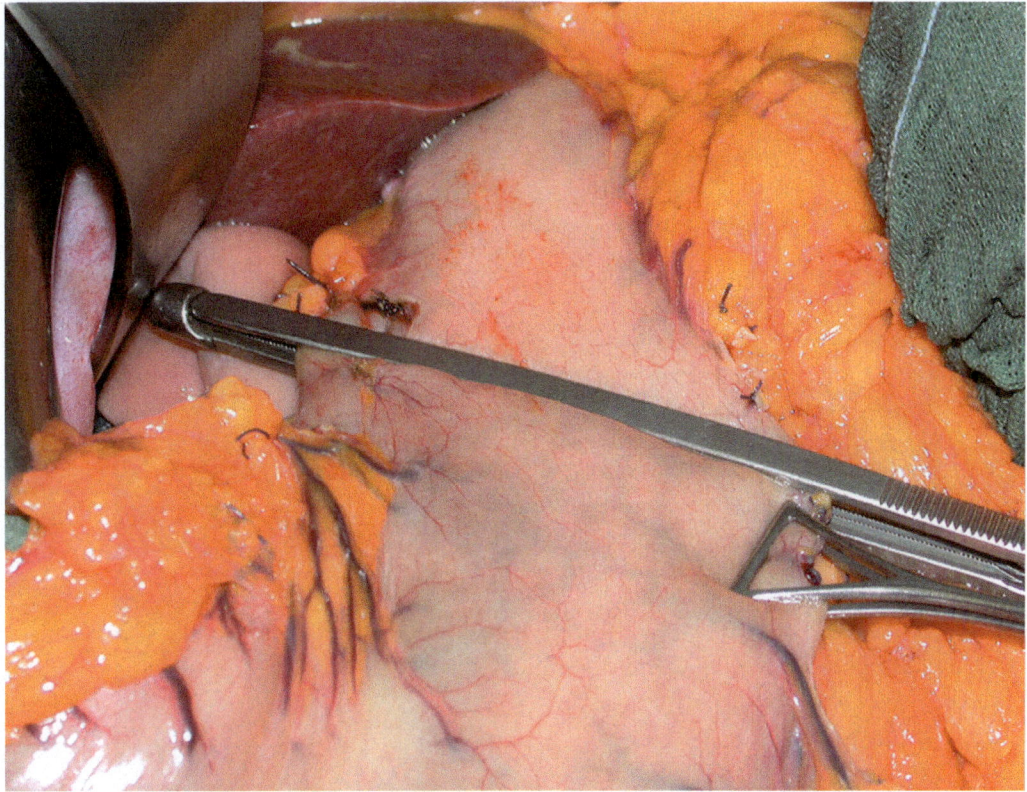

**Fig. 4.8** The gastric tool of the Haberer clamp should be applied to the gastric fundus at an obtuse angle (120–130°) with respect to the lesser curvature. In this way, the transection line affords both macroscopically correct margins and removal of antral G cells (thus avoiding retained antrum syndrome)

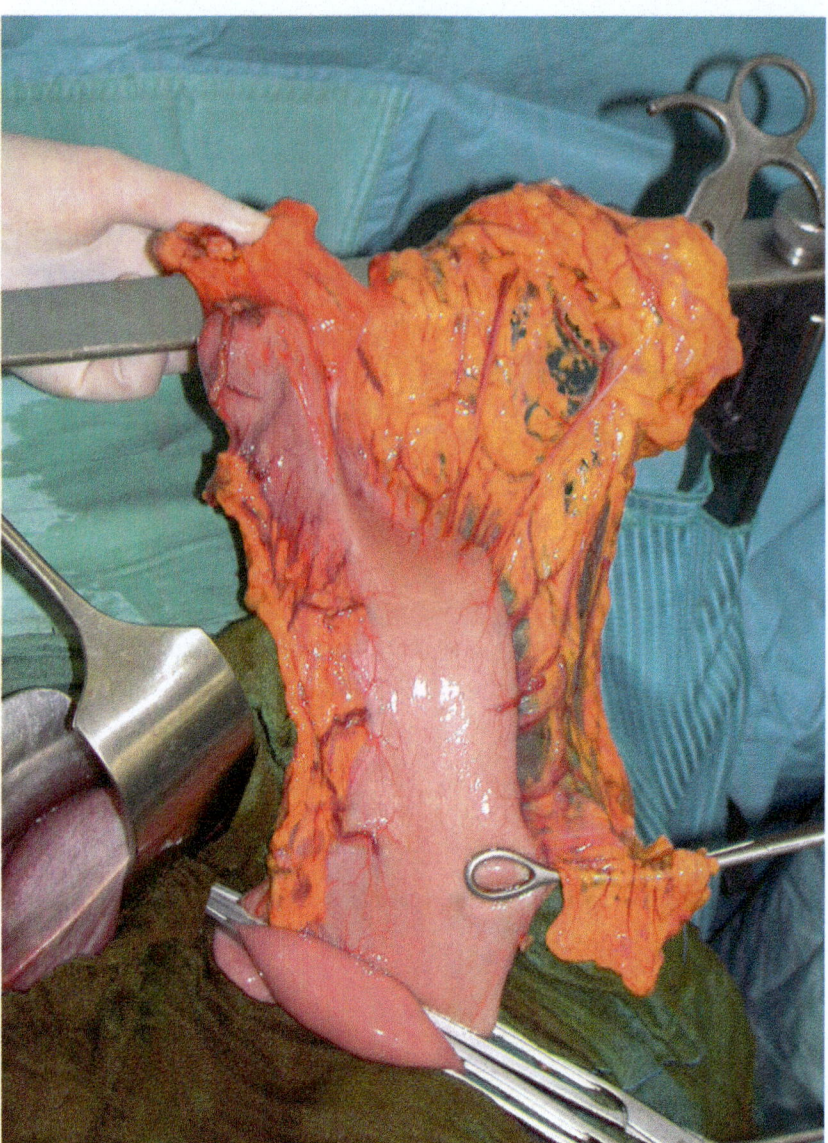

**Figs. 4.9 and 4.10** With the stomach elevated and retracted upward, to expose its posterior wall which is held in slight tension, the first assistant raises the previously prepared closed Roux limb with two forceps, while the surgeon gently tightens the jejunal tool of the clamp at the level of the mesenteric edge. The gastric and jejunal wall are approximated on the lateral side of the greater curvature. The gastric and jejunal clamps are then brought close together and blocked with the third clamp. The latter is locked when the gastric and the jejunal wall are approximated on the lateral side of the greater curvature. Three laparotomy pads, one behind the stomach, another in front of the Roux limb, and the third above the three clamps, are applied prior to execution of the anastomosis, to prevent contamination of the operating field and trapping of the suture threads in the clamp jaws

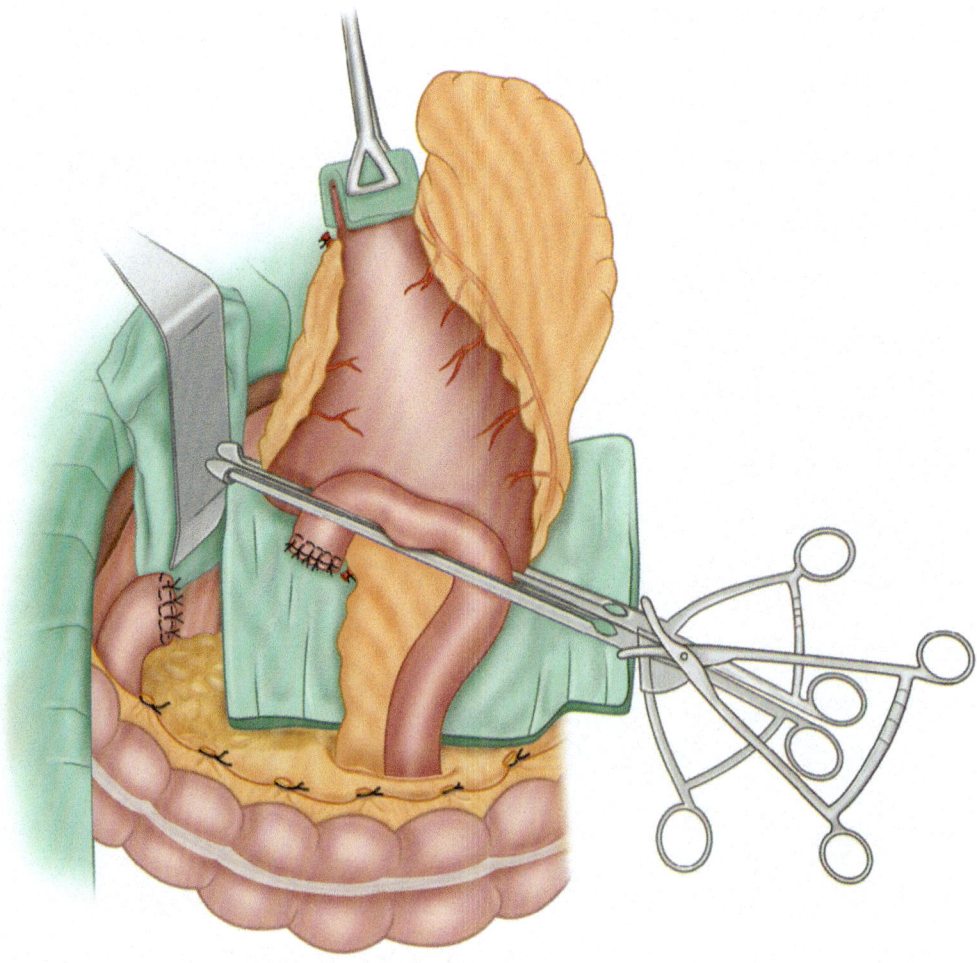

**Figs. 4.9 and 4.10** (continued)

## 4.6    Creation of the Gastrojejunostomy

### 4.6.1    First Layer of the Posterior Wall

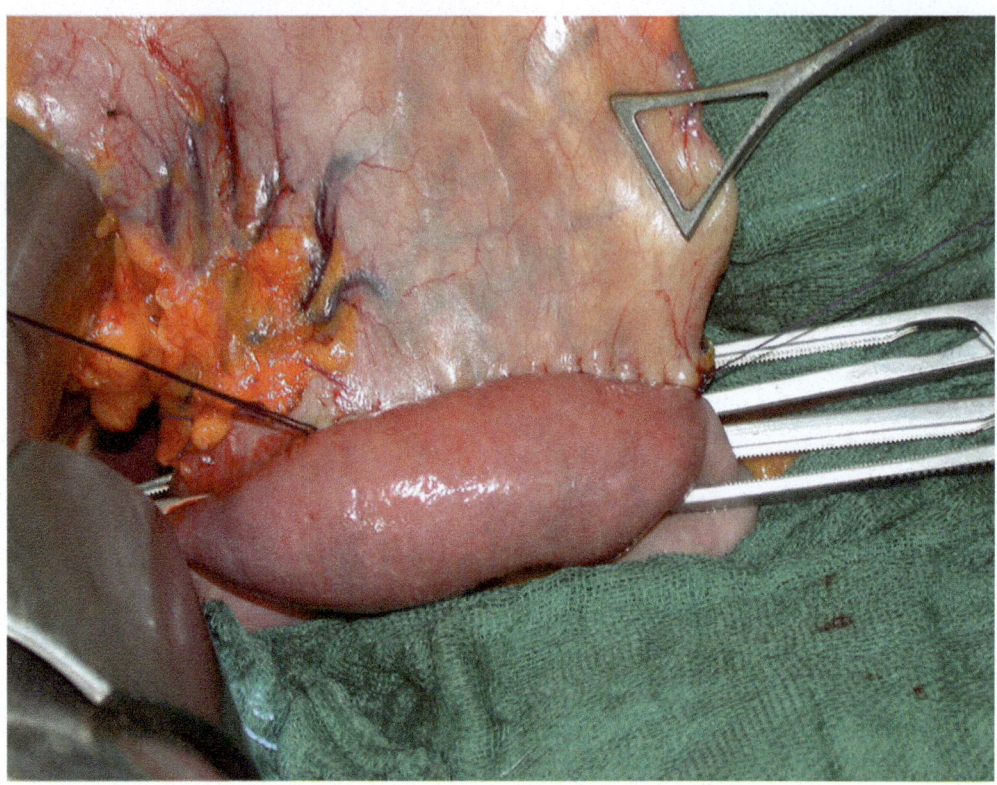

**Figs. 4.11 and 4.12** The first layer of the posterior wall is realized from the lateral portion of the greater curvature toward the lesser curvature using a continuous seromuscular slowly absorbable suture (2-0) and a 30 mm needle. The needle is passed at closely spaced (5–7 mm) intervals through the walls at a 45° angle with respect to the major axis of the suture, taking an abundant portion of the gastric seromuscular layer. Inability to see the suture commonly indicates that the correct amount of tension has been applied. Mosquito forceps are placed at either end of the suture

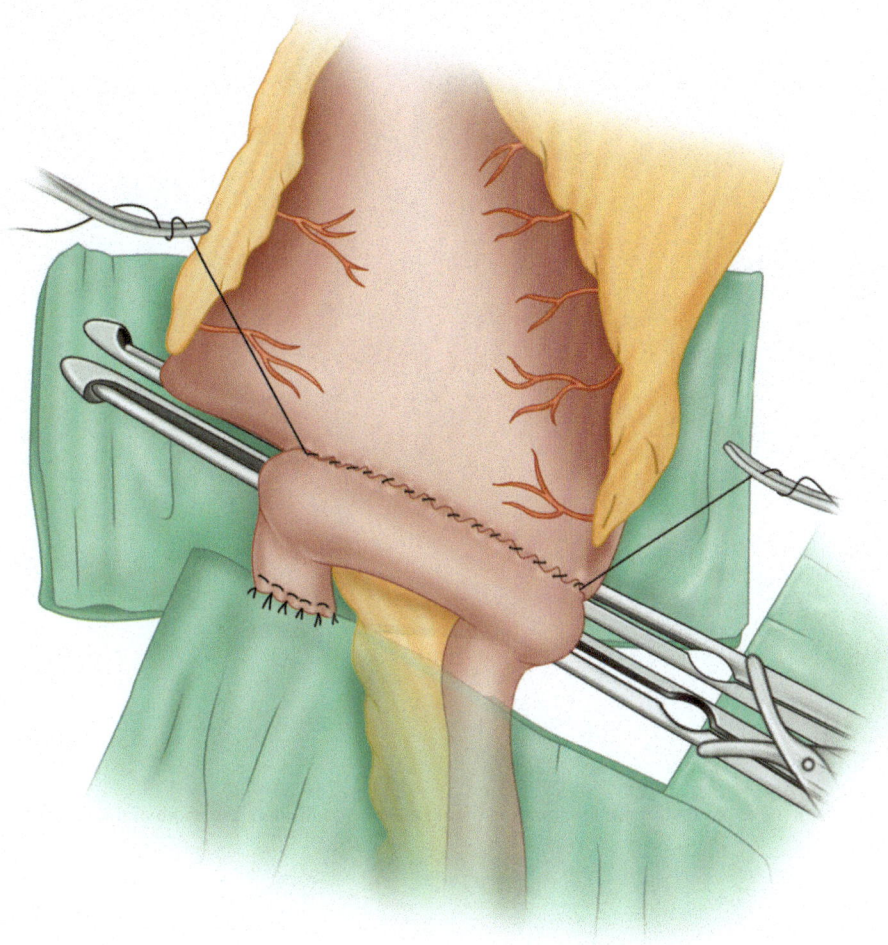

**Figs. 4.11 and 4.12**  (continued)

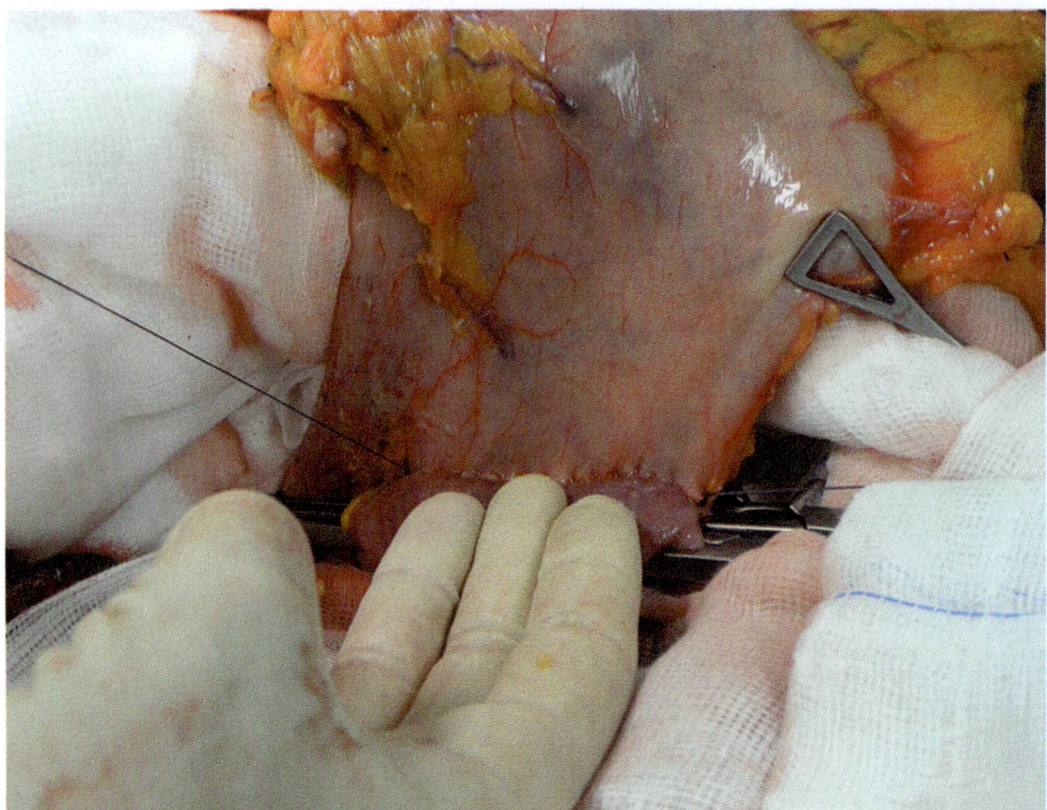

**Fig. 4.13** The mouth of the partial inferior anastomosis should measure ca. 6 cm or the width of three fingers

**Figs. 4.14 and 4.15** A long clamp encompassing the whole stomach is placed upstream of the suture, to avoid operative field contamination; then the posterior gastric wall is resected first, at a distance of 1 cm from the suture on the side of the greater curvature and of 1.5–2 cm on the side of the lesser curvature. The seromuscular layer is excised with electrocautery, and the vessels of the rich submucosal venous plexus are coagulated tangent to the section margin, to avoid leaving excess mucosa, which would complicate the execution of the internal layer of the anastomosis

### 4.6.2    Resection of the Stomach and Intraoperative Consultation

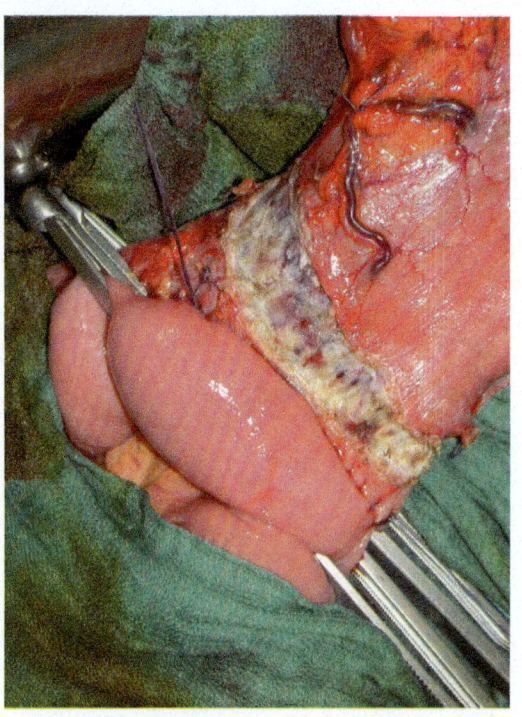

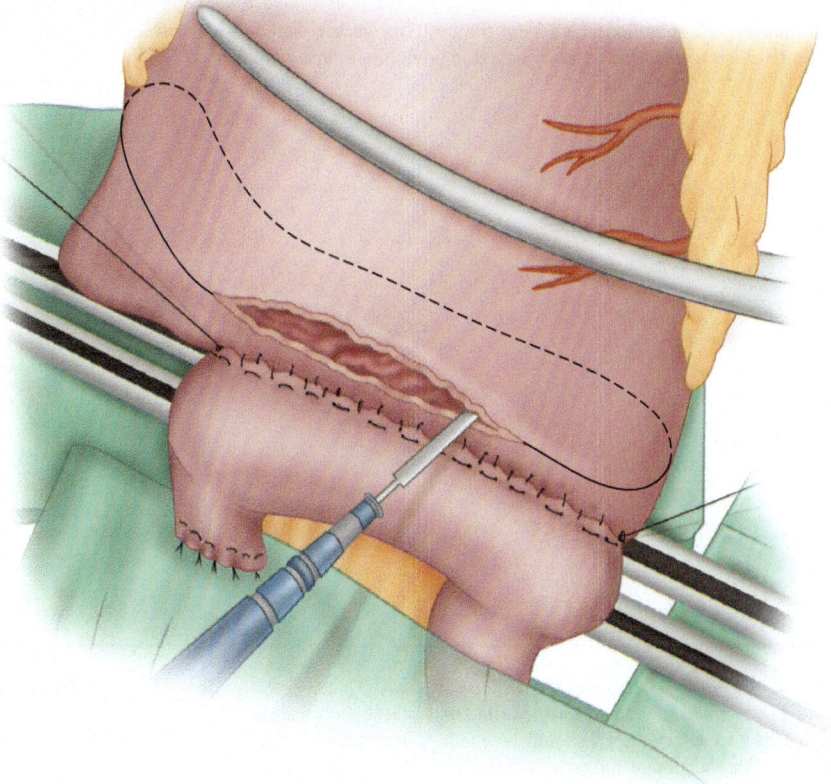

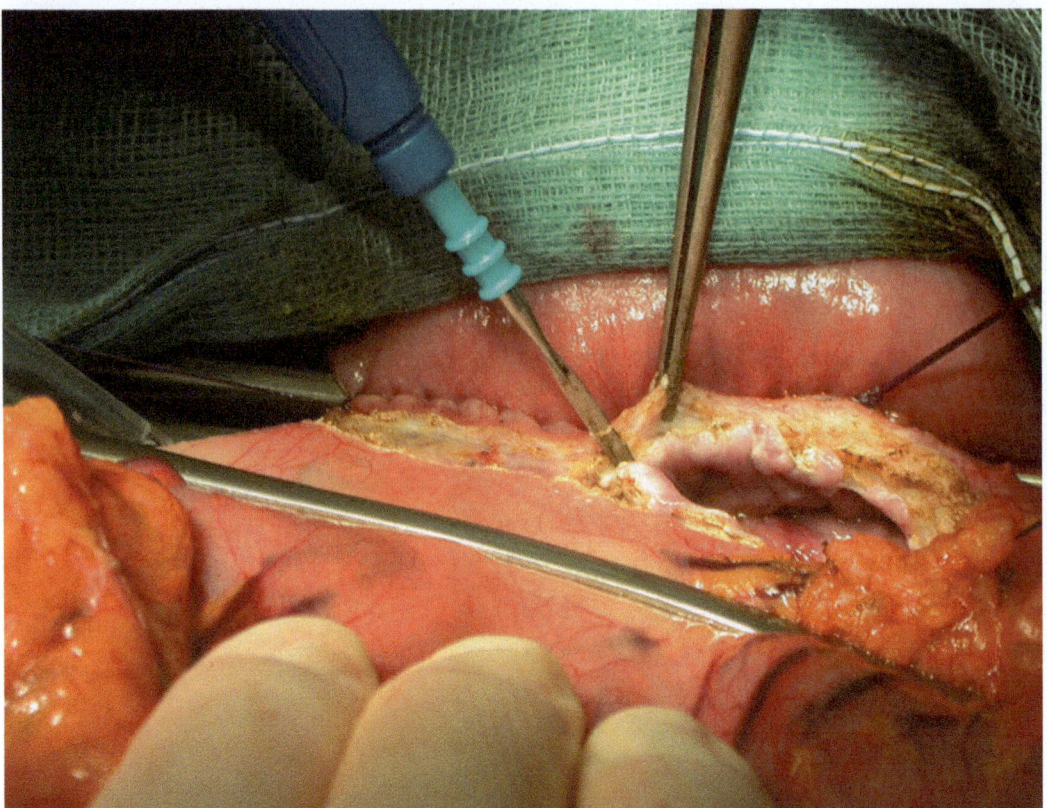

**Fig. 4.16** The mucosal and submucosal layers of the posterior gastric wall are then excised with electrocautery. The open gastric stump is disinfected, and a gauze soaked in povidone-iodine is applied

**Figs. 4.17 and 4.18** The stomach is replaced, excising the anterior wall as described for the posterior wall. Tip: the resection line on the anterior wall should be made 2 cm from the suture on the side of the greater curvature and 3 cm from it on the side of the lesser curvature, to facilitate creation of the anastomosis and oversewing of the medial portion of the gastric stump

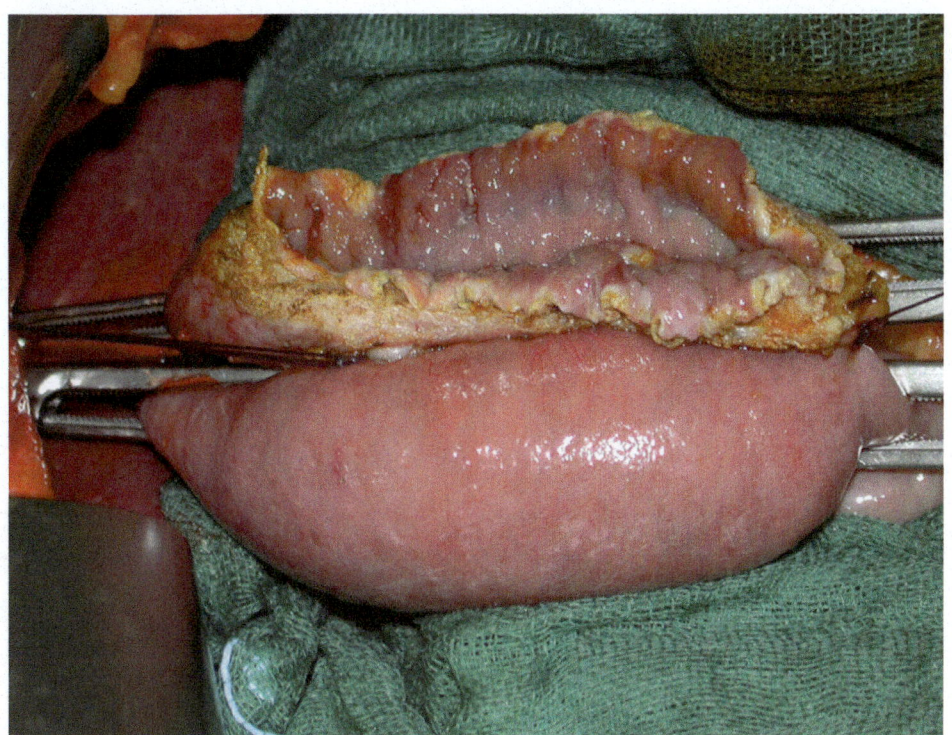

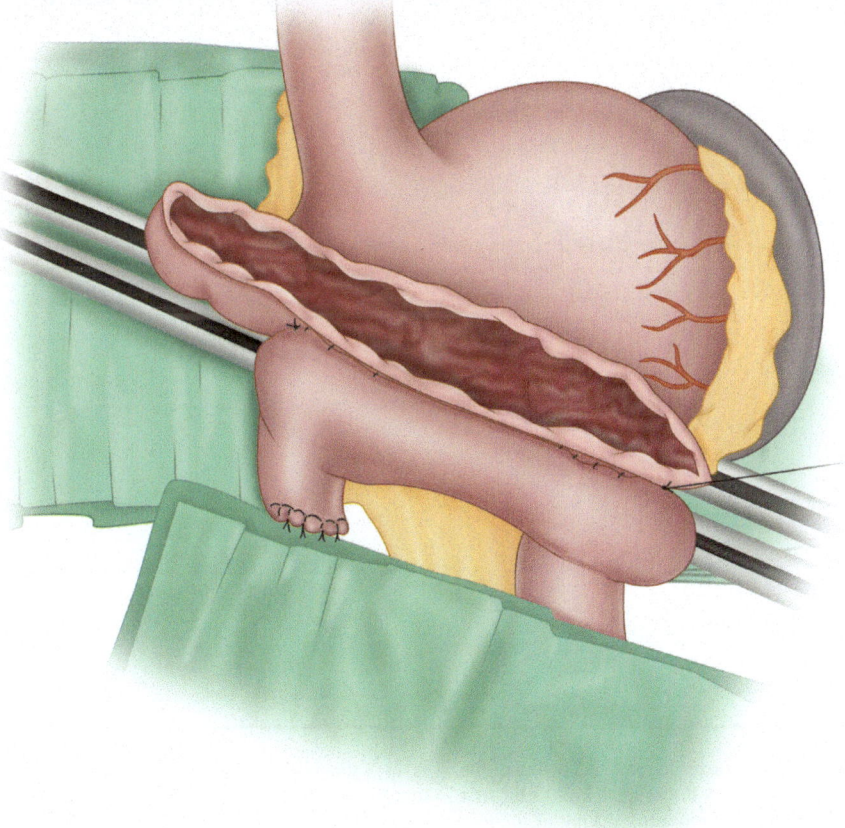

**Fig. 4.19** The specimen is removed and submitted for frozen section assessment of the margins and microscopic evaluation of their negativity

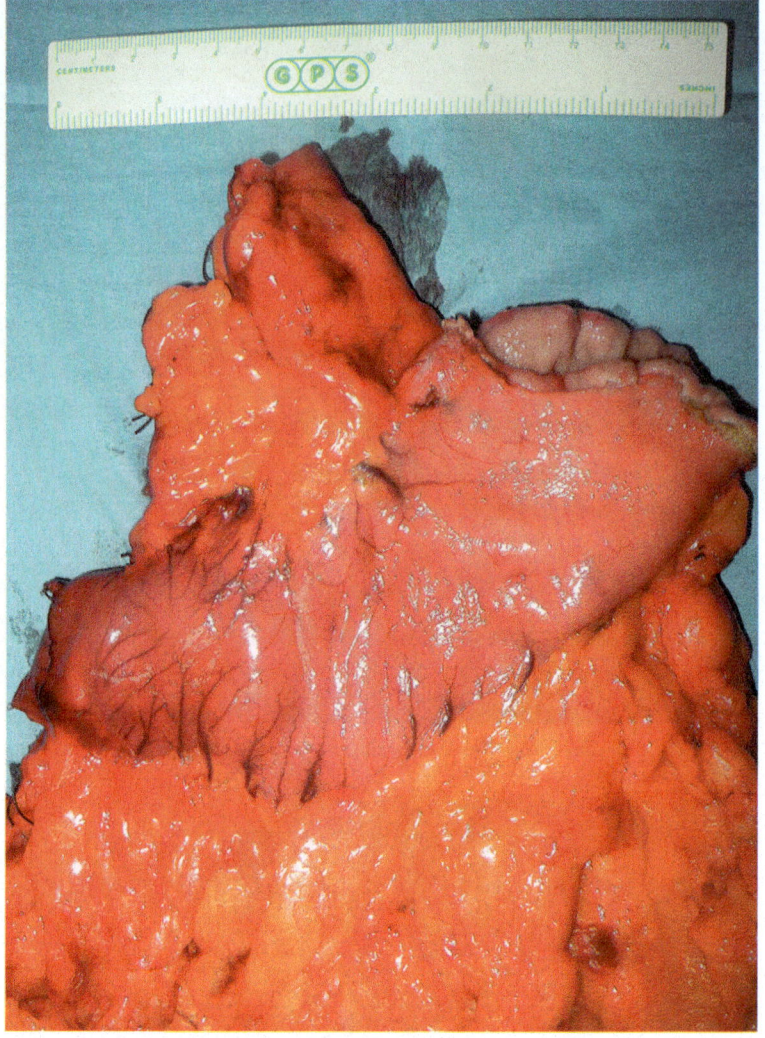

**Figs. 4.20 and 4.21** Closure of the medial portion of the gastric stump not sutured to the jejunal limb. The first stitch is full-thickness and is close to the knot of the first layer of the posterior wall of the anastomosis. This ensures that the mouth of the partial inferior anastomosis is the size of the width of three fingers

### 4.6.3 Closure of the Medial Gastric Stump

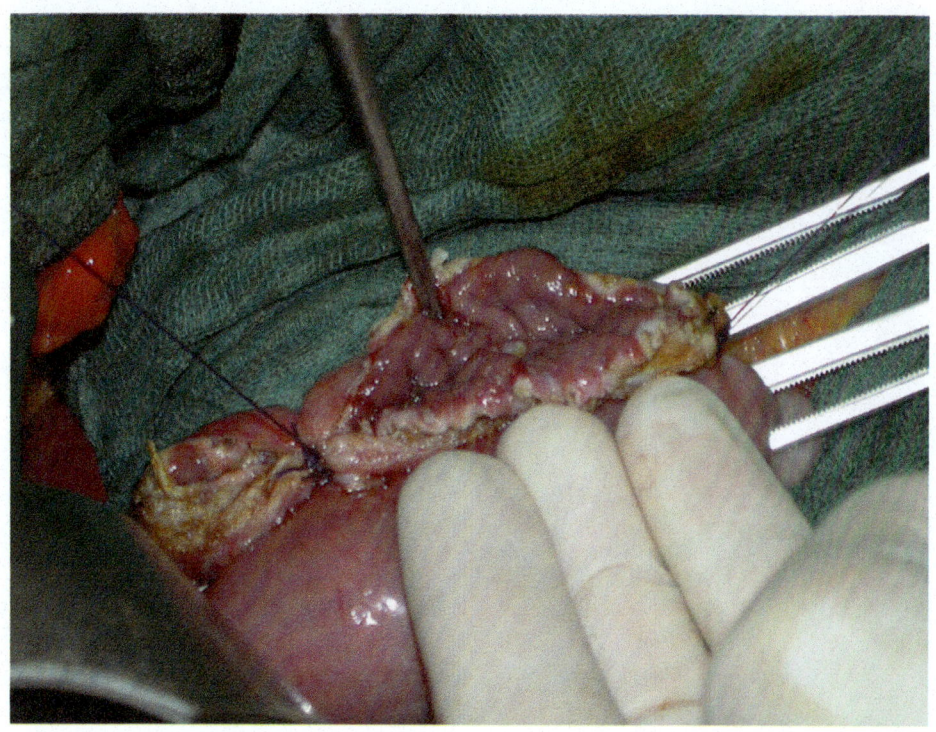

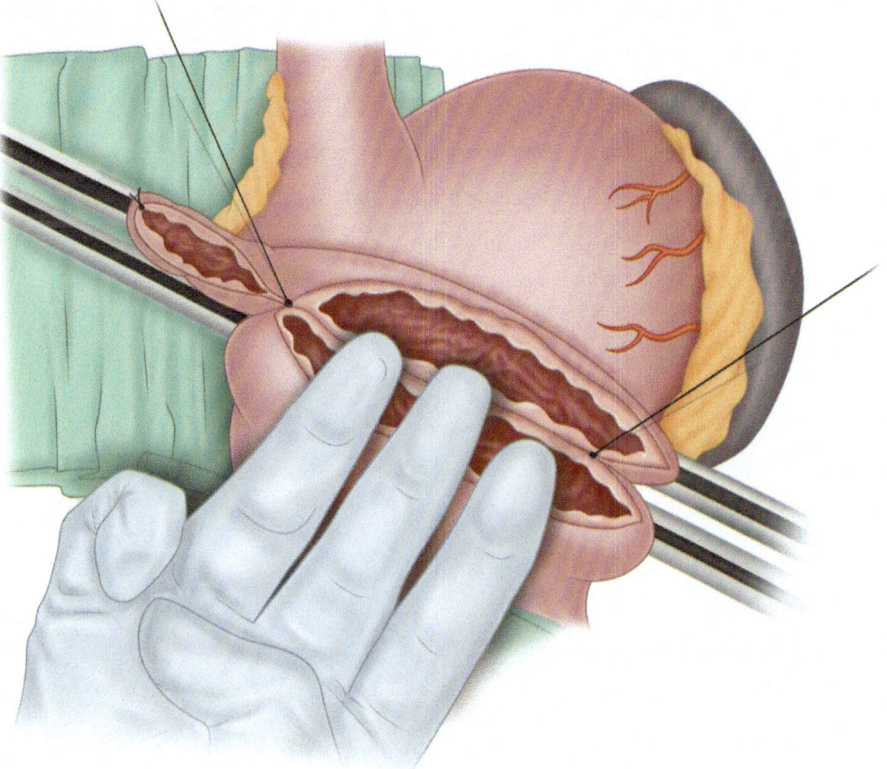

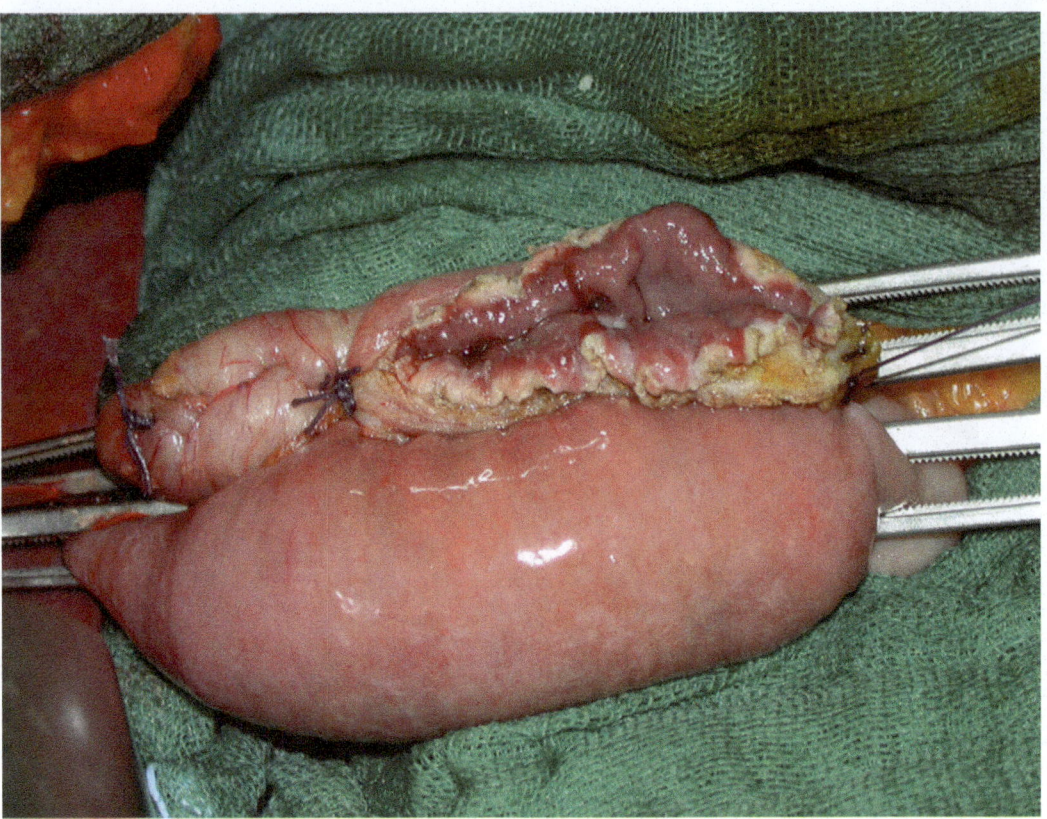

**Fig. 4.22** The medial gastric stump is closed with a continuous slowly absorbable 2-0 suture according to O'Connell

### 4.6.4   Second Posterior Layer and First Anterior One

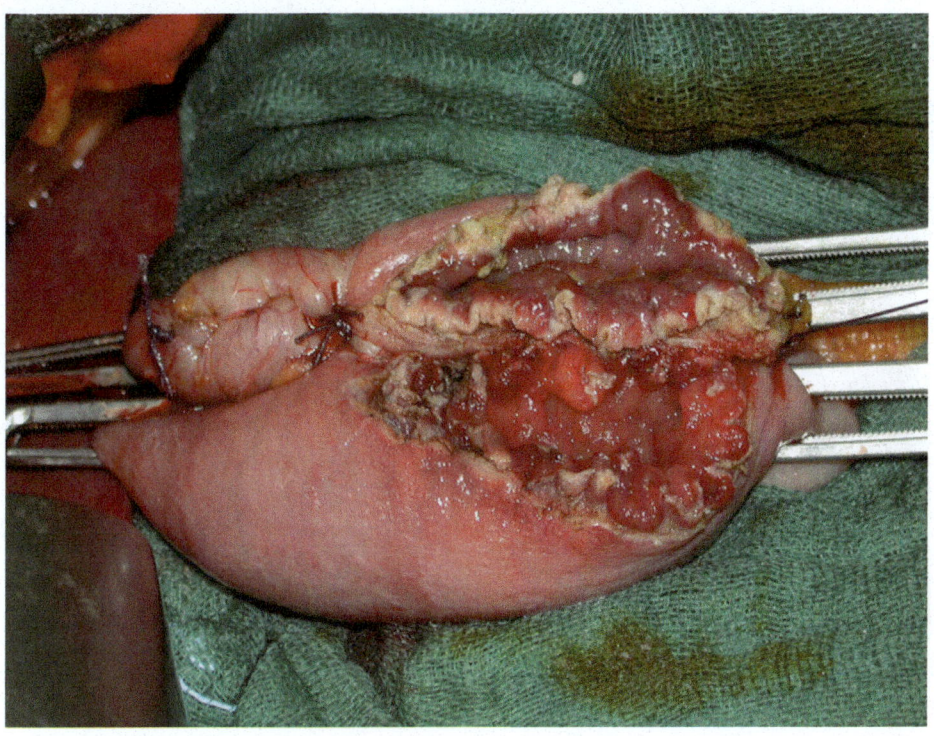

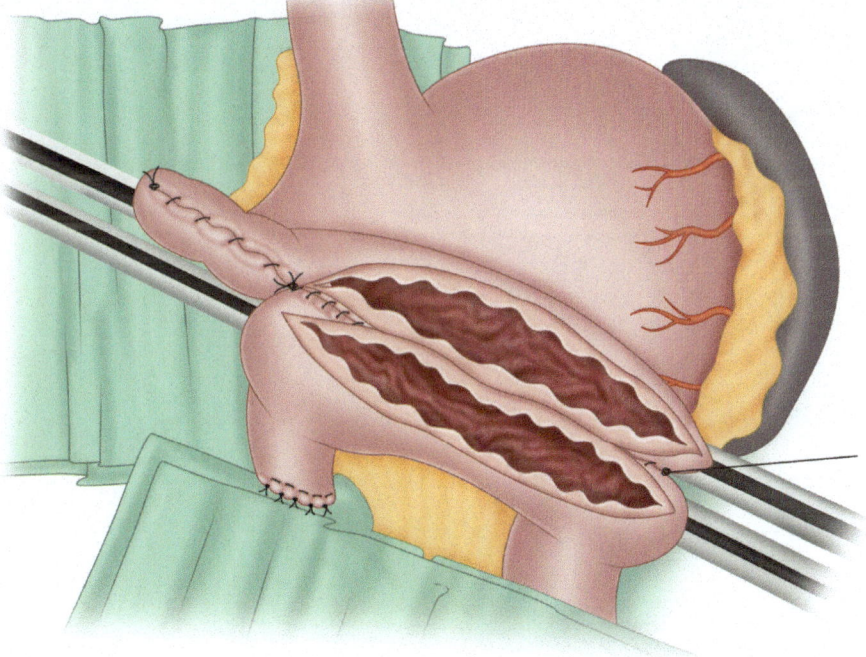

**Figs. 4.23 and 4.24**   Incision of the jejunal loop. The jejunum is incised approximately 1 cm from the posterior suture line for a length corresponding to the width of the anastomosis

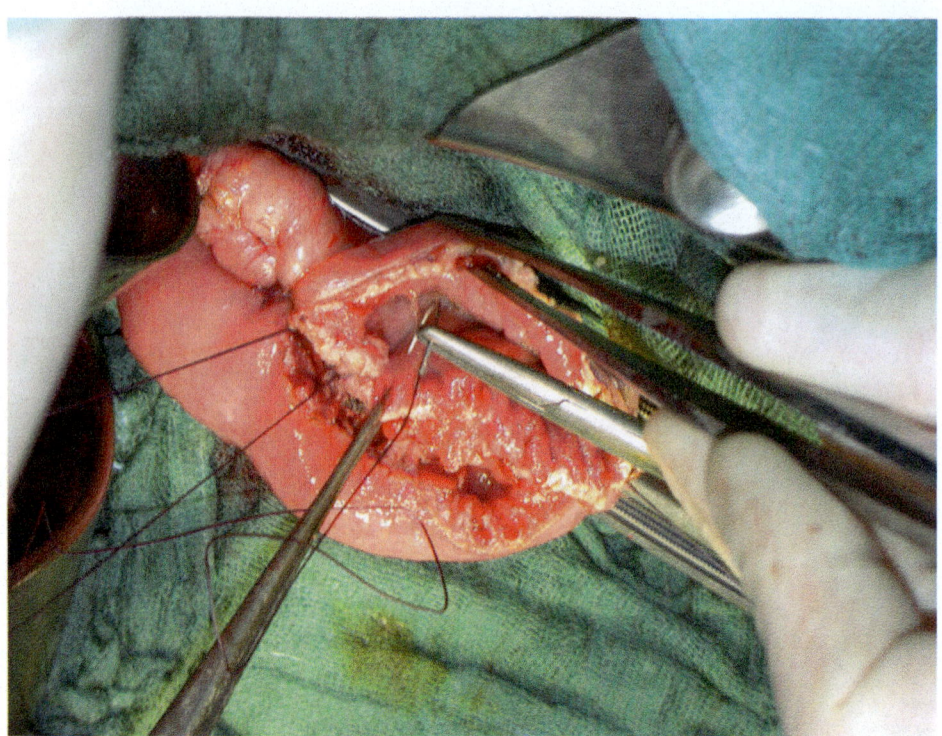

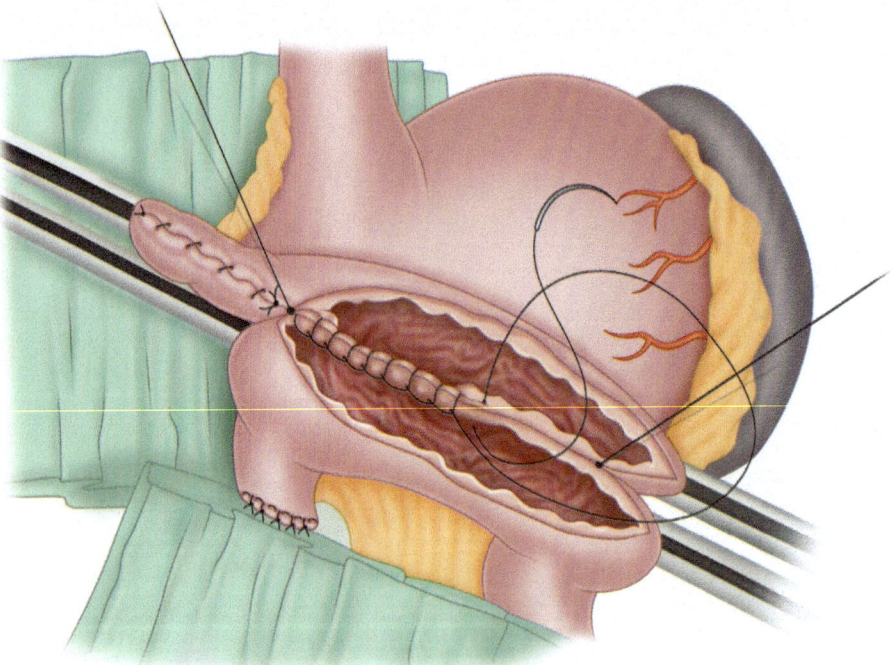

**Figs. 4.25 and 4.26** The second layer of the posterior wall is begun with a continuous running locked slowly absorbable suture (2-0) from the lesser to the greater curvature. The first stitch is inside out, passing first through the gastric wall and then through the medial side of the jejunal wall. While the surgeon tightens the knot, pushing it posteriorly, the first assistant tucks in the excess mucosa using two forceps so as to close and seal the medial corner of the anastomosis. The loose end of this suture is knotted with the thread of the continuous suture of the first layer of the posterior wall and cut

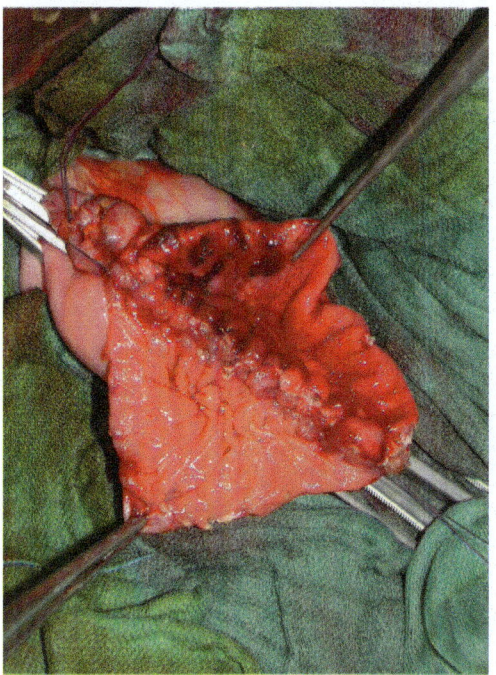

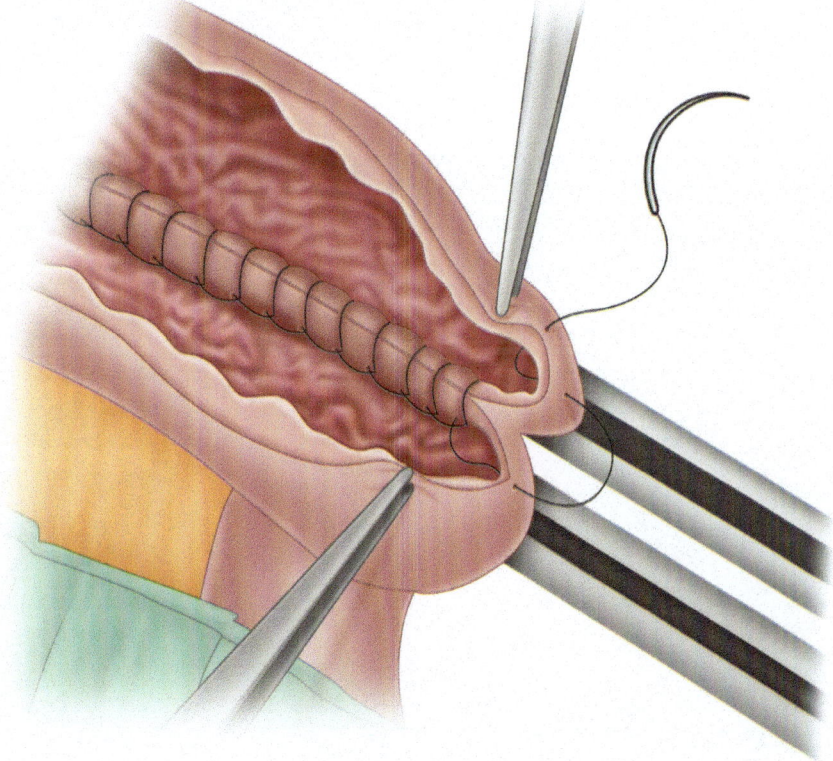

**Figs. 4.27 and 4.28** The running locked suture of the second layer of the posterior wall ensures hemostasis and seals the inner layer. After completion of the second layer of the posterior wall, the needle exits through the jejunal wall and is reintroduced through the end of the anastomosis on the side of the greater curvature. From here the suture is begun again, proceeding from the greater to the lesser curvature, using the same thread

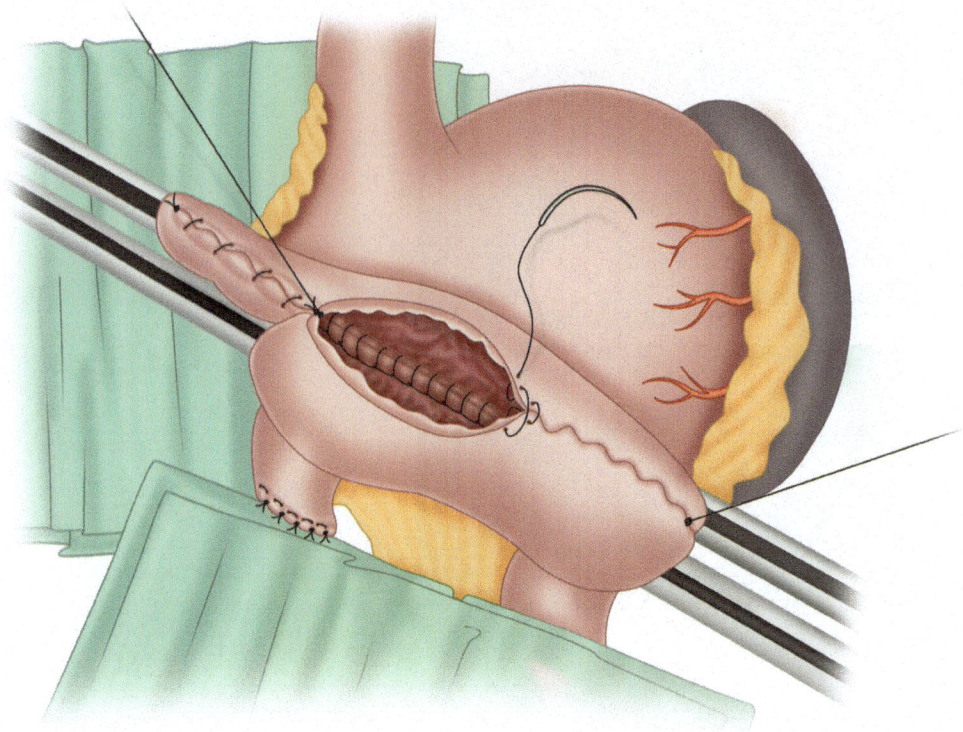

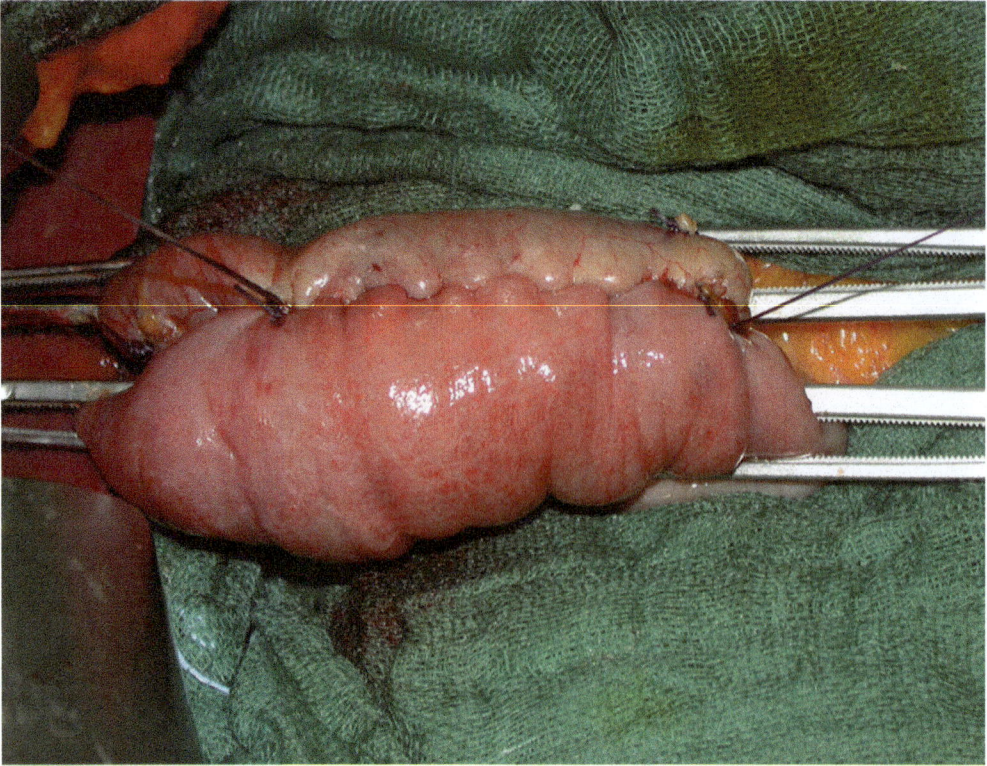

**Figs. 4.29 and 4.30** The first layer of the anterior wall is performed from the gastric to the jejunal wall at 5–7 mm intervals with a full-thickness suture according to O'Connell

### 4.6.5 Oversewing of the Medial Gastric Stump

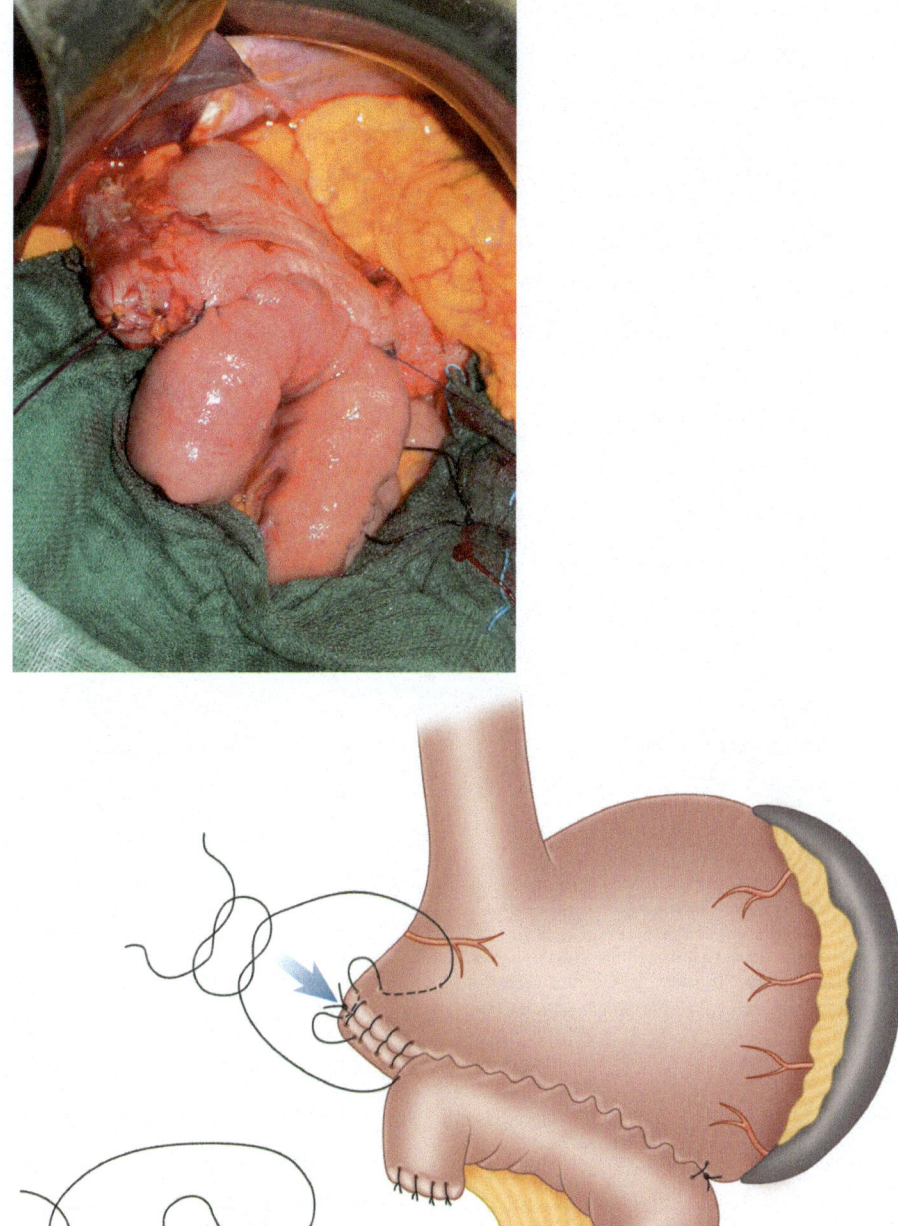

**Figs. 4.31 and 4.32** The non-anastomosed gastric stump, which has been closed with a continuous suture, forms an acute angle that needs to be straightened. A semipouch suture is passed through the seromuscular layer on the anterior gastric wall, 2–3 cm from the angle, through the angle itself, and through the seromuscular layer of the posterior gastric wall. The first assistant oversews then tucks in the angle of the gastric stump

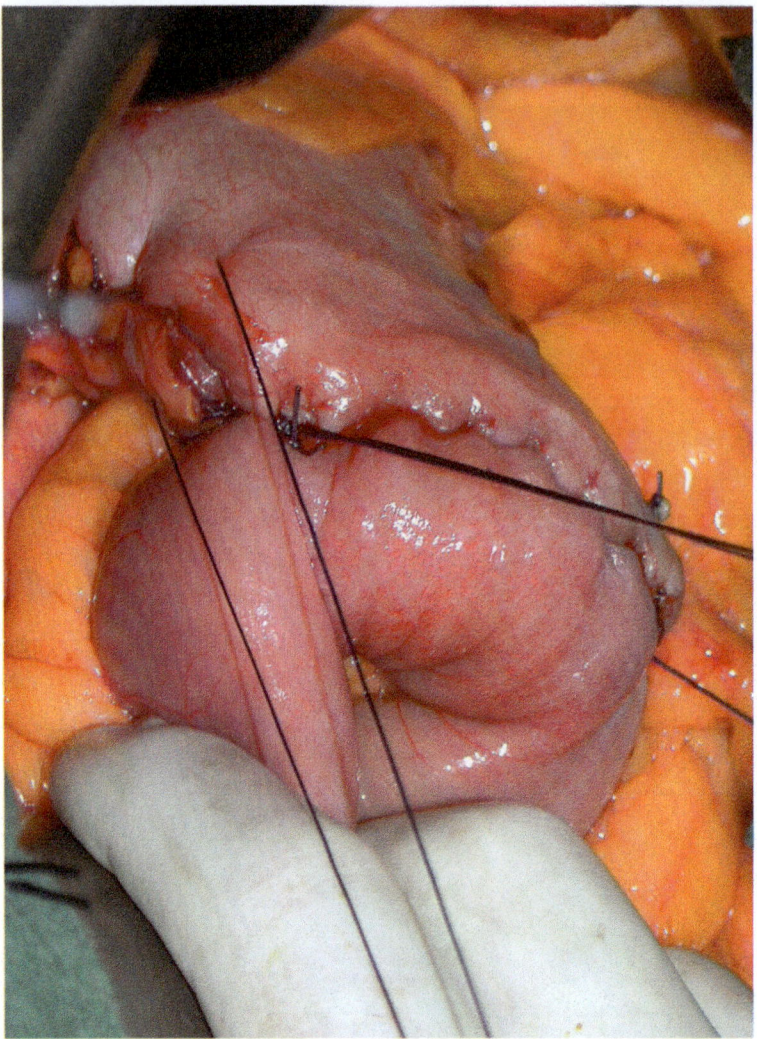

**Figs. 4.33 and 4.34** Two to three interrupted slowly absorbable seromuscular sutures (2-0) are placed upstream and downstream of the semipouch suture. The whole second layer of the non-anastomosed gastric stump is finally achieved; the stump is straightened and reduced to the size of the anastomosis

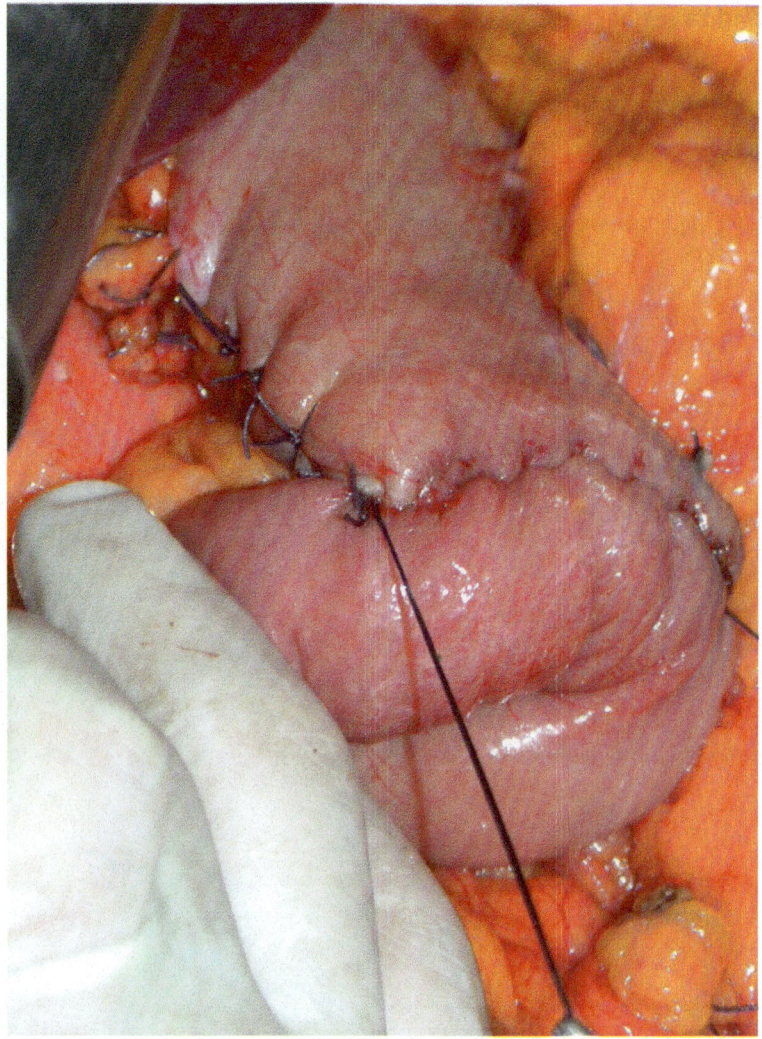

**Figs. 4.33 and 4.34**   (continued)

### 4.6.6    Second Layer of the Anterior Wall

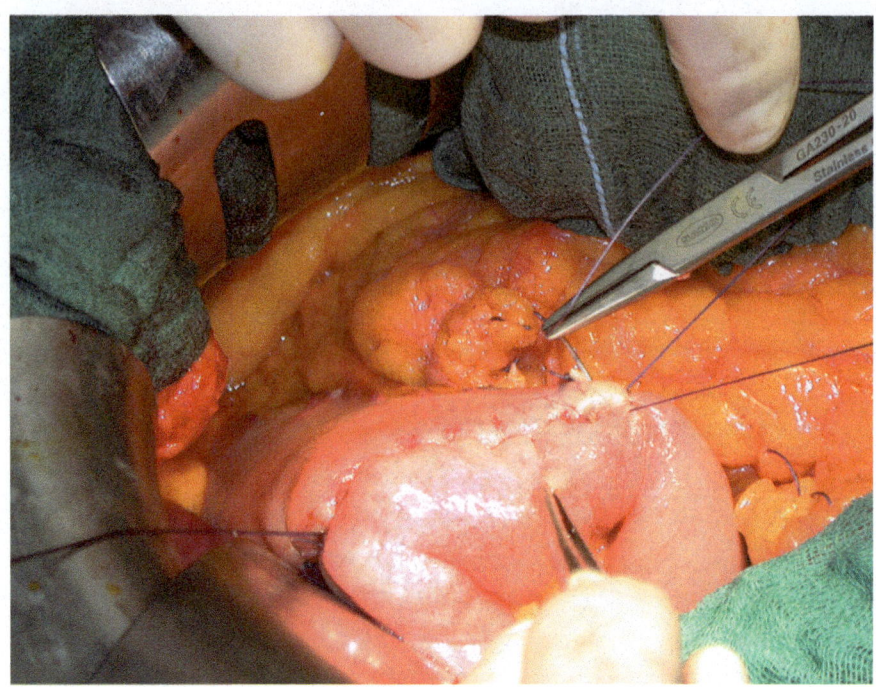

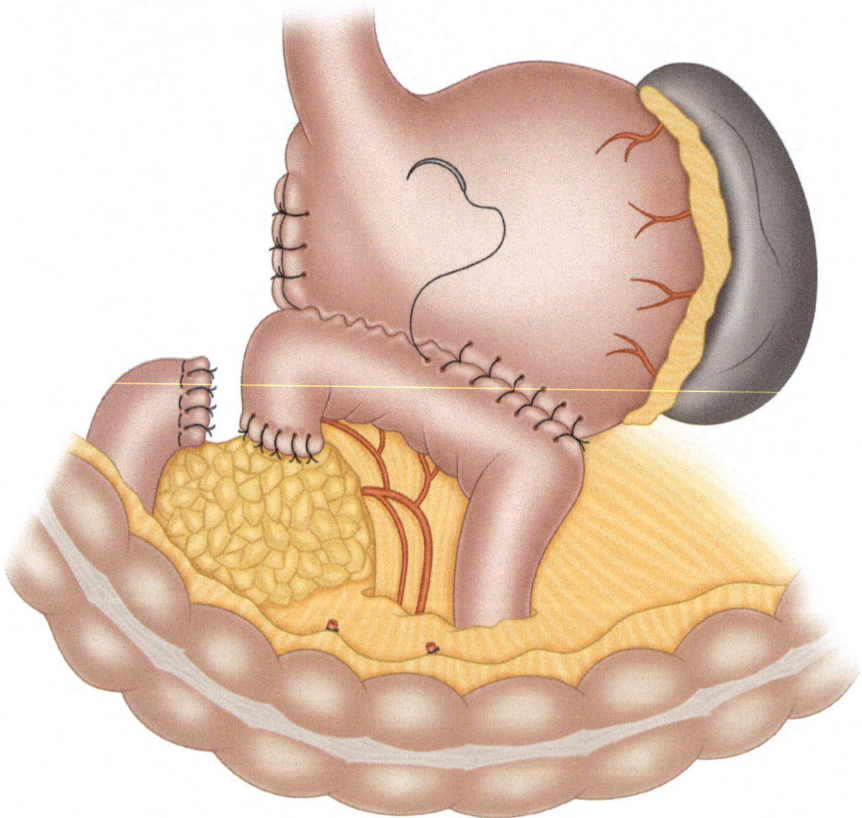

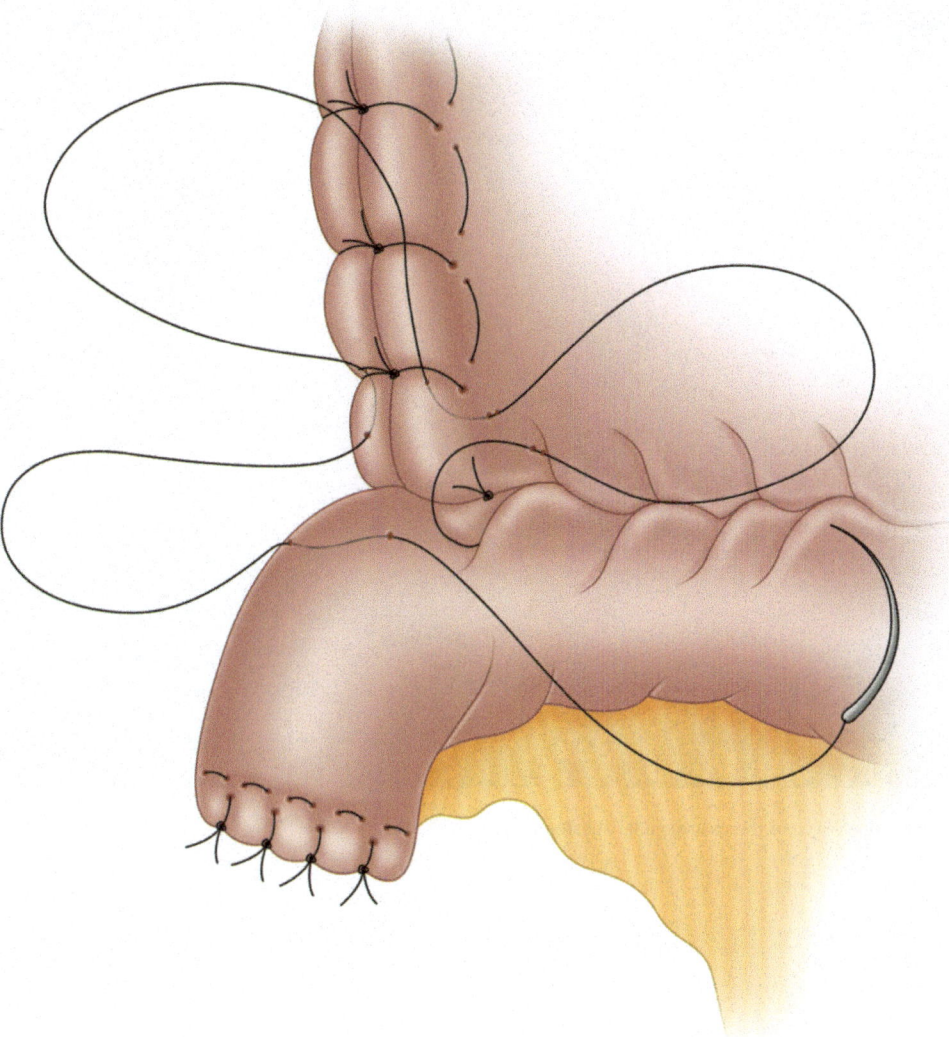

**Fig. 4.37** The thread of the first continuous suture is met and overcome close to the medial corner, which is sealed using a triple stitch encompassing the seromuscular layer of the anterior wall of the non-anastomosed gastric stump, its posterior wall, and the jejunal seromuscular layer

**Figs. 4.35 and 4.36** The second layer of the anterior wall is performed starting laterally from the continuous suture of the first layer of the posterior wall, using a continuous slowly absorbable 2-0 suture, proceeding from the greater to the lesser curvature with seromuscular sutures placed 5–7 mm apart

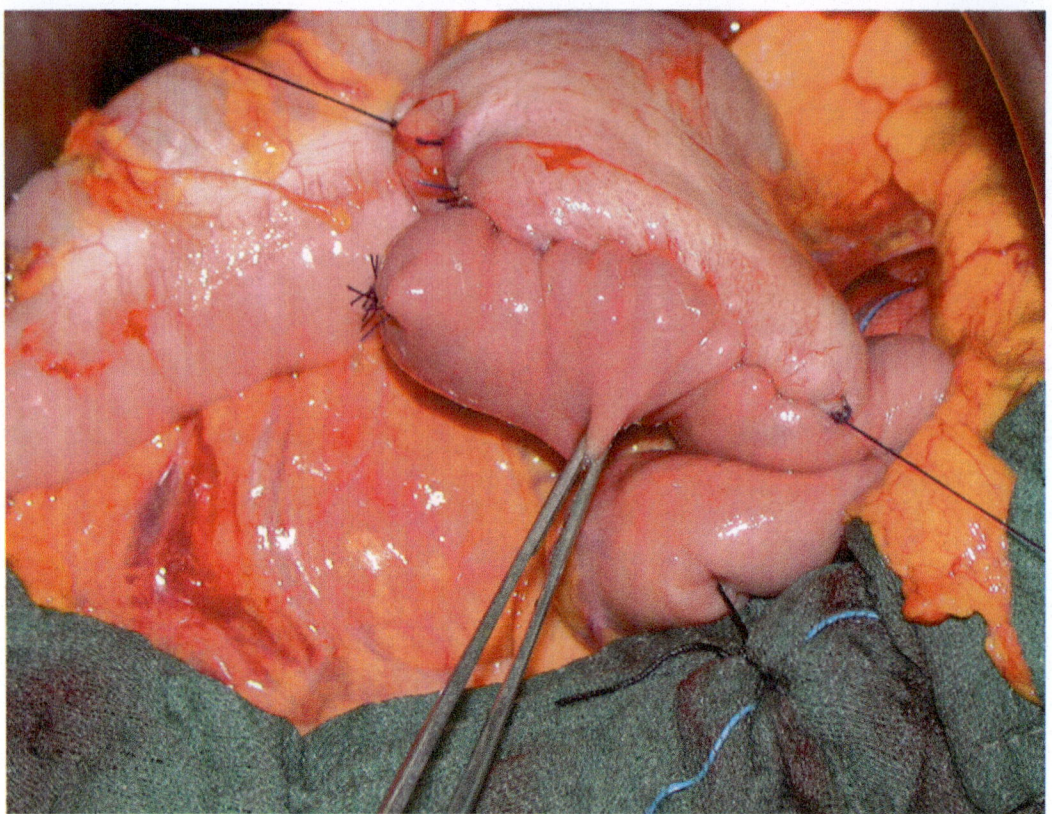

**Fig. 4.38** Final appearance of the gastrojejunal anastomosis

## 4.7    Enteroenterostomy

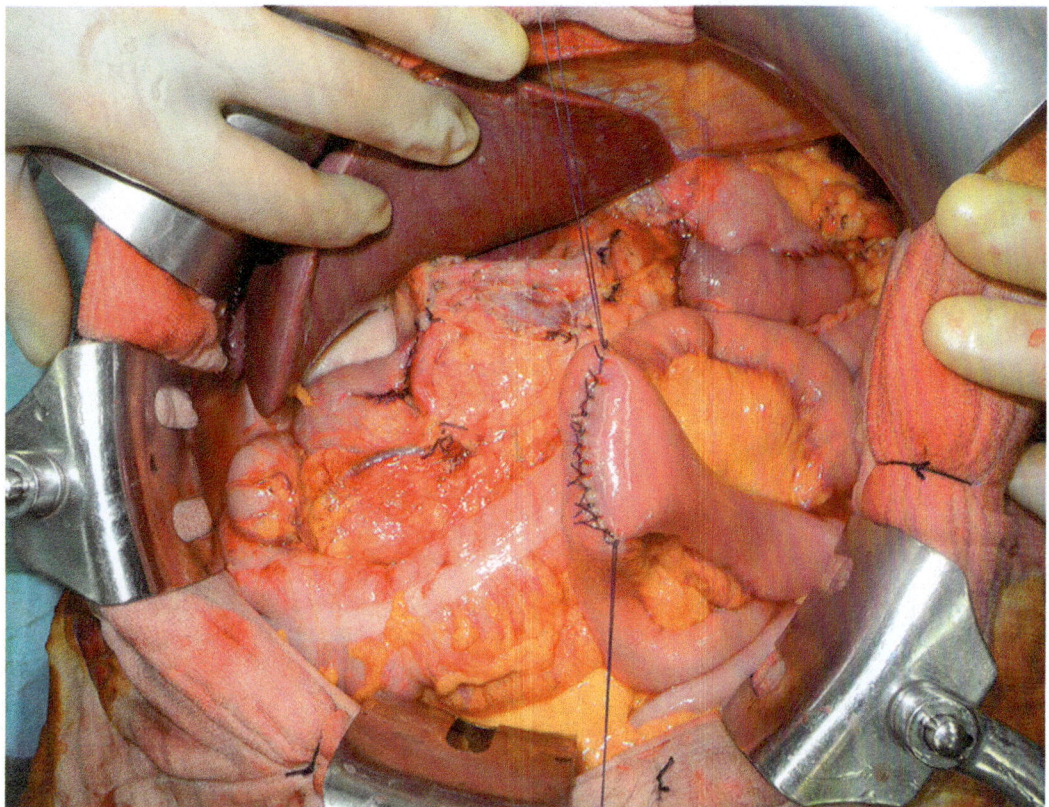

**Fig. 4.39** The afferent jejunal stump is recovered. Intestinal continuity is reestablished by creating a two-layer, end-to-side jejunojejunal anastomosis on the effer-ent jejunal loop 60 cm from the gastrojejunal anastomosis. The mesenteries are carefully closed with interrupted slowly absorbable 3-0 sutures to avoid internal herniation

## Reference

1. Japanese Gastric Cancer Association (2011) Japanese gastric cancer treatment guidelines 2010 (ver. 3). Gastric Cancer 14:113–123. doi:10.1007/s10120-011-0042-4

# Stapled Subtotal Gastrectomy

# 5

Pierpaolo Stortoni, Emilio Feliciotti,
Raffaella Ridolfo, and Walter Siquini

In the eighties staplers determined the reduction of the operative time in esophago-gastric and colorectal surgery.

Staplers are especially used in crafting intracorporeal anastomosis in laparoscopic surgery and are very useful in low rectal and esophago-cardiac resections.

Nowadays staplers are the gold standard devices to perform the esophago-jejunal anastomosis in total gastrectomy. In fact they reduce technique's complexity, operative time and rate of complications, especially anastomotic leaks.

In subtotal gastrectomy the advantage of mechanical anastomosis is reduced compared to the manual technique for the increased accessibility of the operative site.

The mechanical subtotal gastrectomy is definitely a faster, more standardized, and simpler technique than the manual one, although it is more expensive because many stapler refills are needed.

There are many techniques described in literature to perform a stapled gastric resection with Billroth II or Roux-en-Y limb, end-to-side or side-to-side anastomosis, and linear or circular stapler.

We describe the technique of mechanical subtotal gastrectomy with gastric transection performed with multiple linear staplers and reconstruction with Roux-en-Y loop and end-to-side gastrojejunostomy with circular stapler on the greater curvature.

We prefer to oversee all the sutures with interrupted slowly absorbable 3-0 stitches to reduce the risk of leakage and bleeding.

P. Stortoni (✉)
Division of General Surgery,
"A. Murri" Hospital, Fermo, Italy
e-mail: pierpaolostortoni@libero.it

E. Feliciotti
Department of Surgery, "Ospedali Riuniti" University Hospital, Ancona, Italy
e-mail: feliciotti@live.it

R. Ridolfo
Division of General Surgery,
Senigallia General Hospital, Senigallia, Italy
e-mail: raffaella.ridolfo@email.it

W. Siquini
Division of General Surgery,
"Madonna del Soccorso" Hospital,
San Benedetto del Tronto, Italy
e-mail: walter.siquini@sanita.marche.it

W. Siquini (ed.), *Total, Subtotal and Proximal Gastrectomy in Cancer: A Color Atlas*,
DOI 10.1007/978-88-470-5749-4_5, © Springer-Verlag Italia 2015

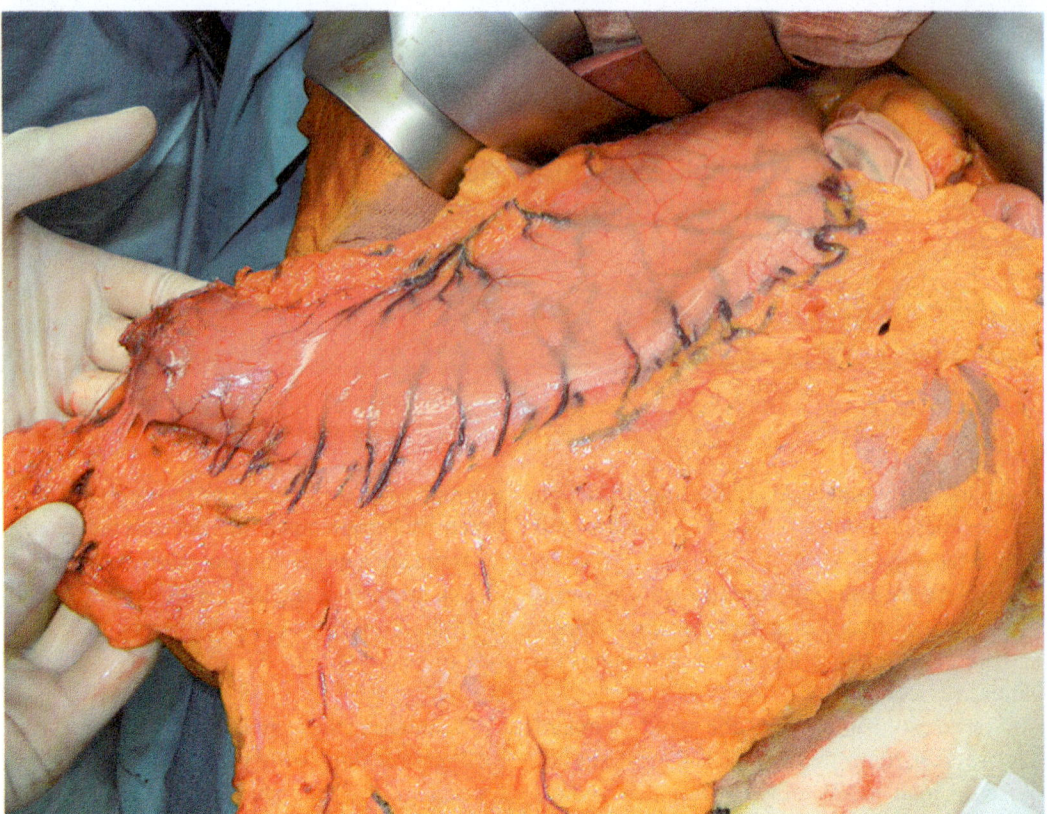

**Fig. 5.1** Subtotal gastrectomy is selected when a satisfactory proximal resection margin can be obtained. There are several techniques to perform a stapled subtotal gastrectomy: total or partial inferior anastomosis, side-to-side anastomosis using a linear stapler (GIA), and circular anastomosis after closure and transection of the gastric stump with a GIA

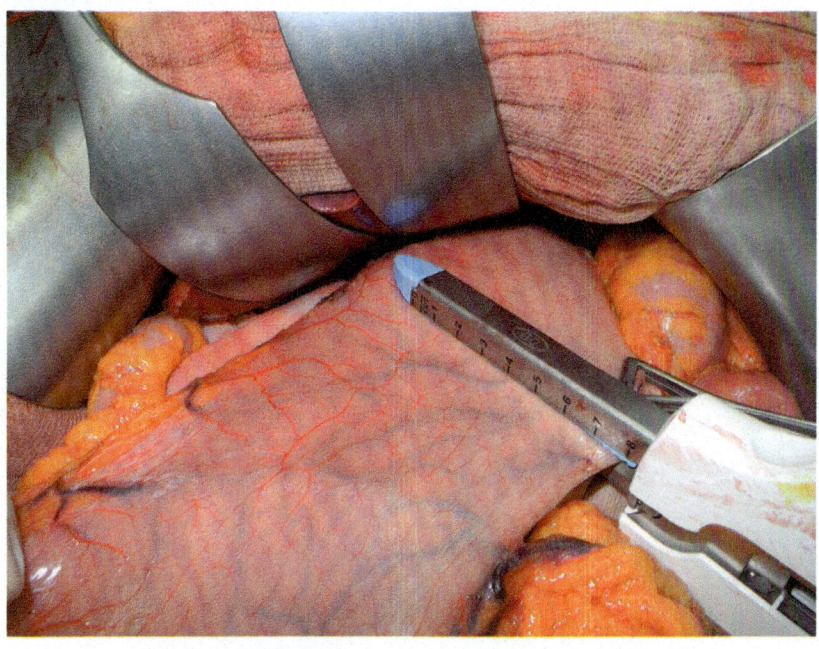

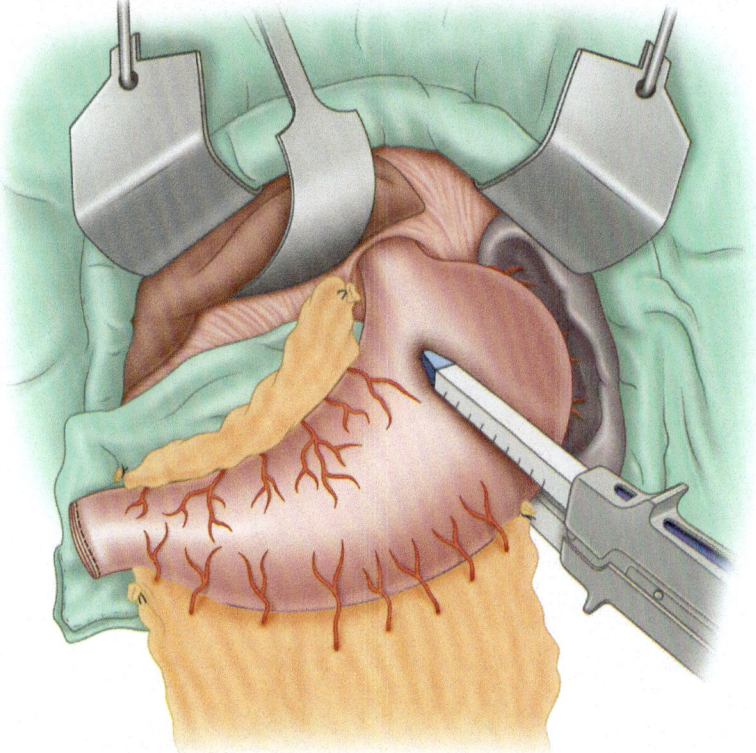

**Figs. 5.2 and 5.3** We prefer to close the gastric stump completely with a GIA stapler and then create a stapled end-to-side gastrojejunal circular anastomosis on defunc-tionalized Roux limb on the low lateral portion of the greater curvature

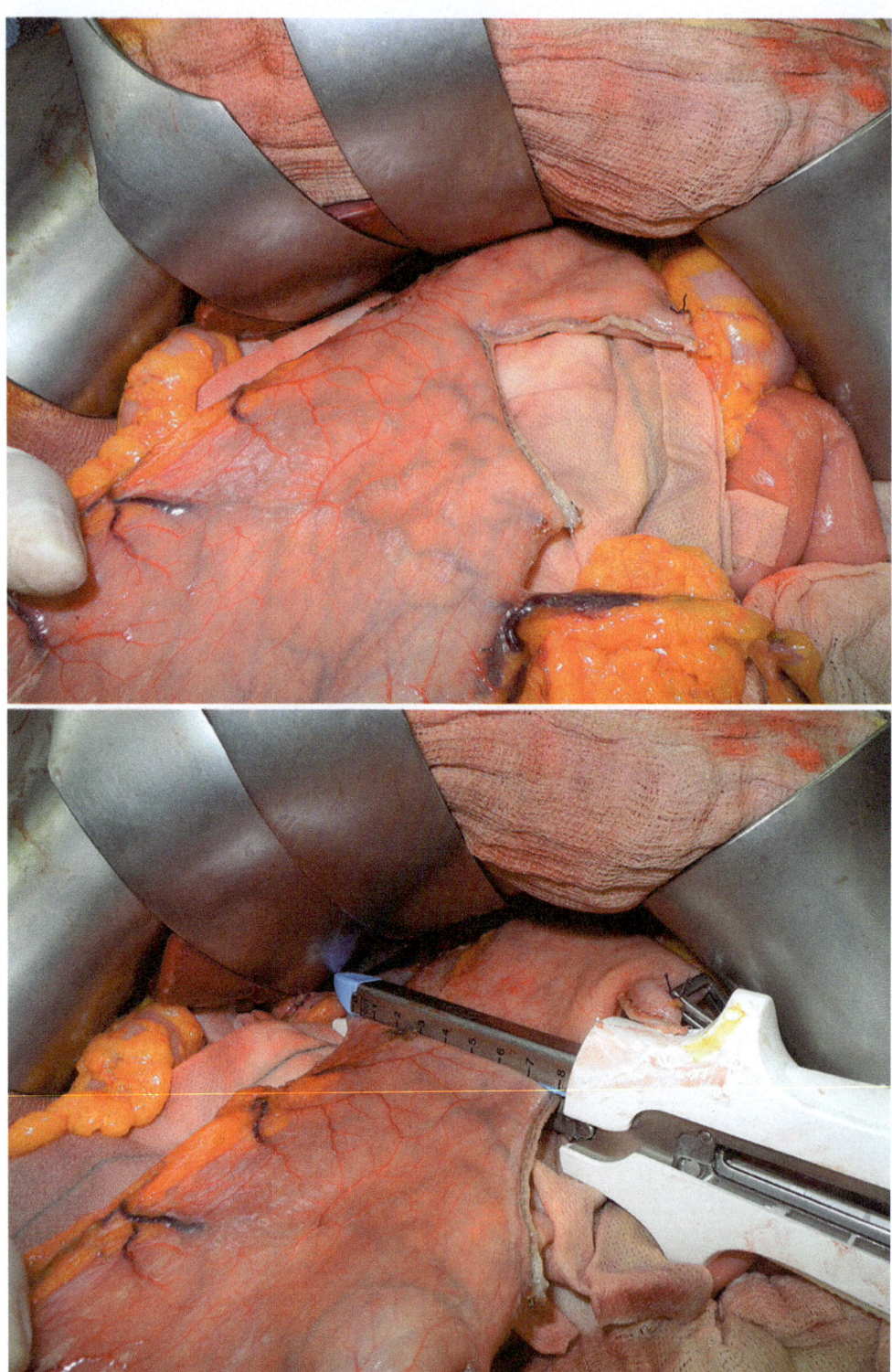

**Figs. 5.4, 5.5 and 5.6** A GIA linear mechanical stapler allows closure and transection of the stomach along the transection line passing through the lesser and greater curvature and forming a 120–130° angle to the lesser curvature. This angle ensures adequate margins and removal of antral G cells. Before locking the stapler jaws, the NGT needs to be drawn back, to avoid inclusion in the staple line

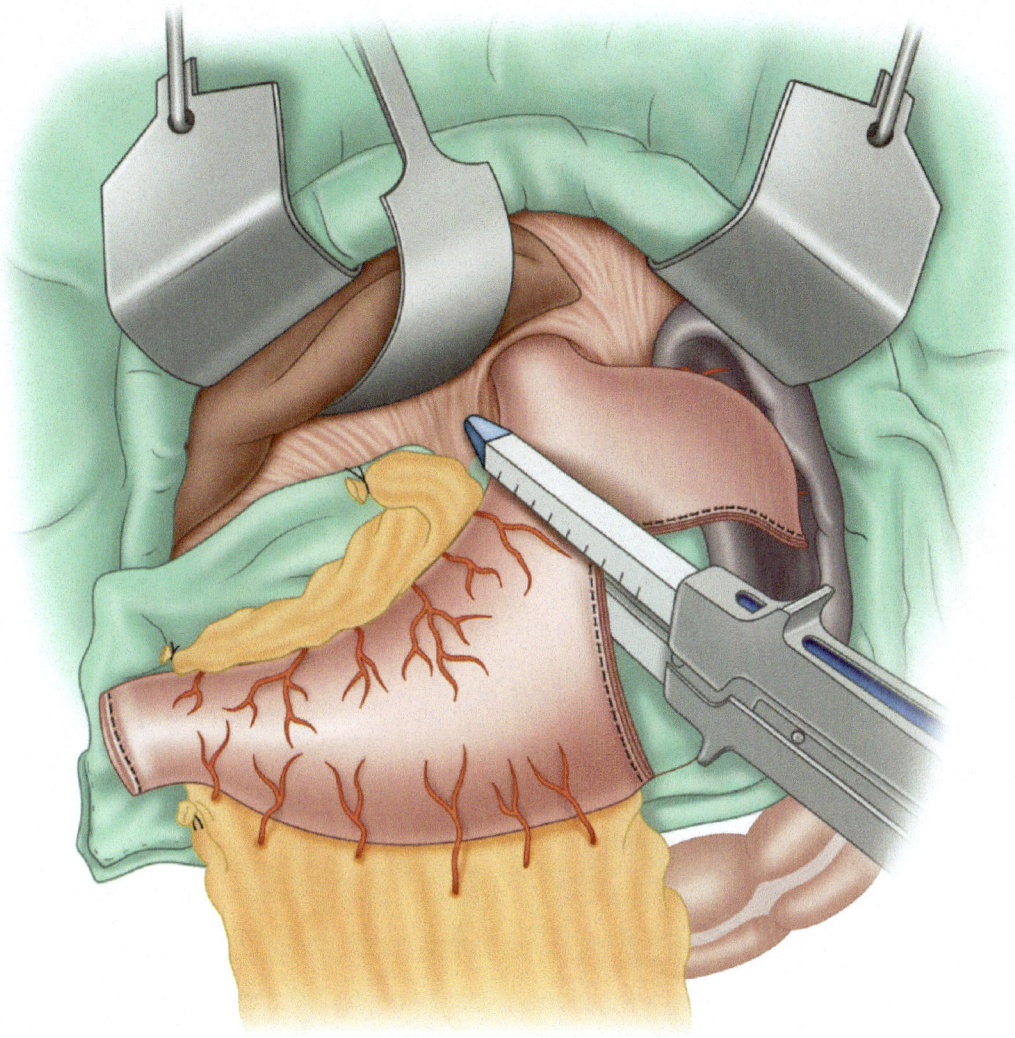

**Figs. 5.4, 5.5 and 5.6**   (continued)

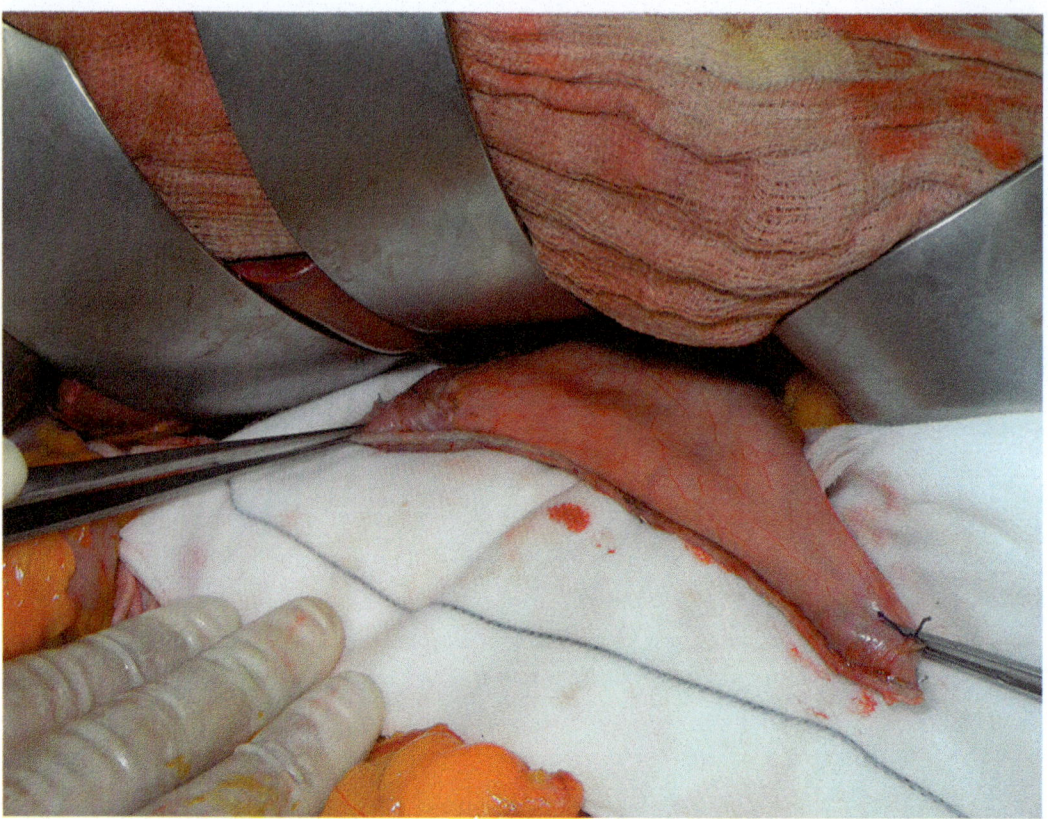

**Fig. 5.7** Final appearance of the residual gastric stump after mechanical transection

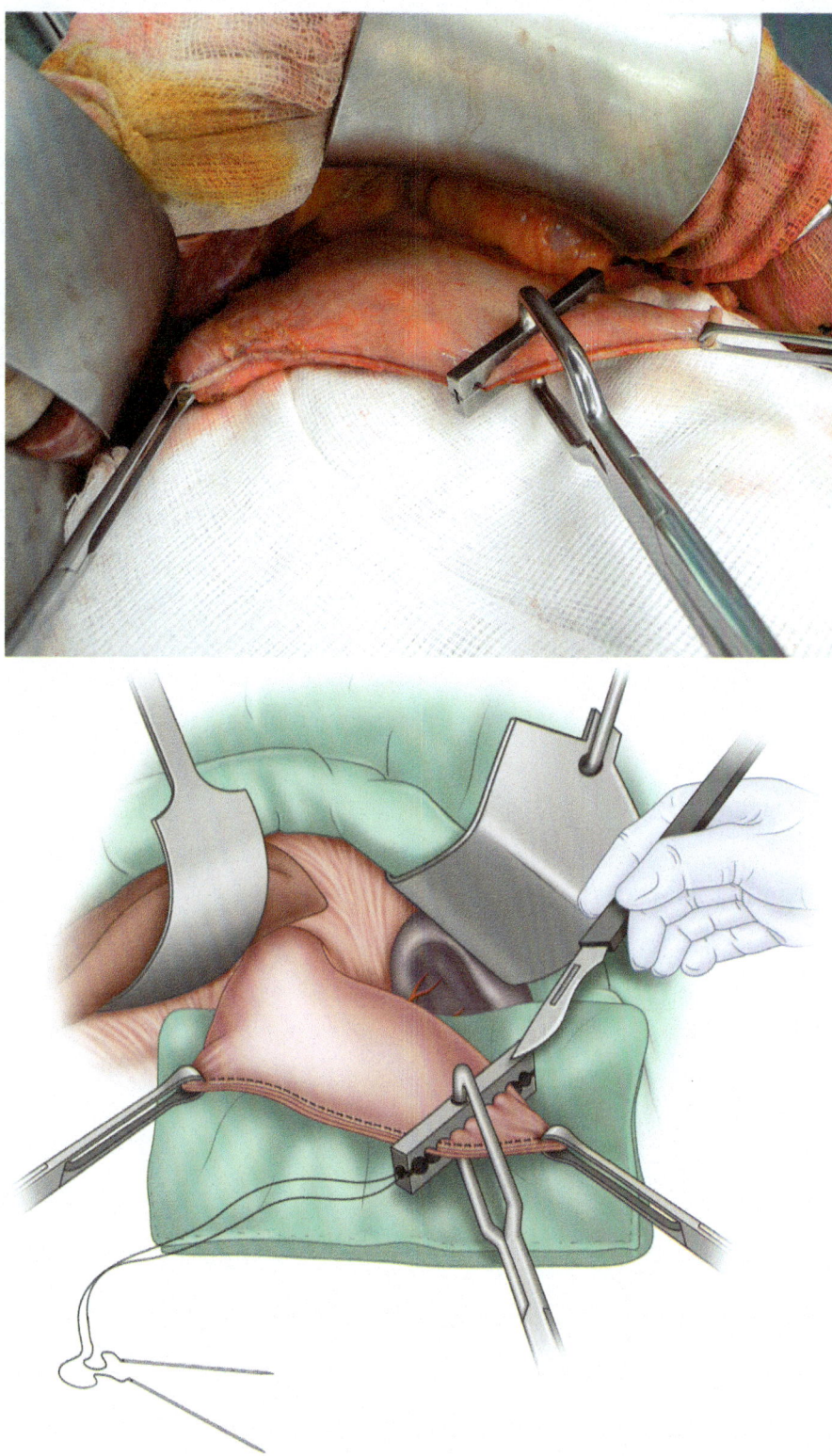

**Figs. 5.8, 5.9, and 5.10**   A rake is placed on the acute angle formed by the suture line and the greater curvature, and then a nonabsorbable monofilament 2-0 purse-string suture is performed. The excess gastric tissue is removed

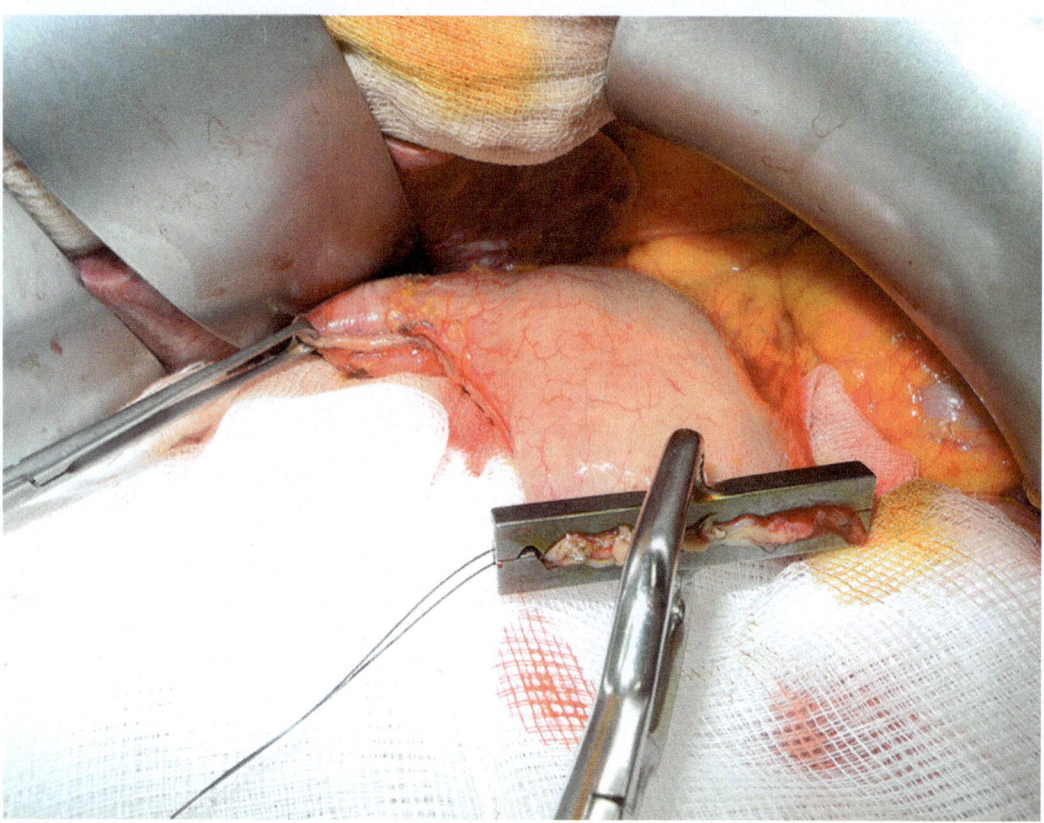

**Figs. 5.8, 5.9, and 5.10**  (continued)

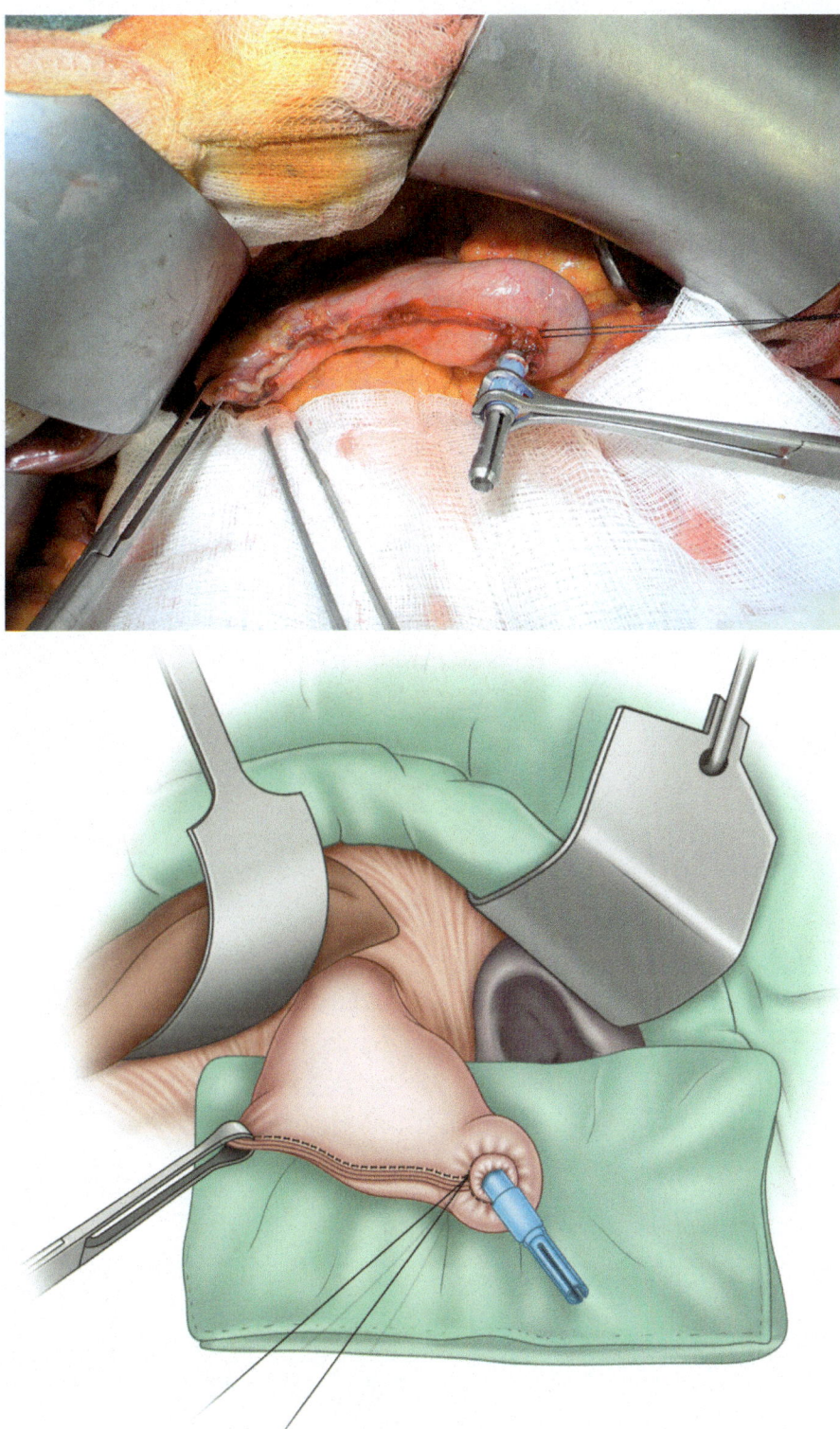

**Figs. 5.11 and 5.12**   A 25 or 31 mm anvil of a circular mechanical stapler is inserted into the gastric stump

**Figs. 5.13 and 5.14** The stapler is introduced into the previously prepared Roux limb to create the end-to-side gastrojejunal anastomosis

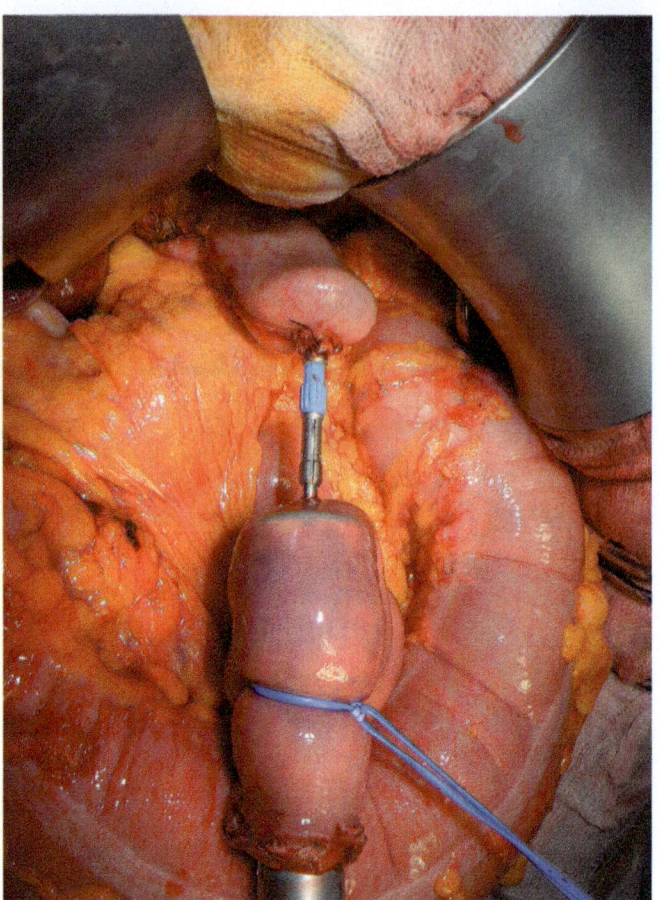

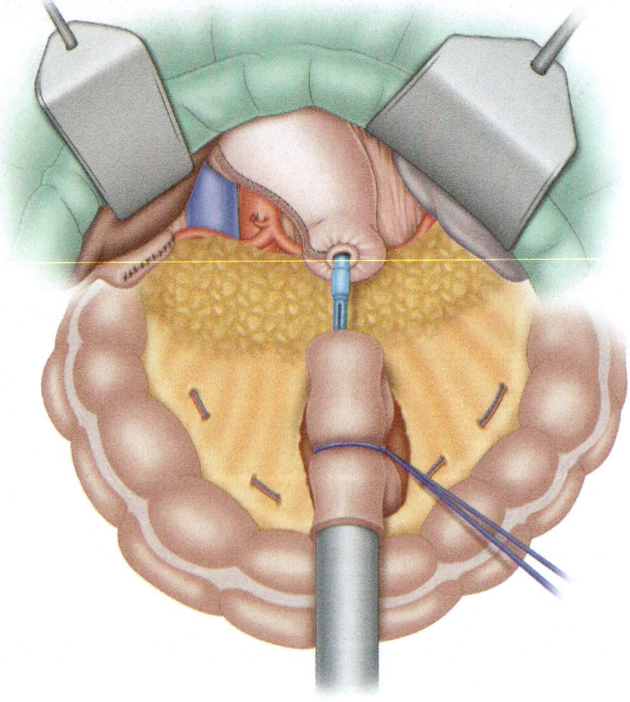

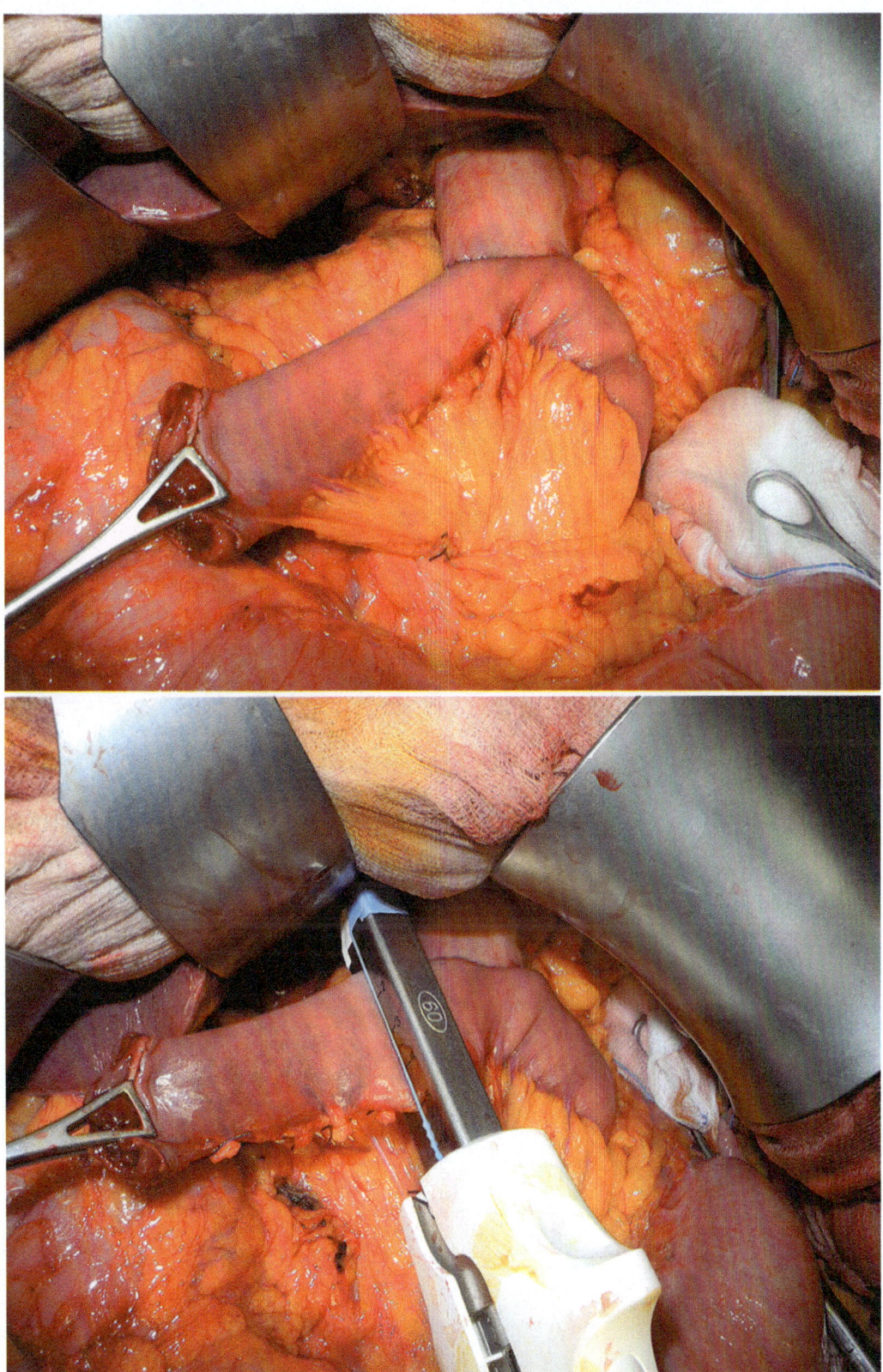

**Figs. 5.15, 5.16, and 5.17**  The lateral jejunal stump is closed with a GIA stapler

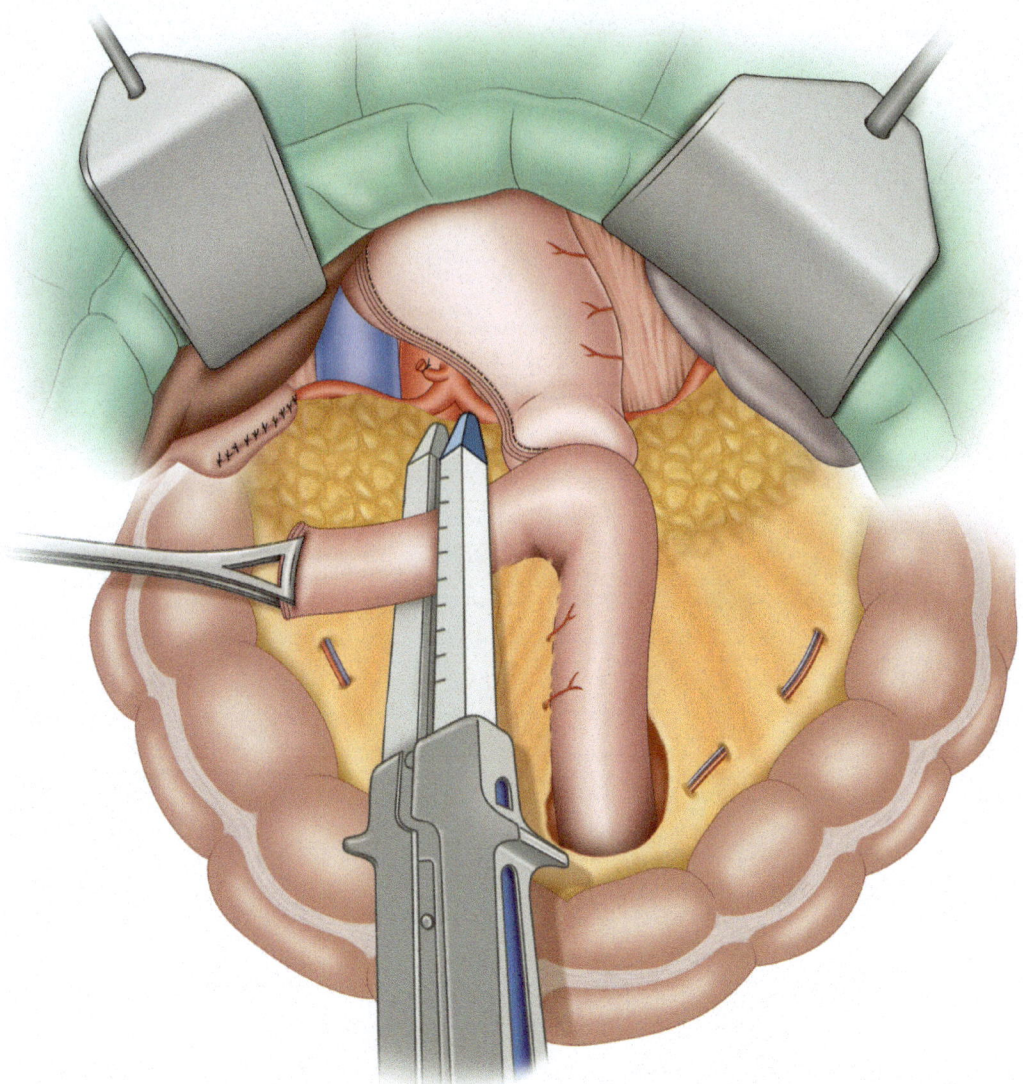

**Figs. 5.15, 5.16, and 5.17** (continued)

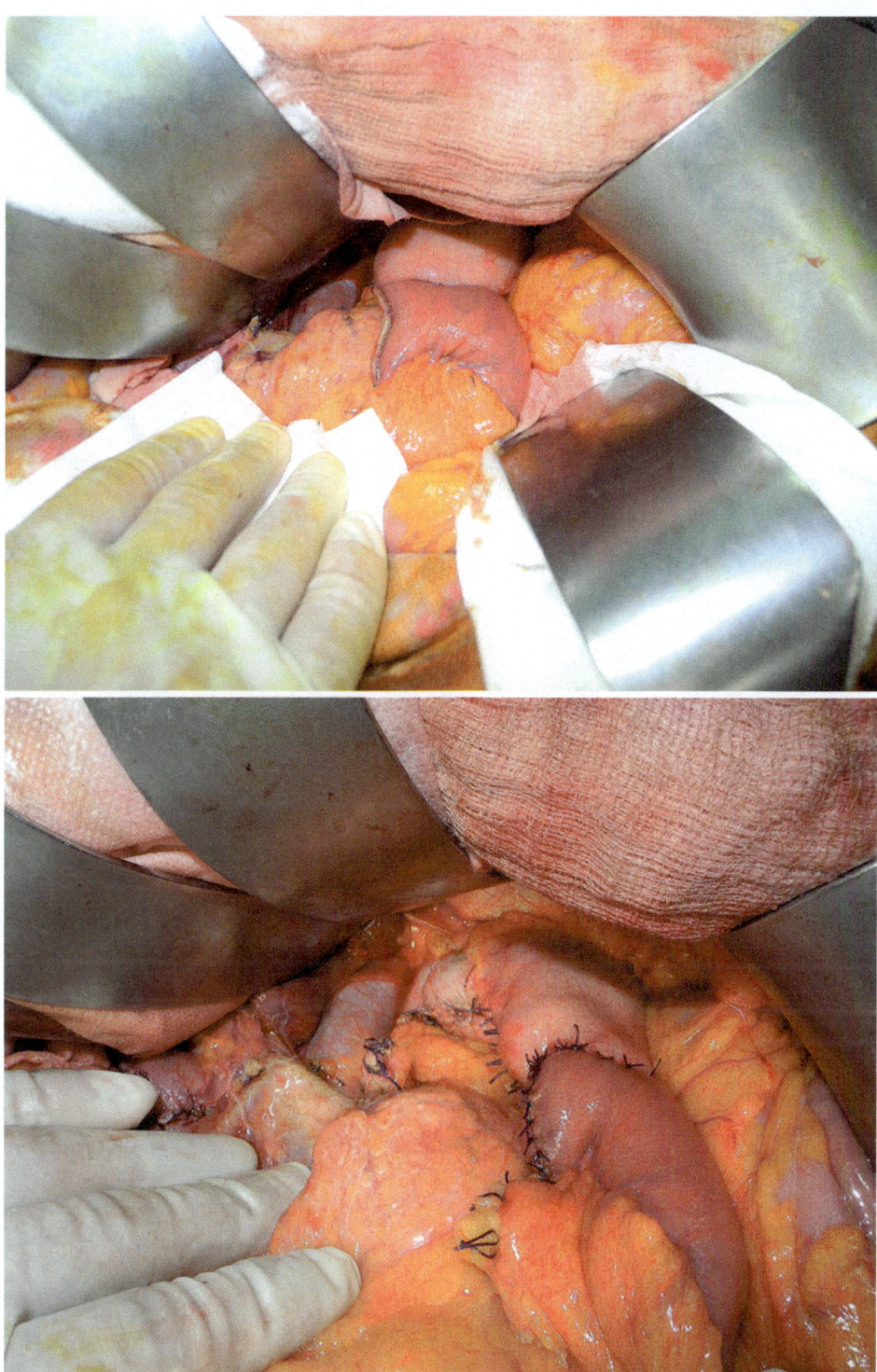

**Figs. 5.18, 5.19 and 5.20** The short residual lateral jejunal stump and the anastomosis are oversewn with interrupted slowly absorbable 3-0 sutures. The staple line closing the whole gastric stump is also strengthened by oversewing with interrupted sutures or with a continuous slowly absorbable 2-0 suture. The surgical procedure ends with the execution of the end-to-side enteroenterostomy, suturing of the mesenteries, and placement of a drain, as in the manual procedure

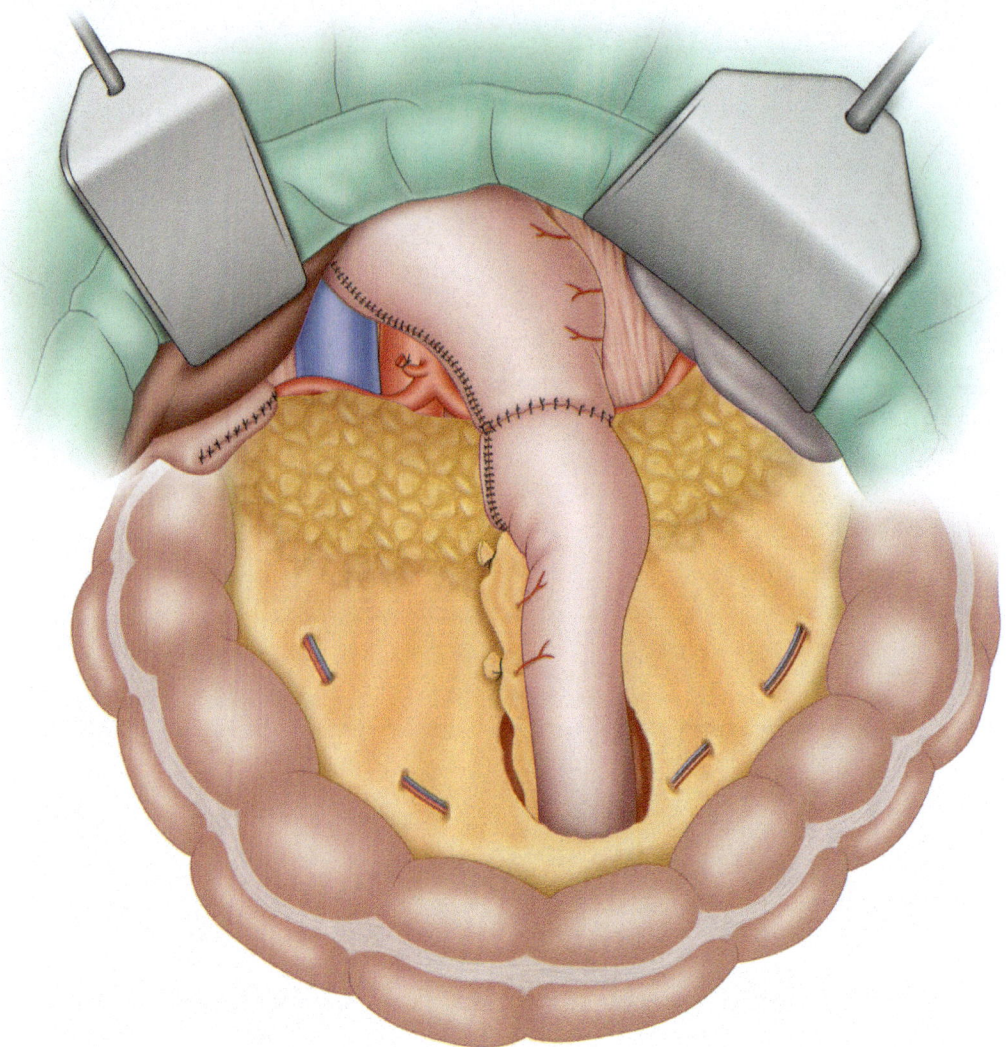

**Figs. 5.18, 5.19 and 5.20** (continued)

# Proximal Gastrectomy

Walter Siquini, Raffaella Ridolfo, Emilio Feliciotti,
Pierpaolo Stortoni, Alessandro Cardinali, and
Giovanni de Manzoni

Esophagogastric junction adenocarcinomas are tumors located in the border zone of the esophagus and stomach. In the new TNM system (7th edition), the tumors of the esophagogastric junction (EGJ) are classified as esophageal cancer.

Several operative techniques are acceptable for esophagogastrectomy in patients with resectable EGJ cancer. Transthoracic esophagogastrectomy and transhiatal esophagogastrectomy are the two most common surgical approaches.

Patients fit for surgery, with Sievert type I tumors, should be treated with Ivor-Lewis esophagogastrectomy with two-level lymph node dissection. It is performed with median laparotomy and right thoracotomy with upper thoracic esophagogastric anastomosis (at or above the azygos vein level).

The gastric conduit is preferred for esophageal reconstruction by the majority of gastroesophageal surgeons. The esophageal reconstruction is made according to the technique proposed by Cordiano. In order to craft the gastric conduit, the stomach is mobilized by the dissection of the celiac and the left gastric lymph nodes, division of the left gastric artery, and preservation of the gastroepiploic and right gastric artery.

Sievert type III tumors are considered as gastric cancers, and the surgical approach for these tumors is the transabdominal, transhiatal approach with Roux-en-Y esophago-jejunal anastomosis.

Sievert type II tumors could be treated with Ivor-Lewis procedure or with transabdominal, transhiatal approach with Pinotti's phrenotomy and intrathoracic anastomosis, evaluating case by case.

W. Siquini
Division of General Surgery,
"Madonna del Soccorso" Hospital,
San Benedetto del Tronto, Italy
e-mail: walter.siquini@sanita.marche.it

R. Ridolfo (✉)
Division of General Surgery,
Senigallia General Hospital, Senigallia, Italy
e-mail: raffaella.ridolfo@email.it

E. Feliciotti
Department of Surgery, "Ospedali Riuniti" University
Hospital, Ancona, Italy
e-mail: feliciotti@live.it

P. Stortoni
Division of General Surgery, "A. Murri" Hospital,
Fermo, Italy
e-mail: pierpaolostortoni@libero.it

A. Cardinali
Division of General Surgery, "Madonna del
Soccorso" Hospital, San Benedetto del Tronto, Italy
e-mail: alessandro.cardinali@sanita.marche.it

G. de Manzoni
Department of Surgery,
General Surgery and Surgery of Esophagus
and Stomach, Verona, Italy
e-mail: giovanni.demanzini@univr.it

W. Siquini (ed.), *Total, Subtotal and Proximal Gastrectomy in Cancer: A Color Atlas*,
DOI 10.1007/978-88-470-5749-4_6, © Springer-Verlag Italia 2015

## 6.1 Abdominal Stage: Cardial Resection and Gastric Tube Construction

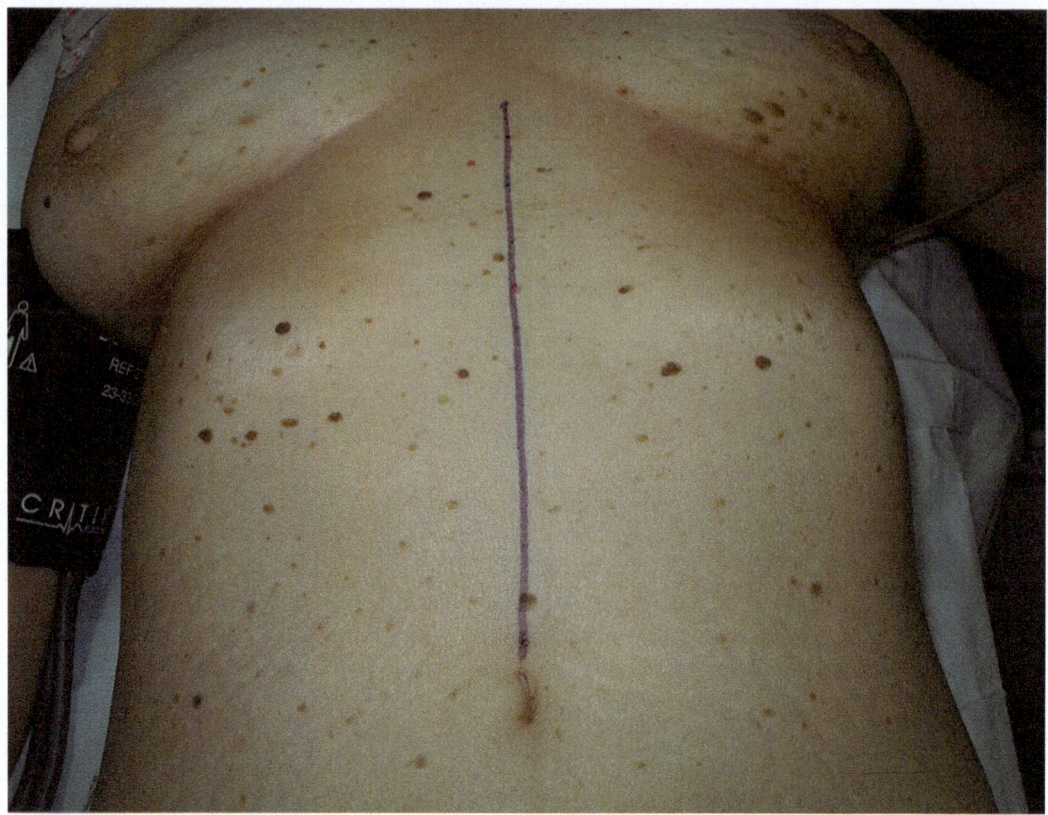

**Fig. 6.1** The abdomen is entered via a midline xipho-umbilical incision

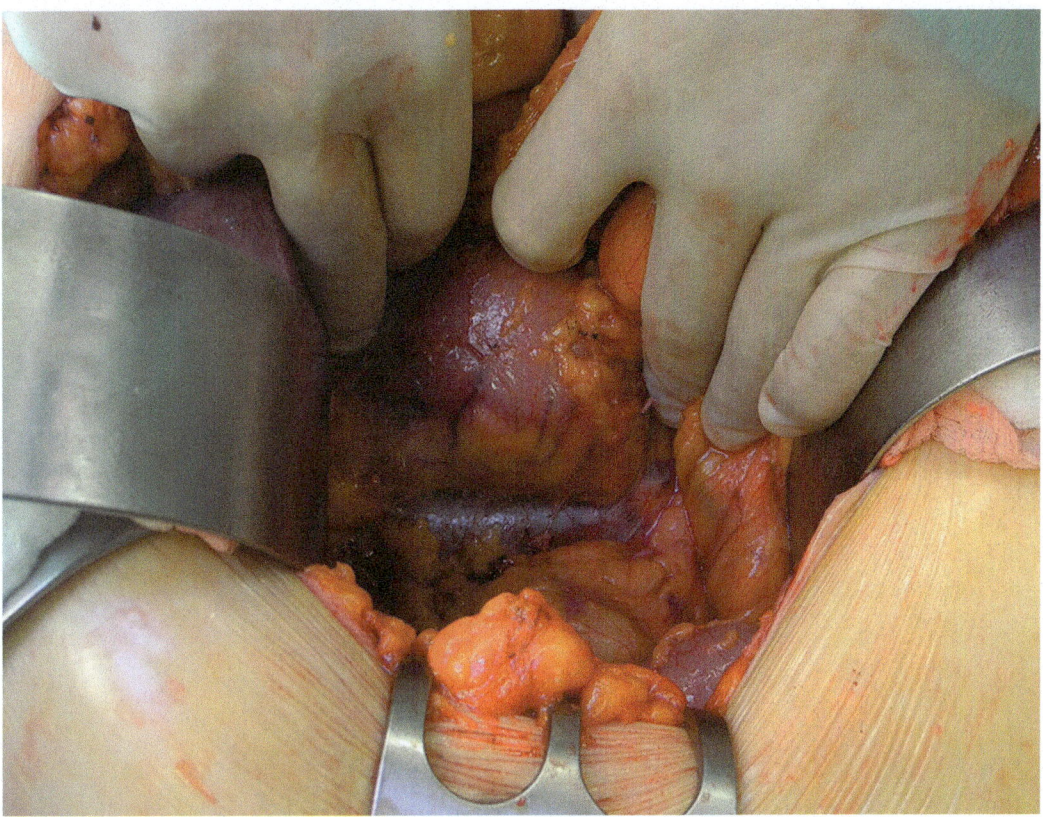

**Fig. 6.2** After separation of the greater omentum, a Kocher maneuver is performed to ensure a better mobilization of the gastric tube

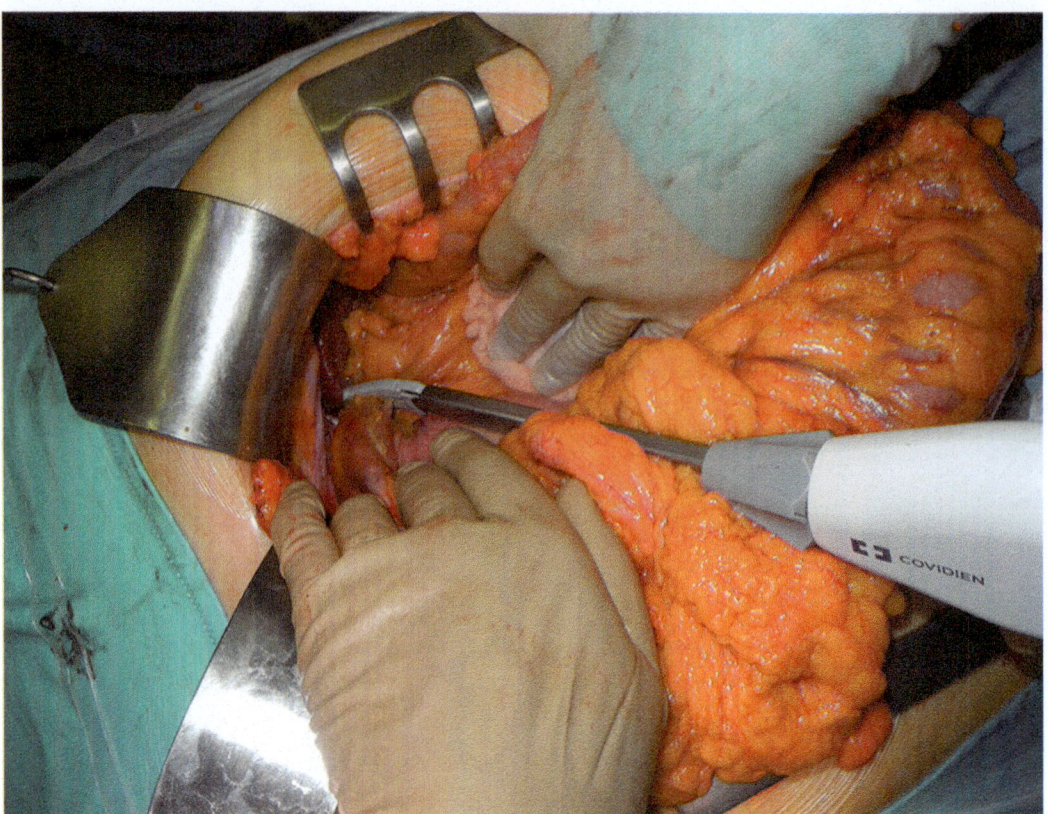

**Fig. 6.3** Short gastric vessels are divided using a radiofrequency device (LigaSure™), obtaining a complete mobilization of the greater curvature of the stomach

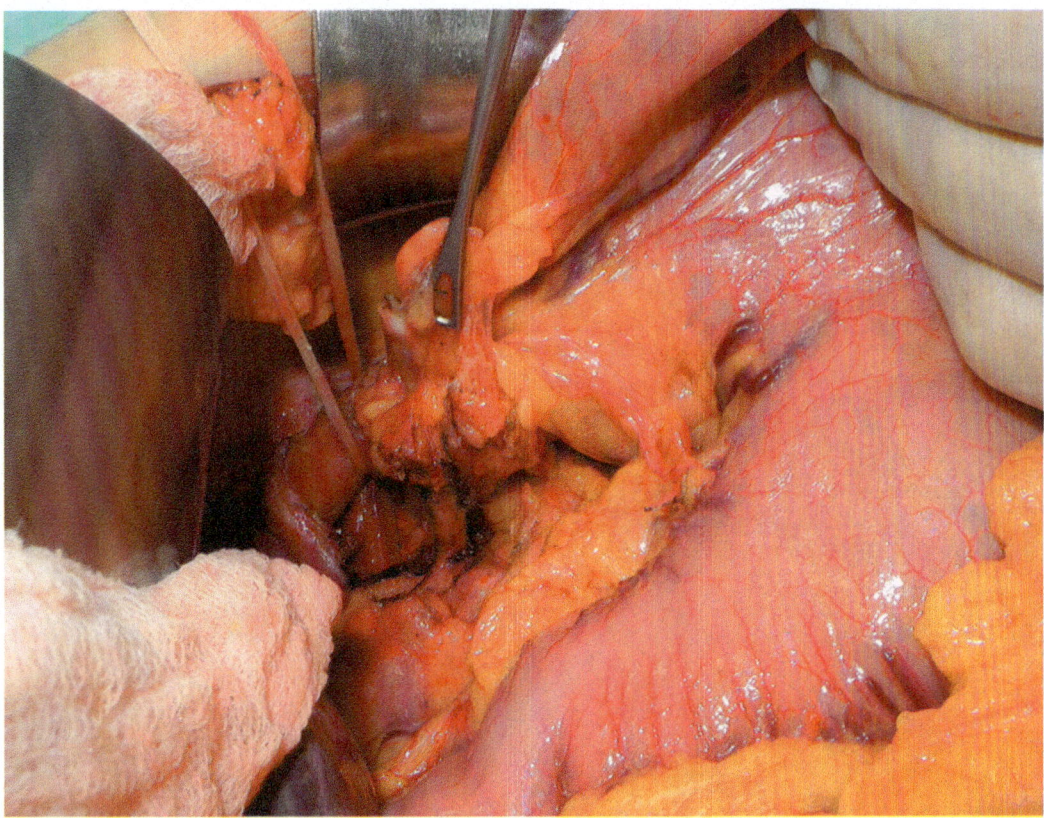

**Fig. 6.4** The abdominal esophagus is completely exposed and encircled. The left gastric artery is dissected and lymphadenectomy at this level (station n. 7) is performed

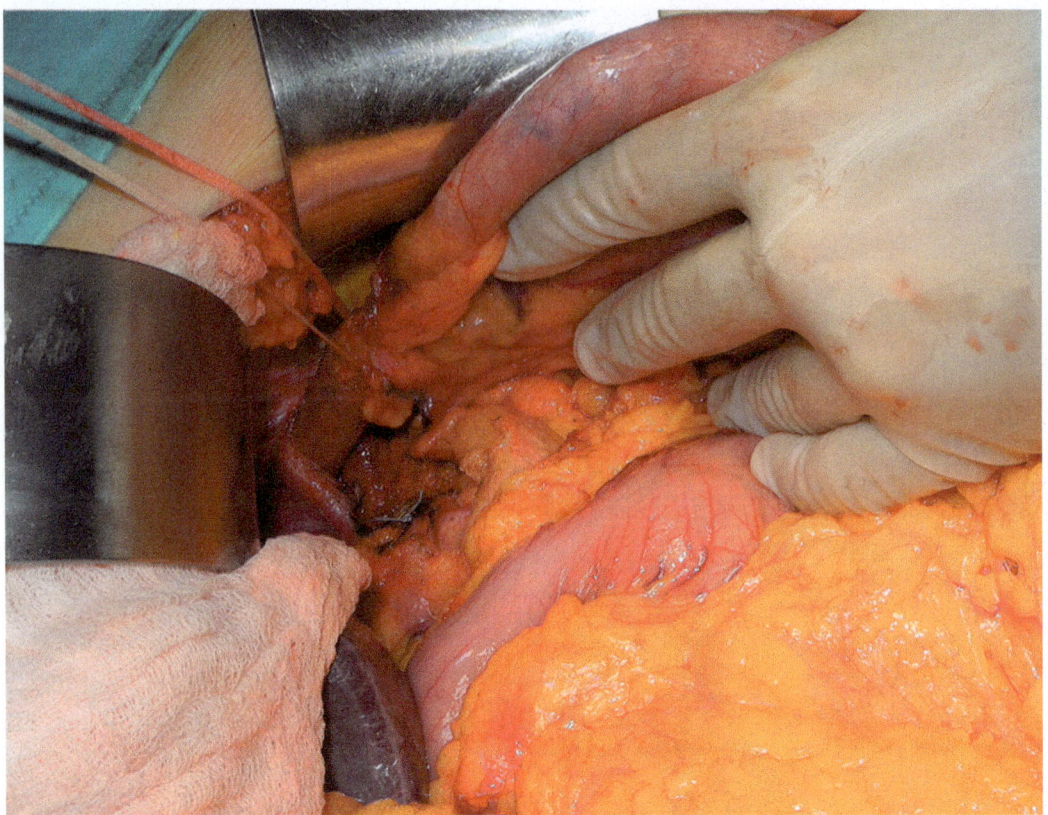

**Fig. 6.5** The left gastric artery is divided at its origin

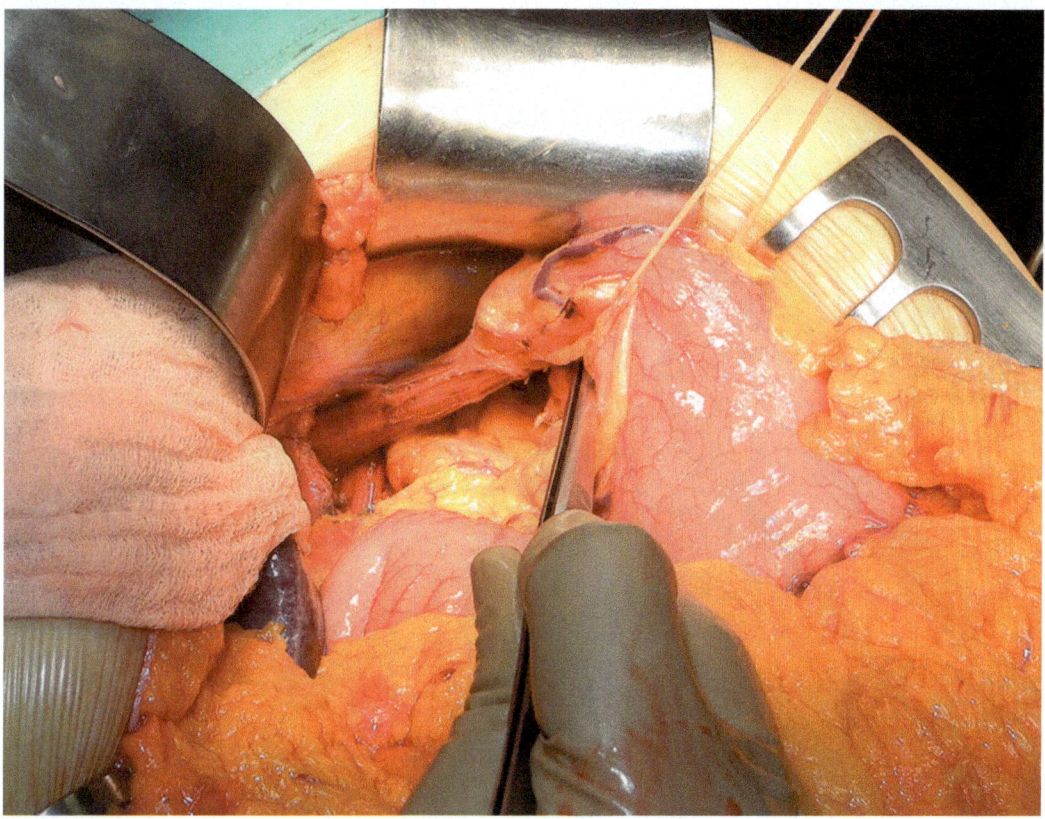

**Fig. 6.6** Section of the anterior and posterior trunks of the vagus nerve with complete mobilization of the abdominal esophagus

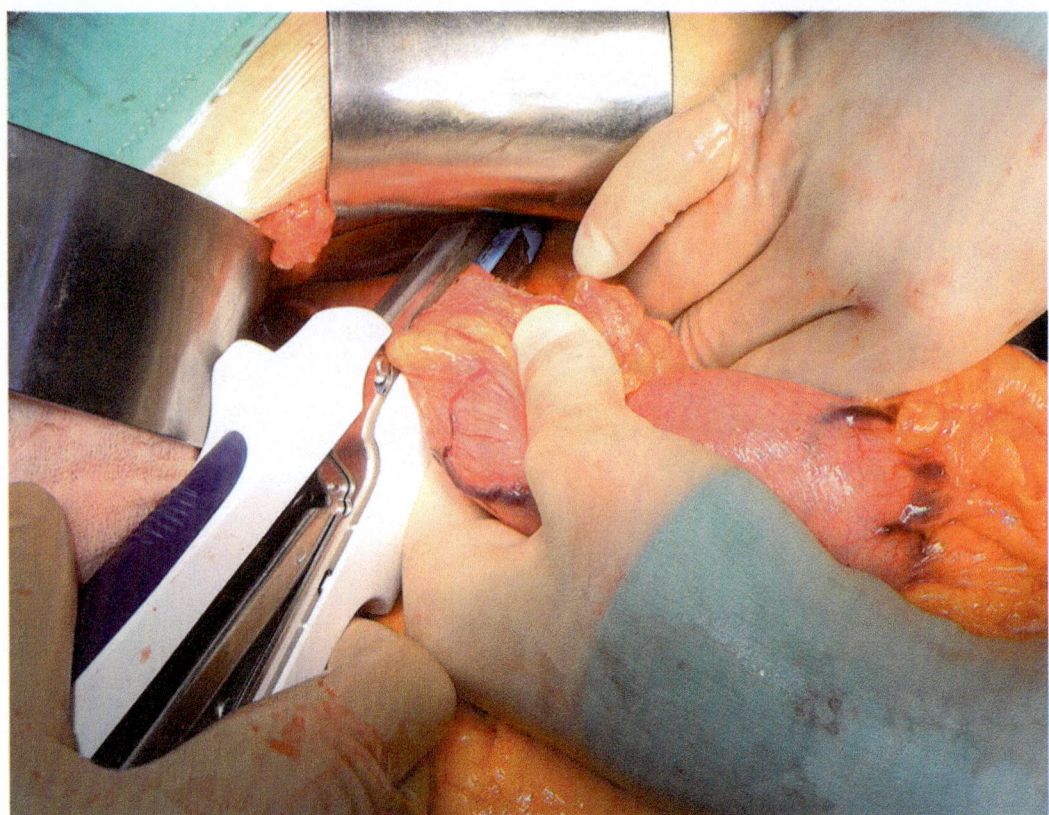

**Fig. 6.7** The esophagus is divided with GIA 60 linear stapler above the level of the esophagogastric junction (EGJ), at least 2 cm above the upper pole of the EGJ tumor

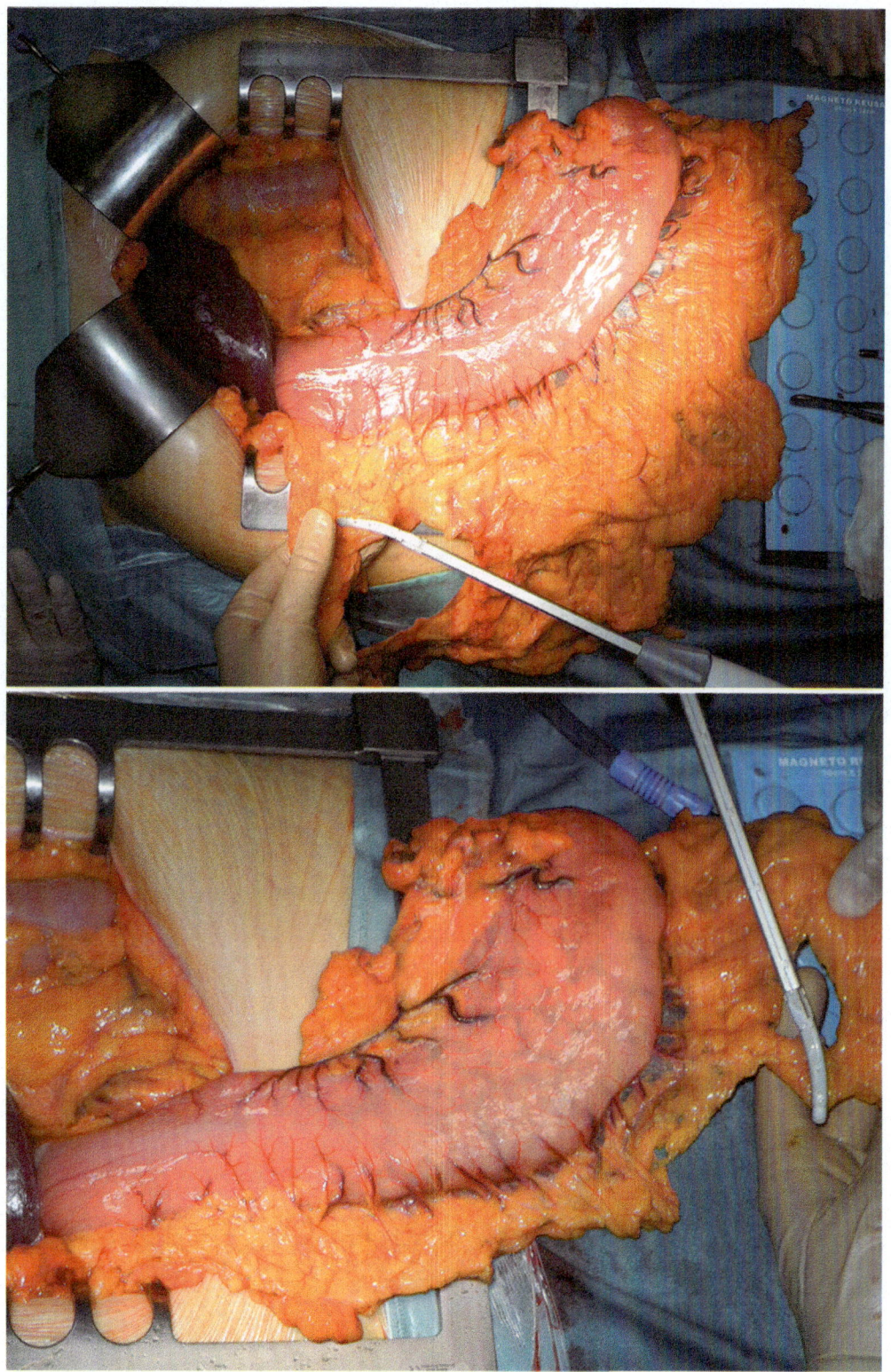

**Figs. 6.8 and 6.9**  The stomach is exposed outside the abdominal cavity and the omentum is resected preserving the gastroepiploic arch

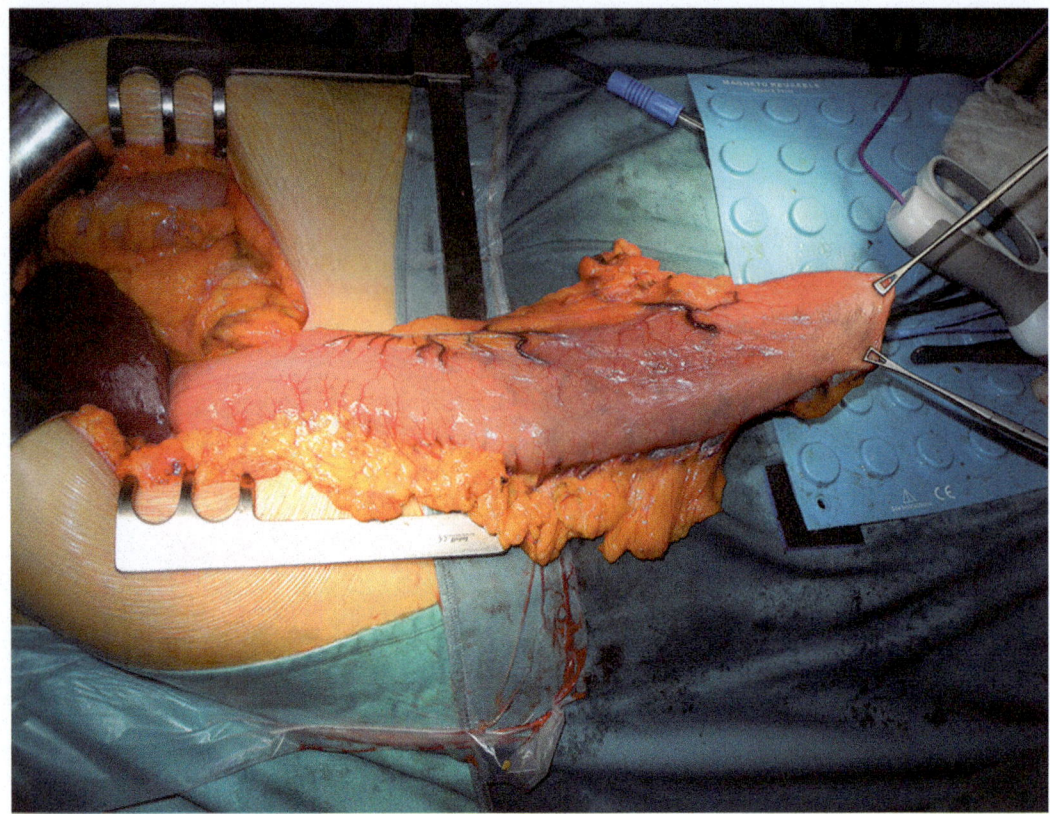

**Fig. 6.10** Two Allis clamps are placed at the level of the gastric fundus to straighten the greater curvature of the stomach

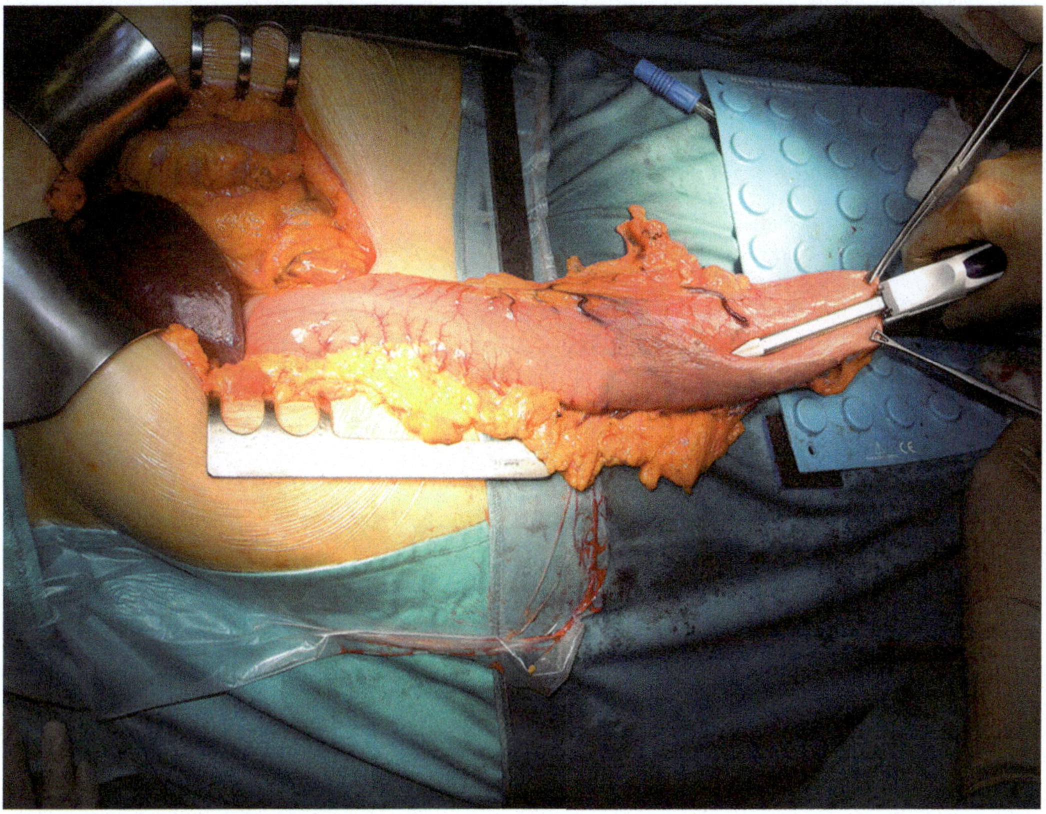

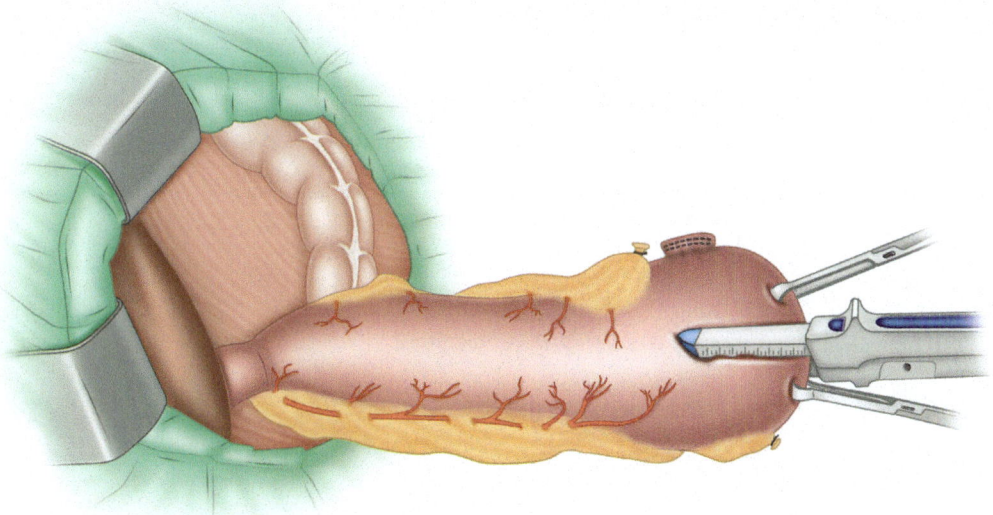

**Figs. 6.11 and 6.12**  The surgeon constructs the gastric tube along the greater curvature using multiple serial firings of linear staplers (GIA 60 and GIA 80). The procedure starts at the top, at the angle of His, with division of the stomach parallel to the greater curvature. The transverse diameter of the gastric conduit should not be more than 4 cm to ensure a good vascularization of the organ

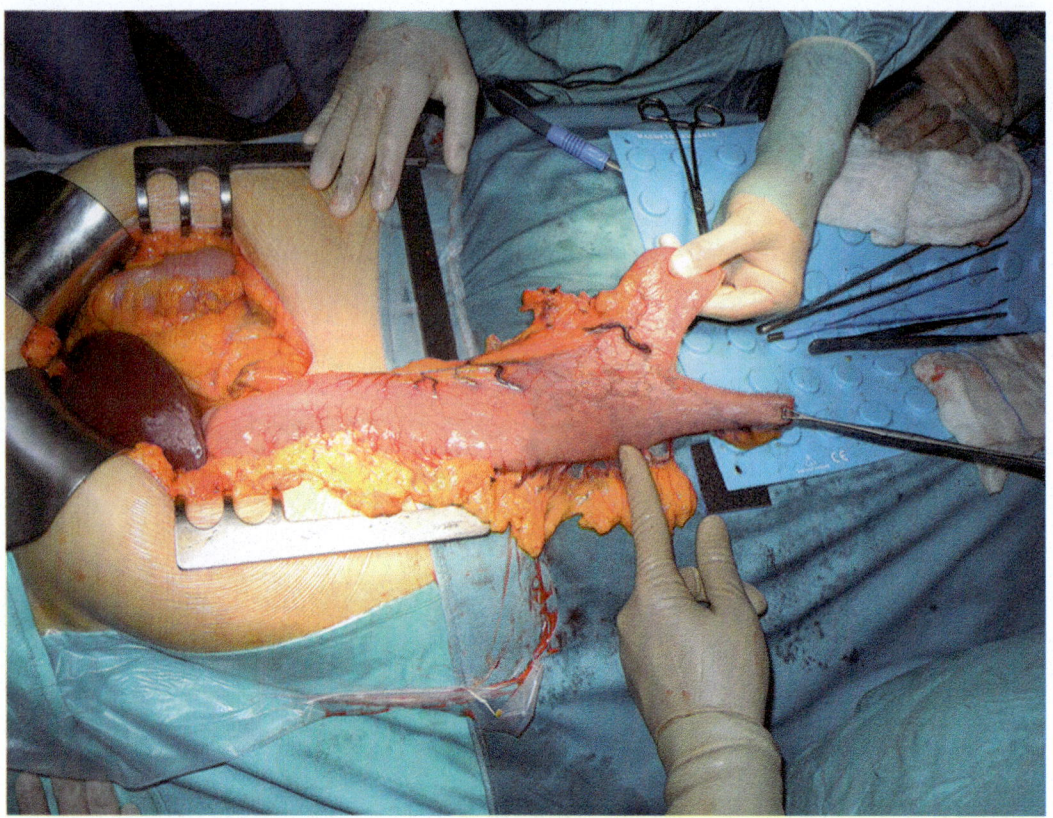

**Fig. 6.13** The appearance after the first firing

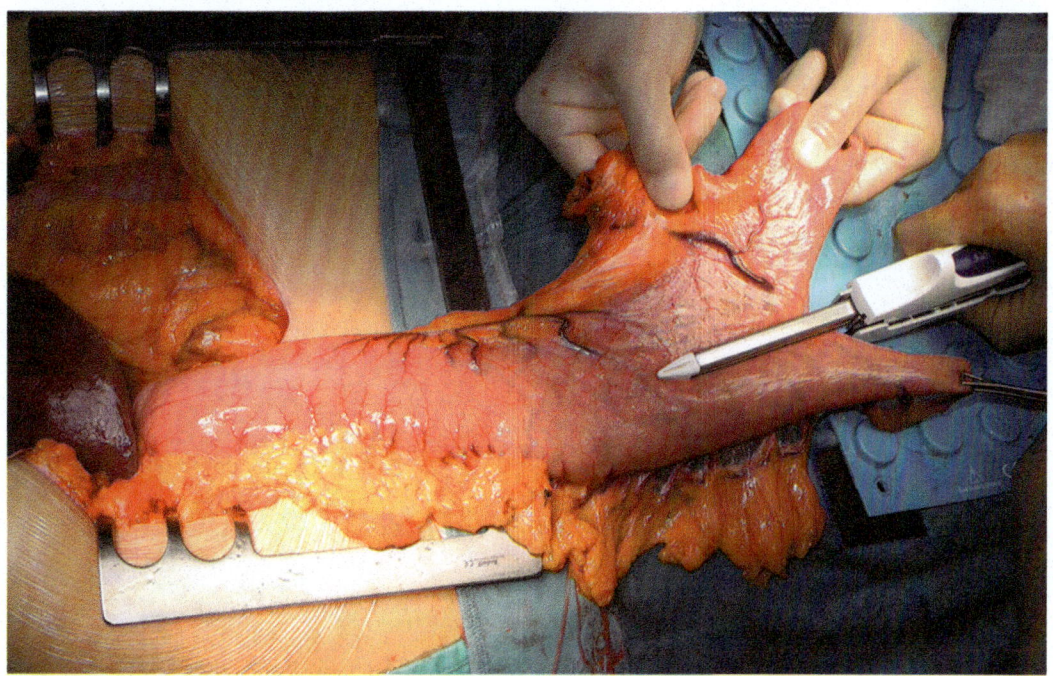

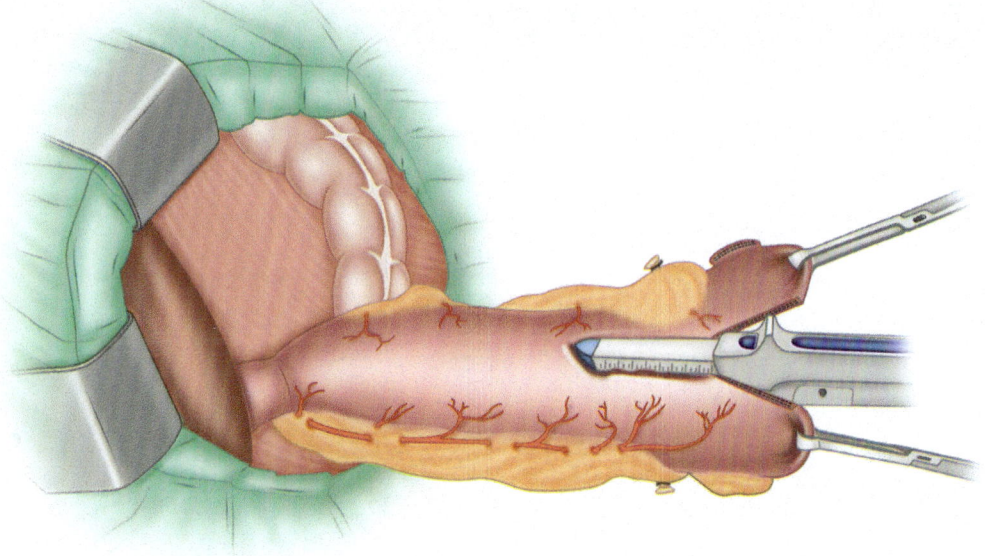

**Figs. 6.14 and 6.15**   The second firing with GIA 80 follows the same direction of the previous firing, maintaining a 4 cm distance from the greater curvature

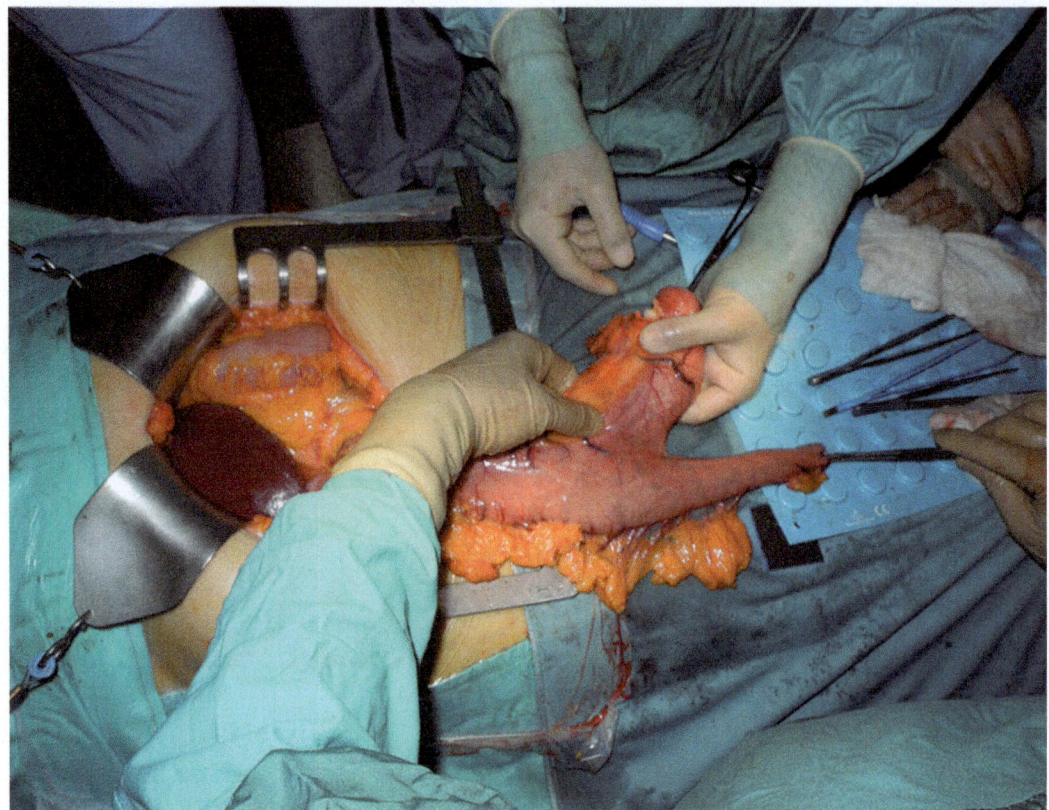

**Fig. 6.16** The appearance after the second firing

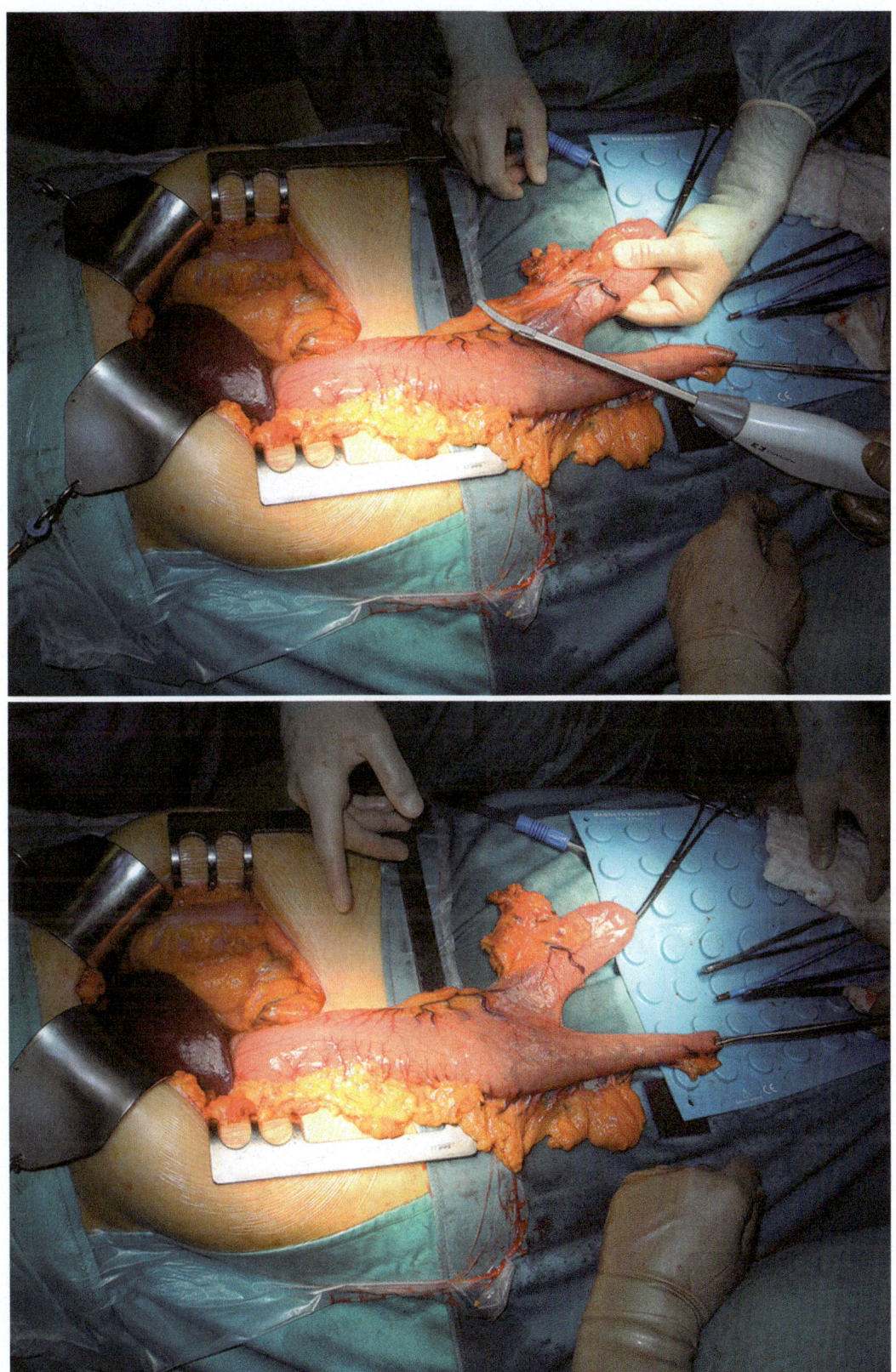

**Figs. 6.17 and 6.18** Preparation of the lesser curvature of the stomach with radiofrequency device

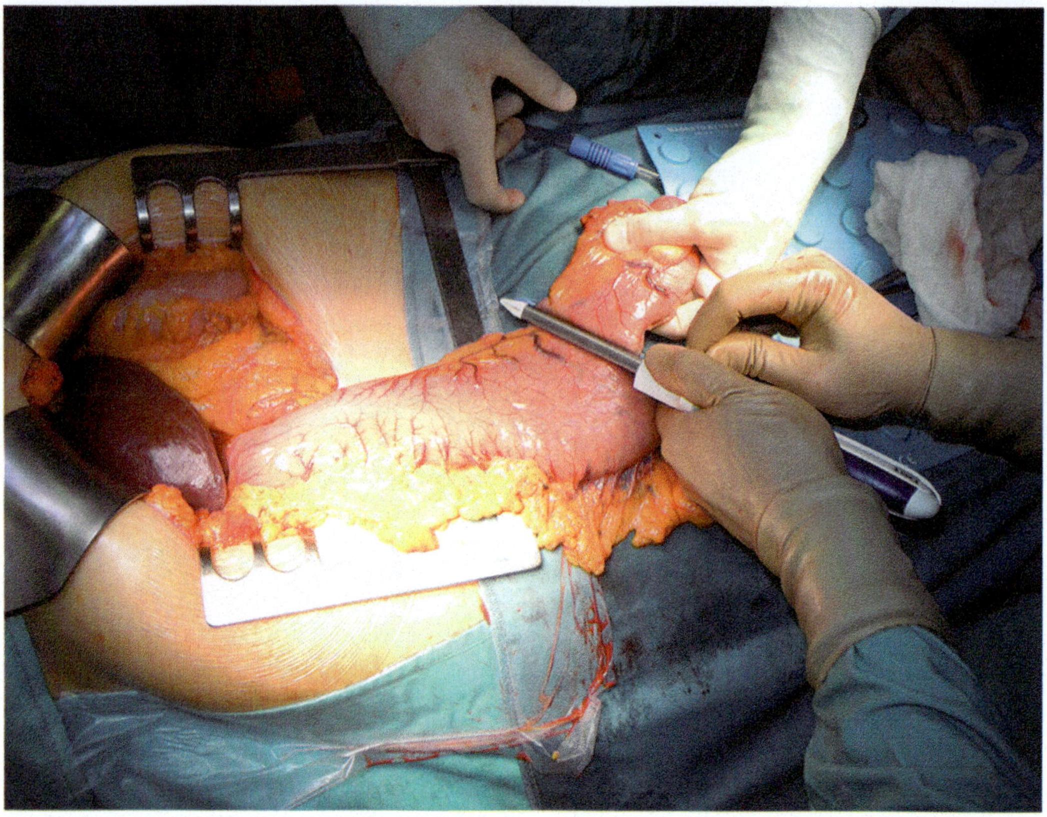

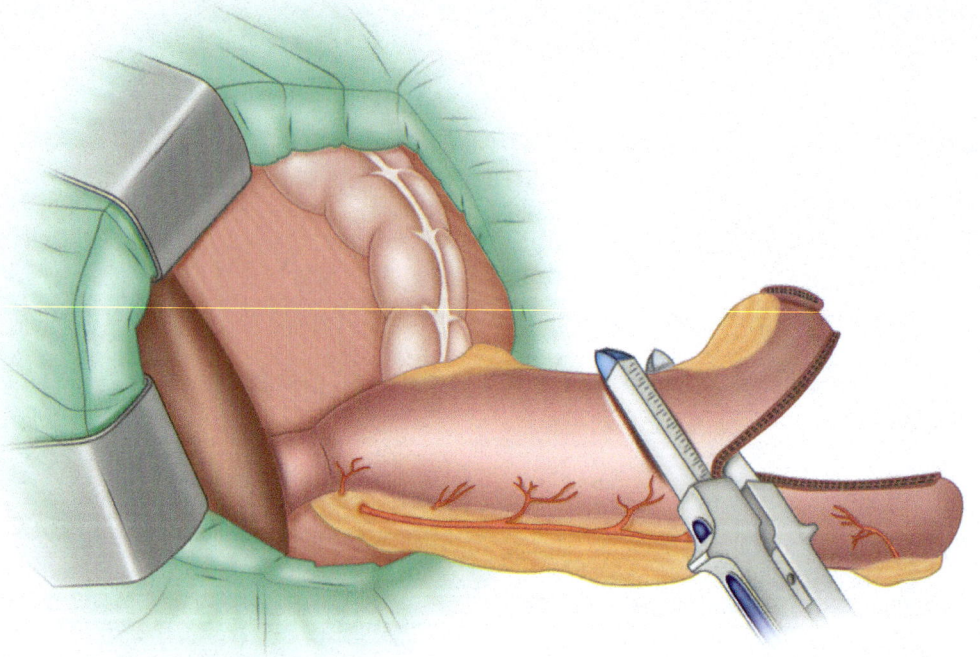

**Figs. 6.19 and 6.20** The third firing is performed moving toward the lesser curvature. The specimen is removed; it consists of the esophagogastric junction, the gastric fundus, the upper portion of the lesser gastric curvature with right paracardial and proximal lesser curvature lymph nodes

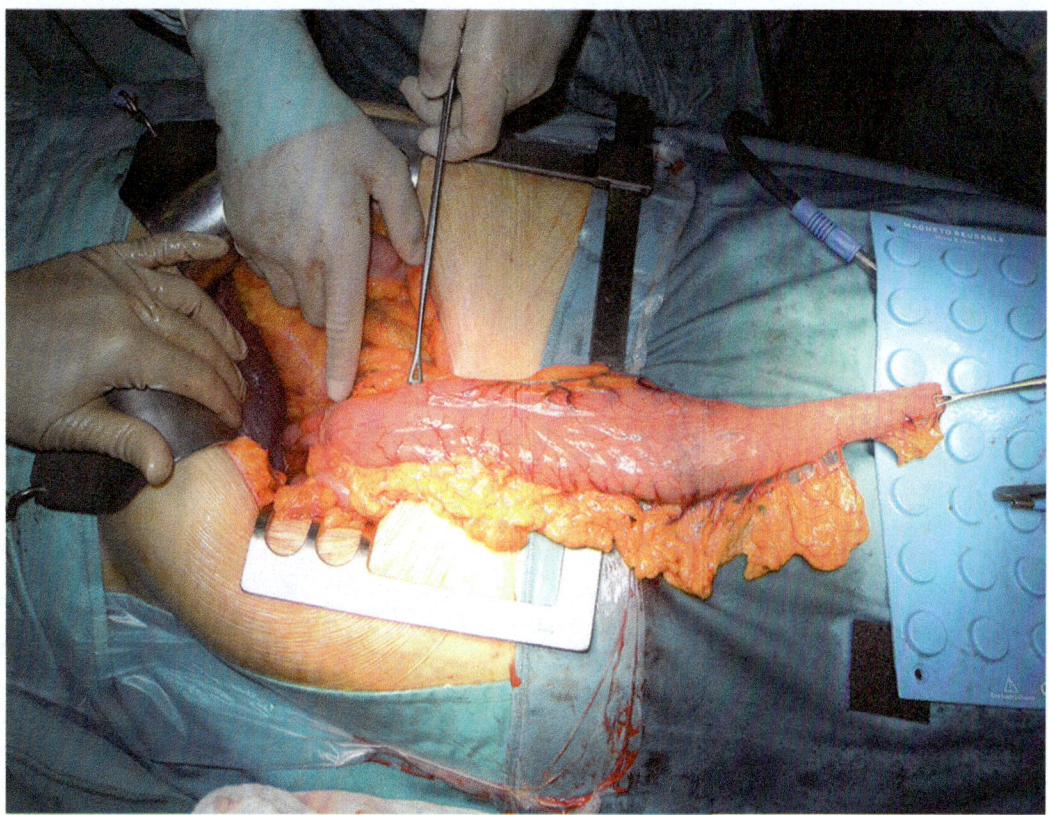

**Fig. 6.21** The appearance after the third firing. The surgeon's finger indicates the pylorus while the Duval clamp is applied 3 cm above. At this level the second step of gastric tube creation will begin

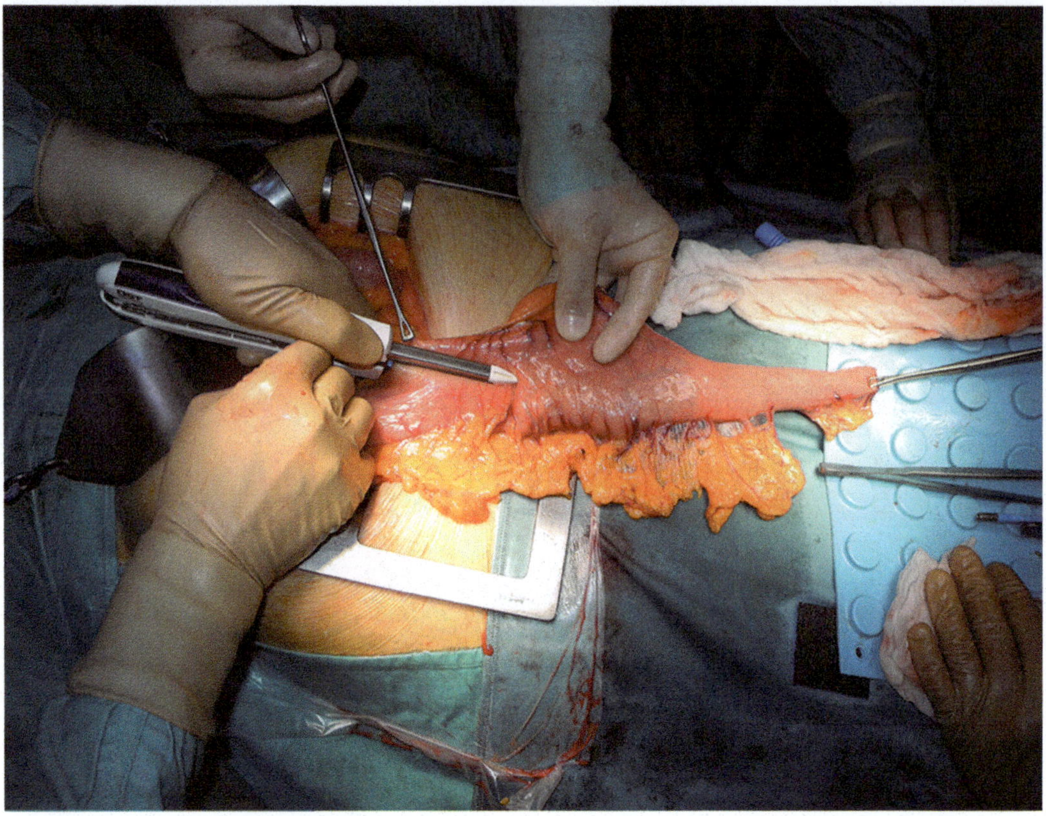

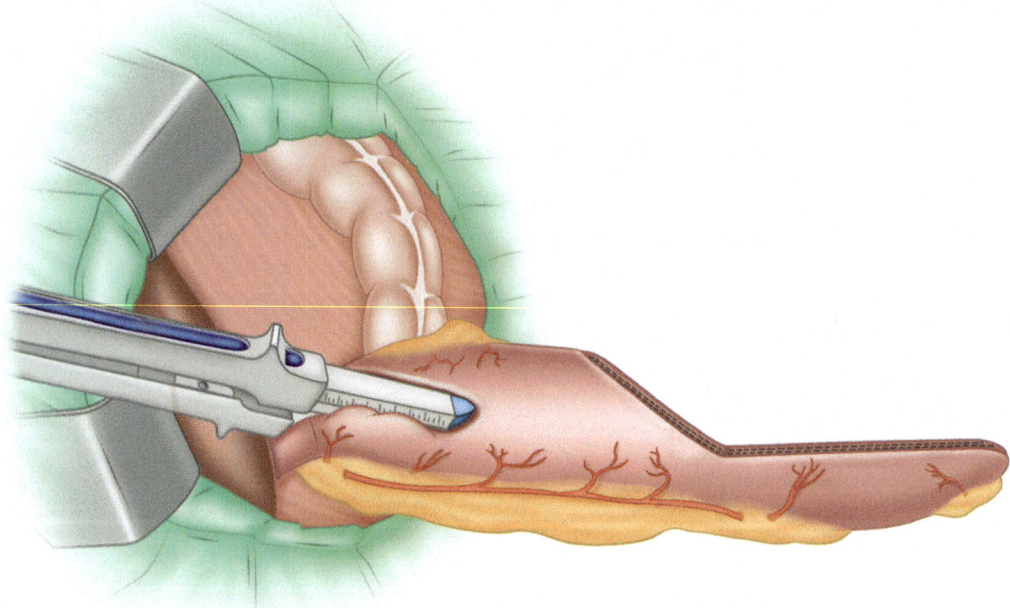

**Figs. 6.22 and 6.23** The fourth firing is started at the distal part of the lesser curvature, parallel to the greater curvature and always distant 4 cm from it

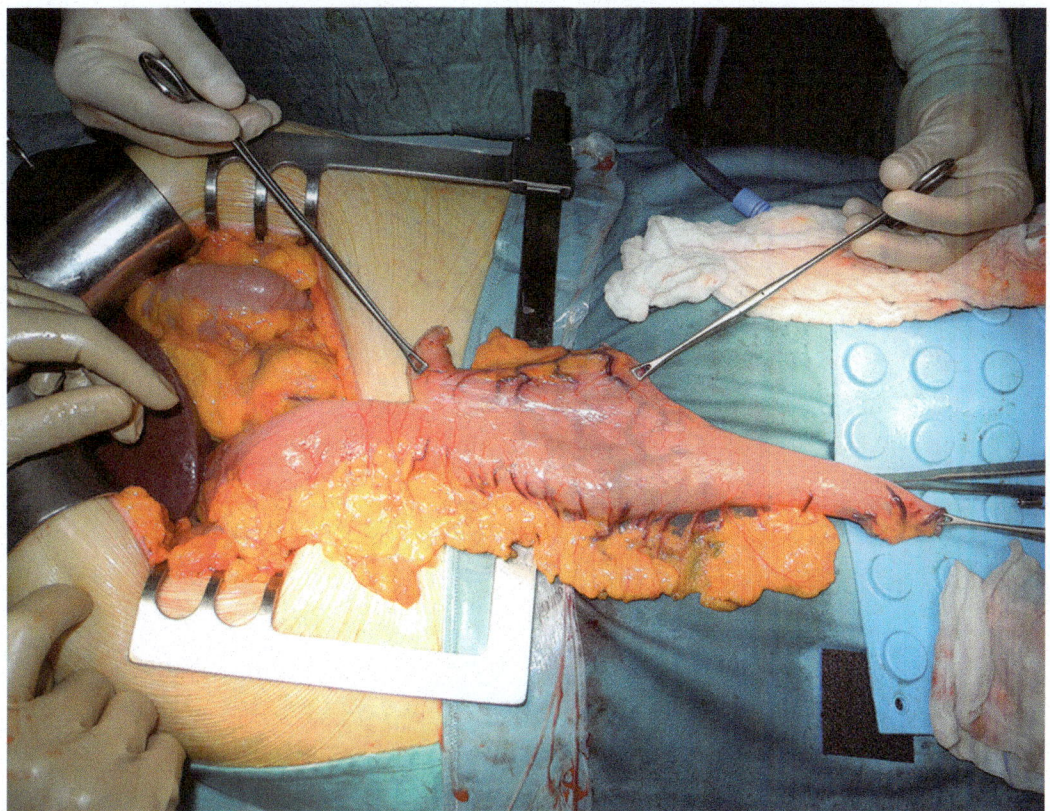

**Fig. 6.24** The appearance after the fourth firing. The gastric conduit creation is going on

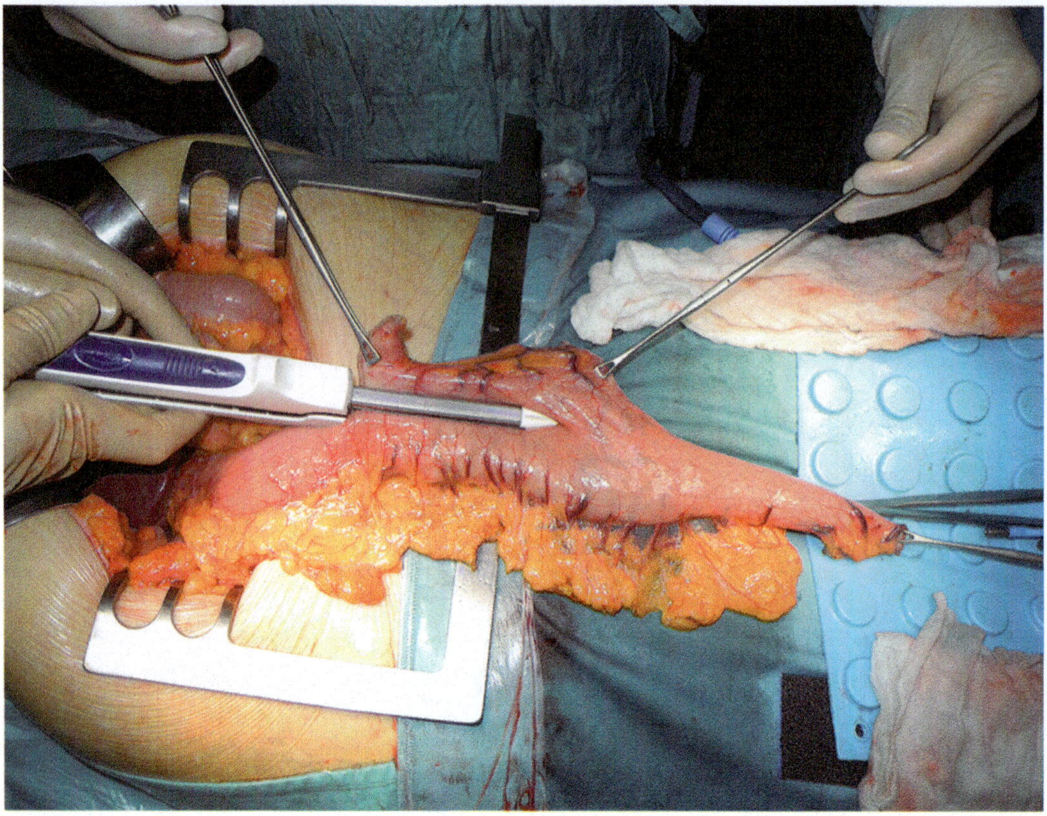

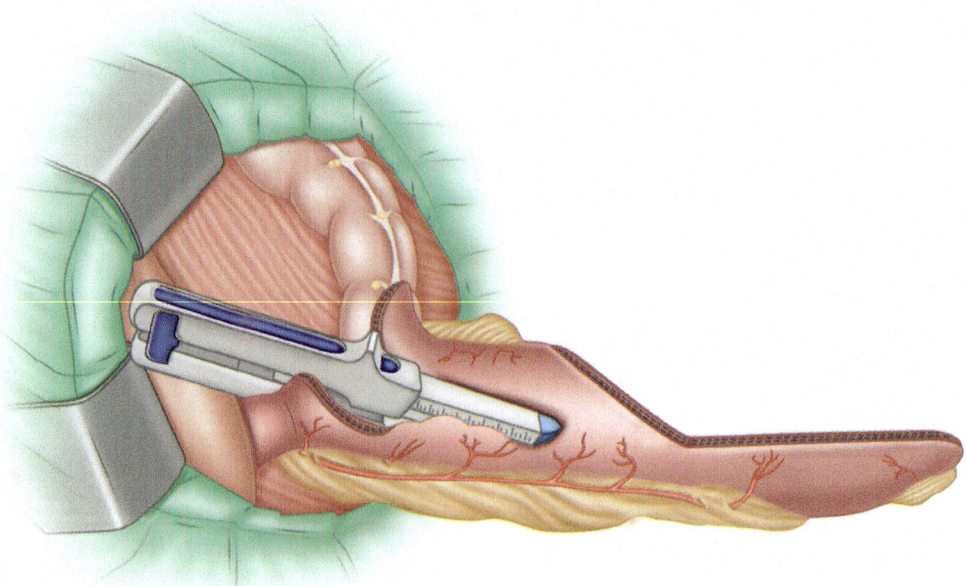

**Figs. 6.25 and 6.26** The fifth firing continues on the same direction of the previous distal section arriving up to 5 cm from the upper section

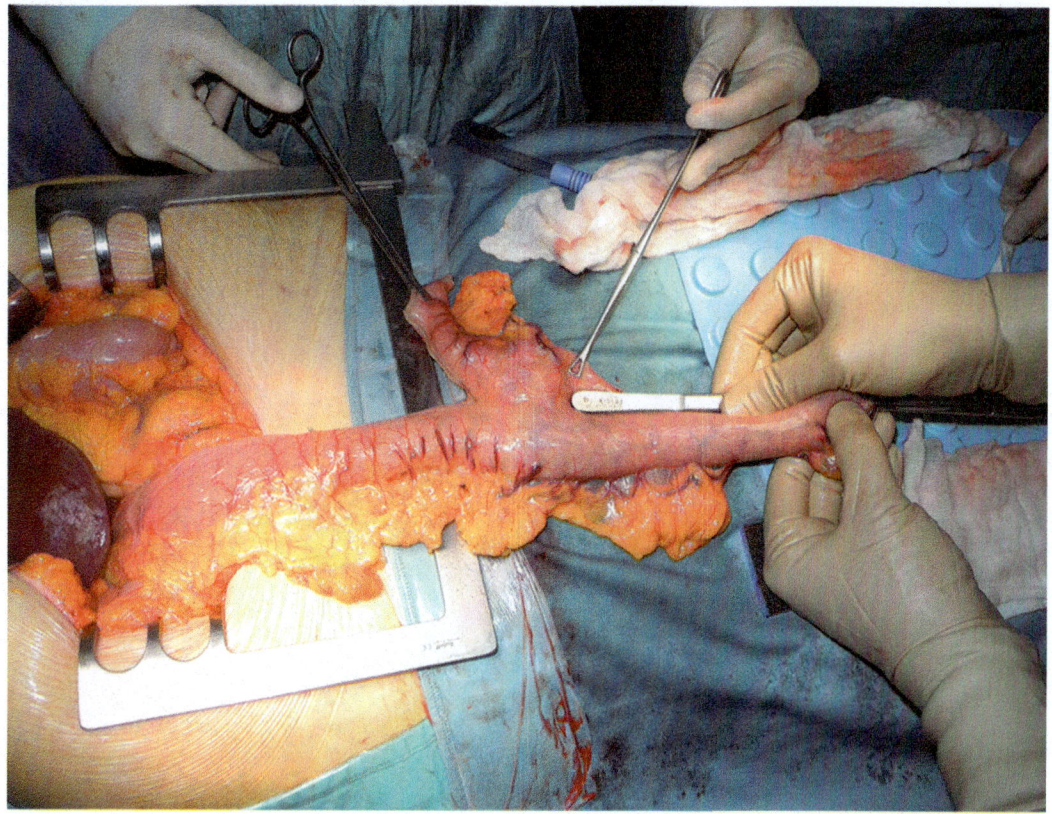

**Fig. 6.27** The appearance after the fifth firing. A pouch is created on the lesser curvature of the stomach

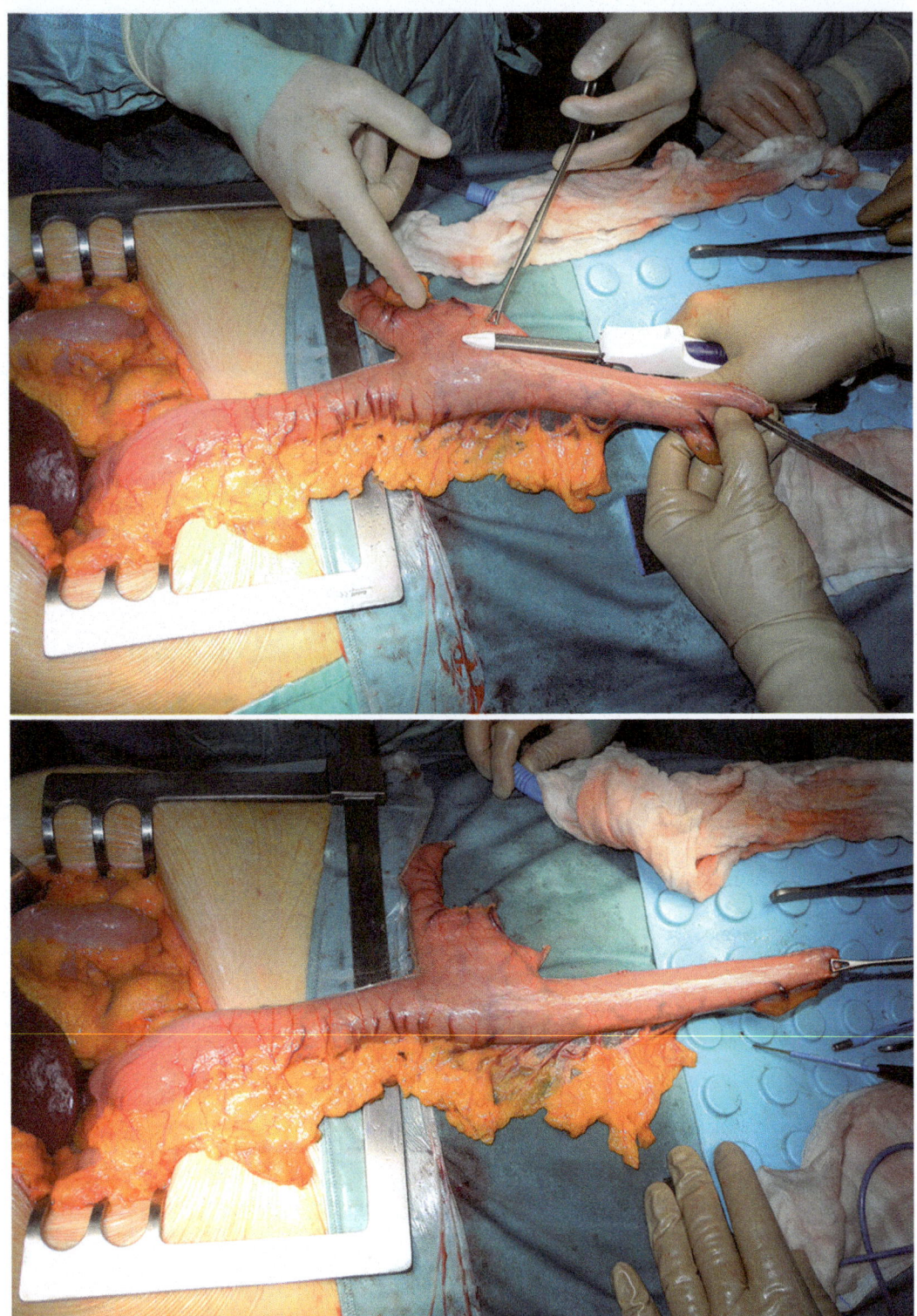

**Figs. 6.28 and 6.29** The sixth firing is performed to reduce the width of the pouch. This results in a gastric tube about 30–35 cm in length and 4 cm in width, with an access pouch that will be used for entry of the circular stapler

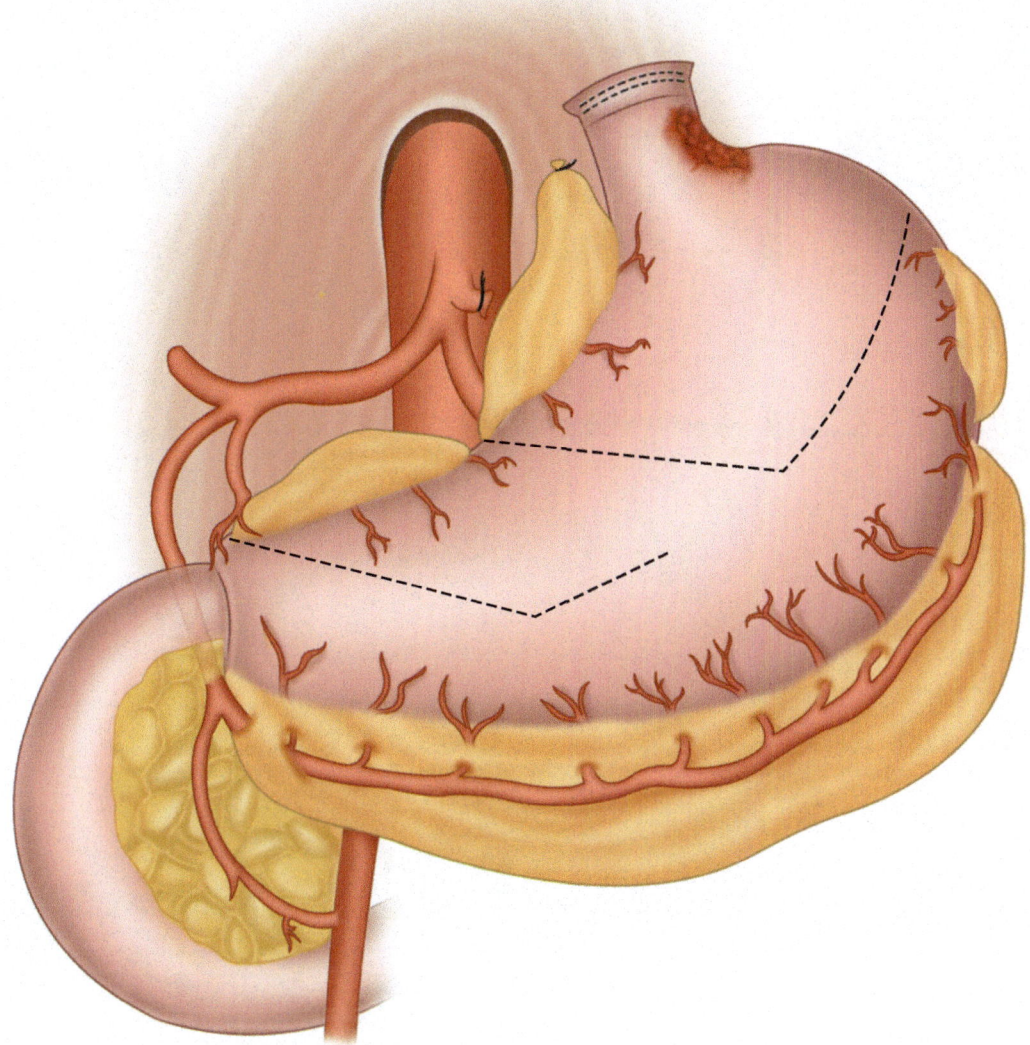

**Fig. 6.30** Scheme of the gastric conduit construction with multiple GIA firings

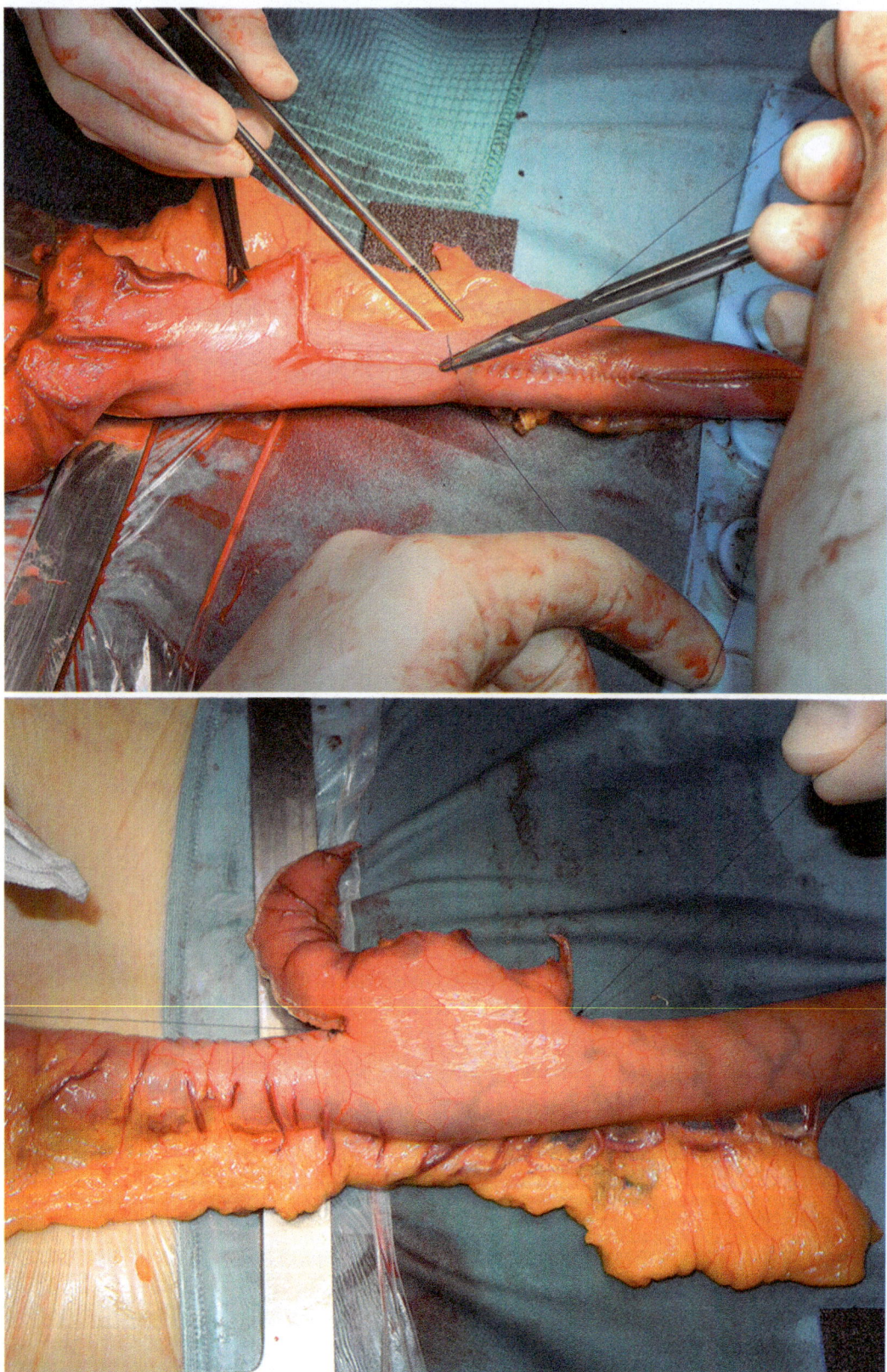

**Figs. 6.31 and 6.32** The linear stapler sutures are oversewn with a PDS 4-0 running suture

**Fig. 6.33** The created gastric tube is long enough to reach the neck of the patient. A D2 lymph node dissection is performed and the esophageal hiatus is opened to free the lower esophagus and to complete lower mediastinal node dissection

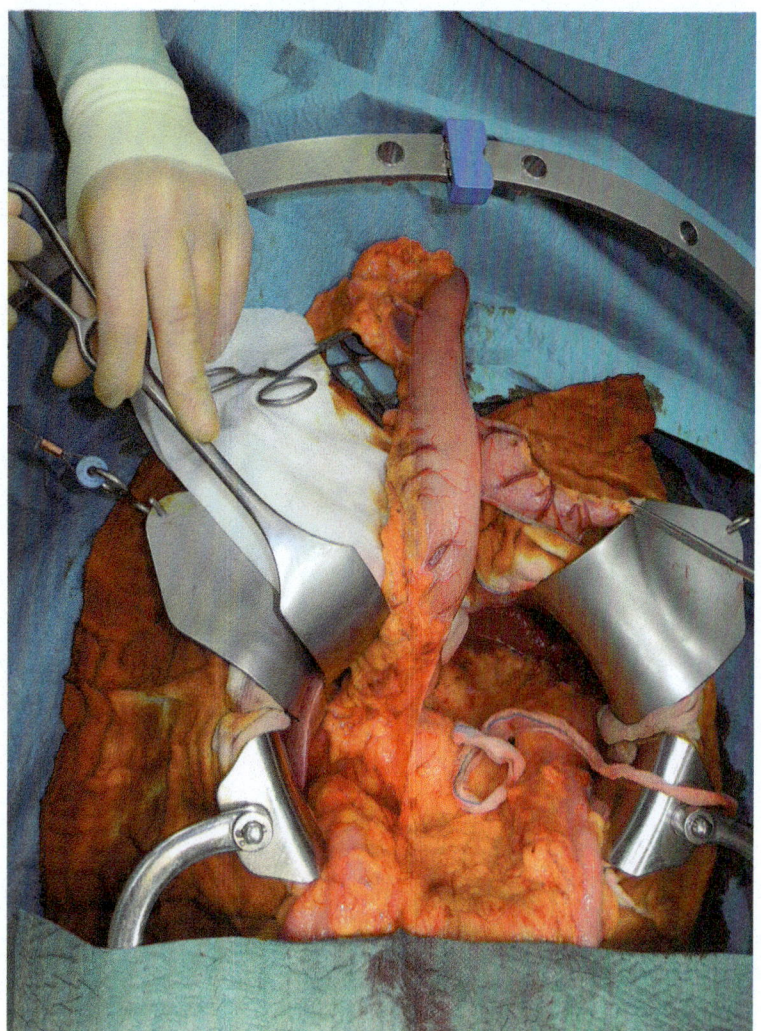

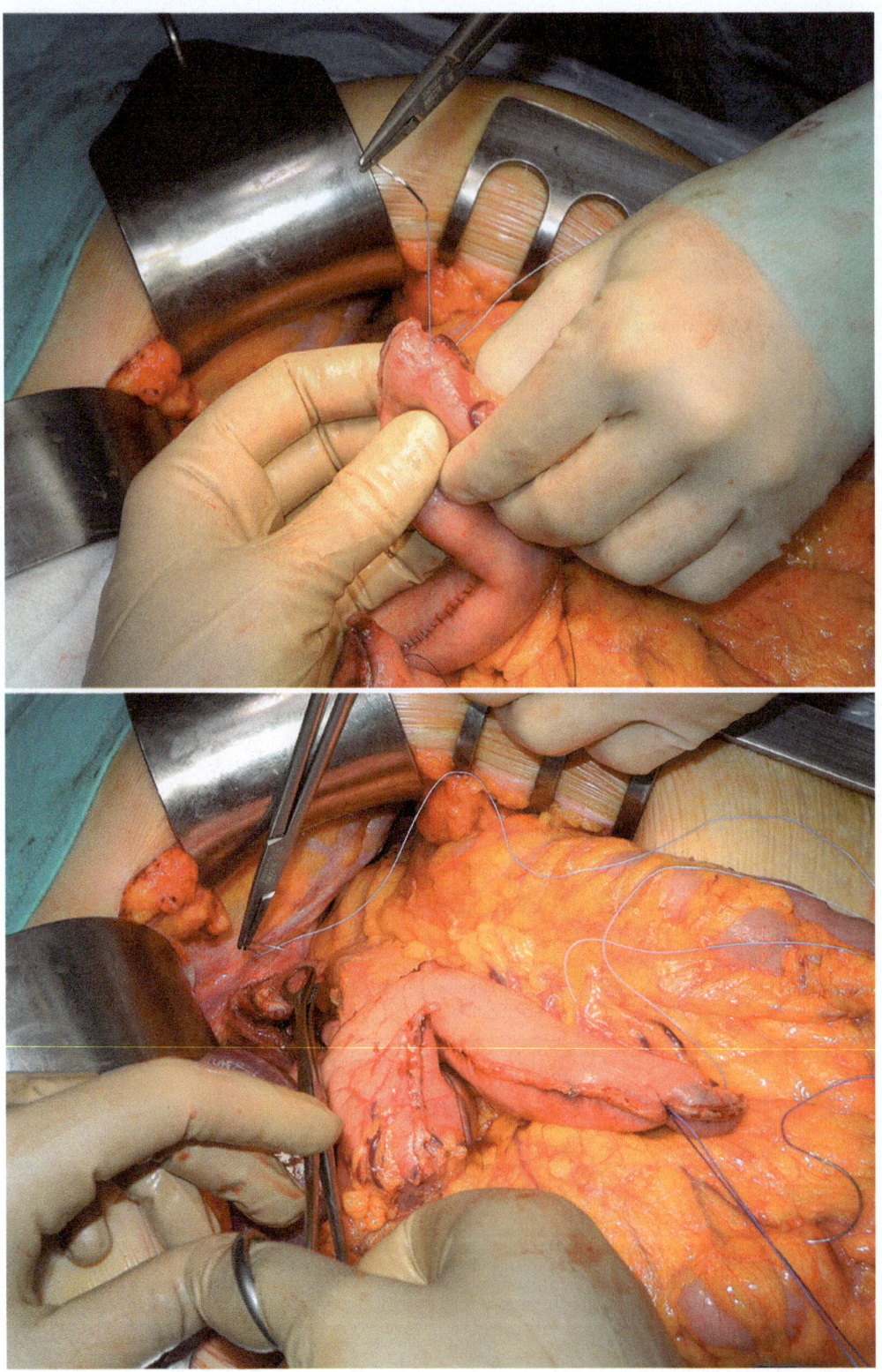

**Figs. 6.34 and 6.35** The gastric tube is ligated with the esophageal stump using two nonabsorbable sutures. This enables the recovery of the gastric conduit during the thoracic phase

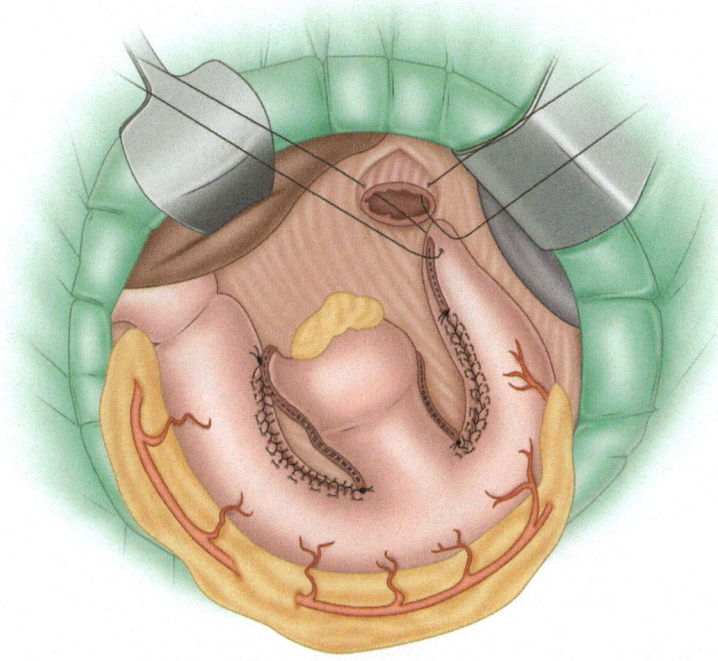

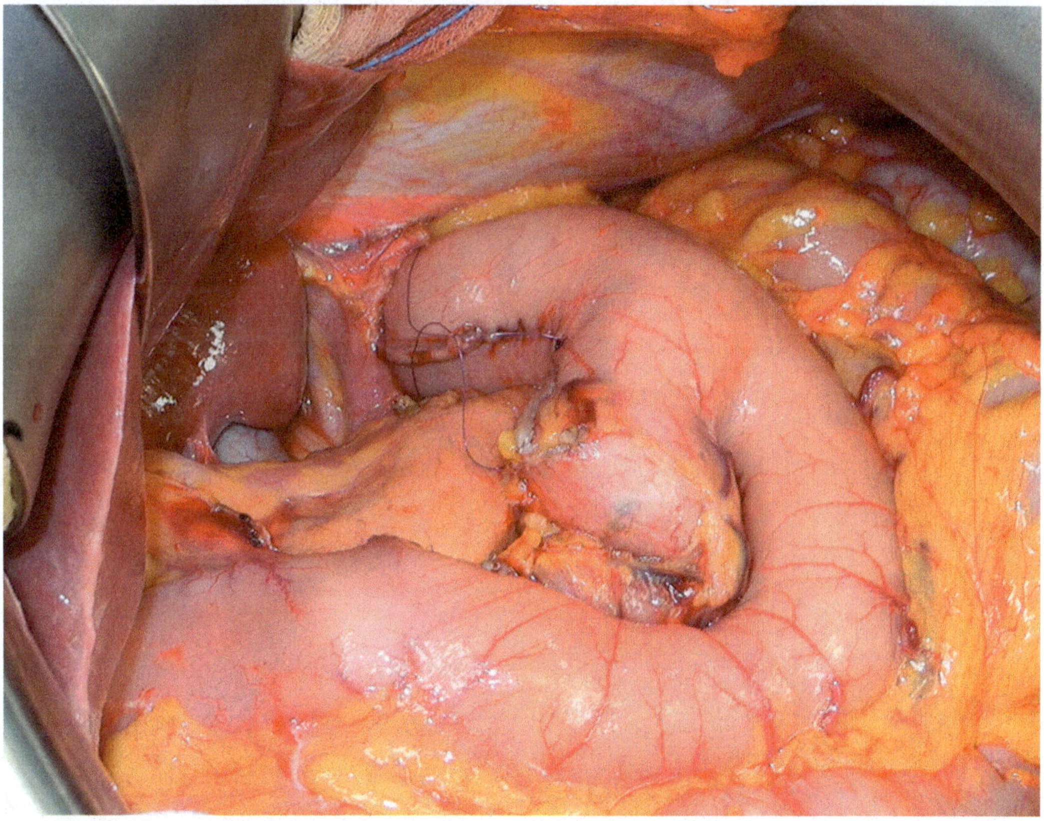

**Figs. 6.36 and 6.37** Final aspect of the gastric tube attached to the esophageal stump. The abdominal cavity is closed and a drainage is usually placed in the right subhepatic space. The patient is positioned in left lateral decubitus

## 6.2    Thoracic Stage: Esophagectomy and Esophagogastric Anastomosis Fabrication

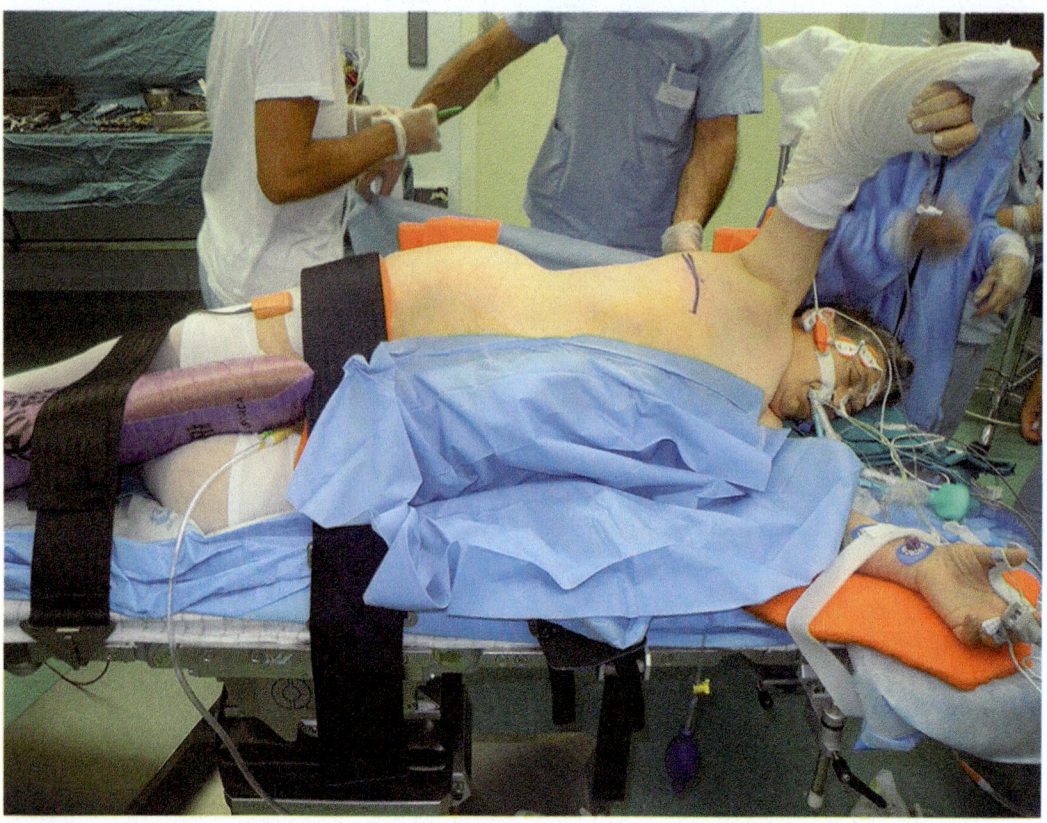

**Fig. 6.38** A right lateral thoracotomy is performed at the fifth intercostal space to enter the chest

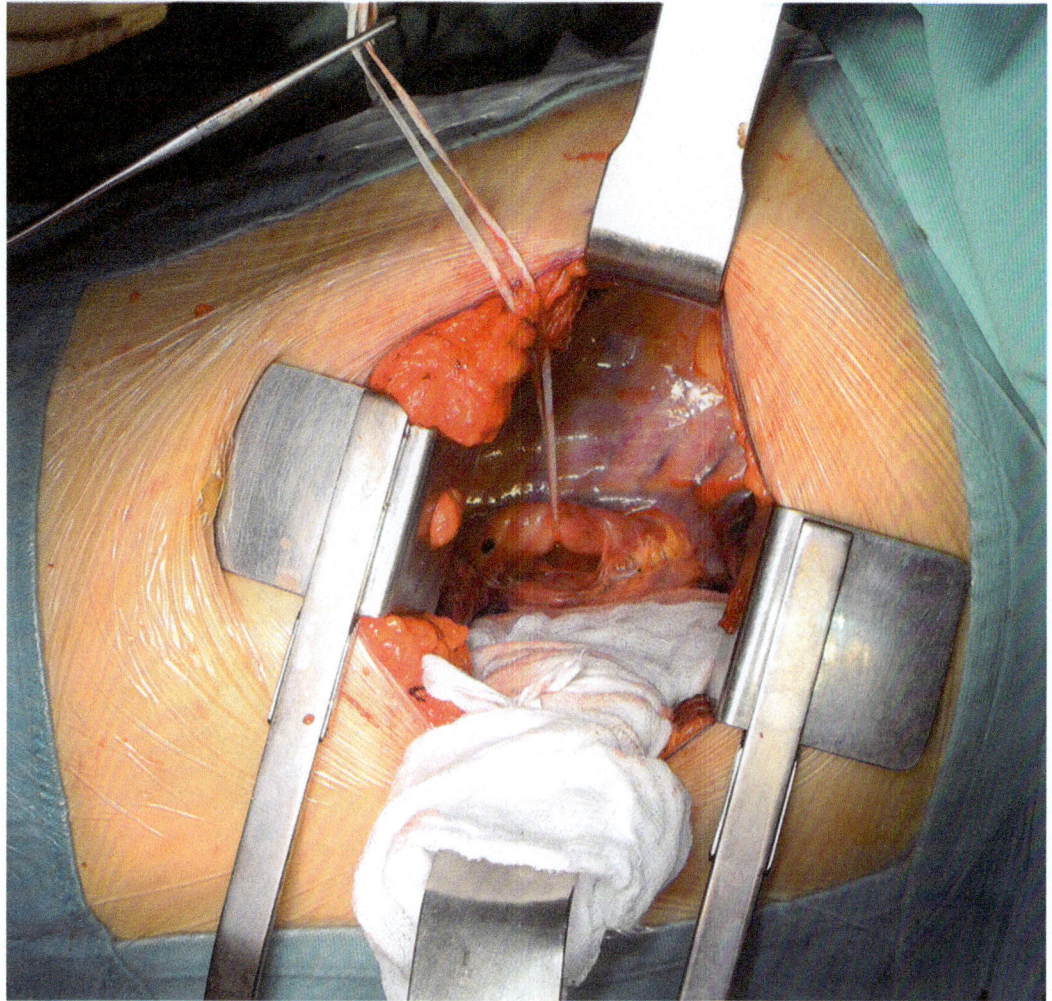

**Fig. 6.39** The mediastinal pleura is incised and the esophagus is encircled with a vascular tape

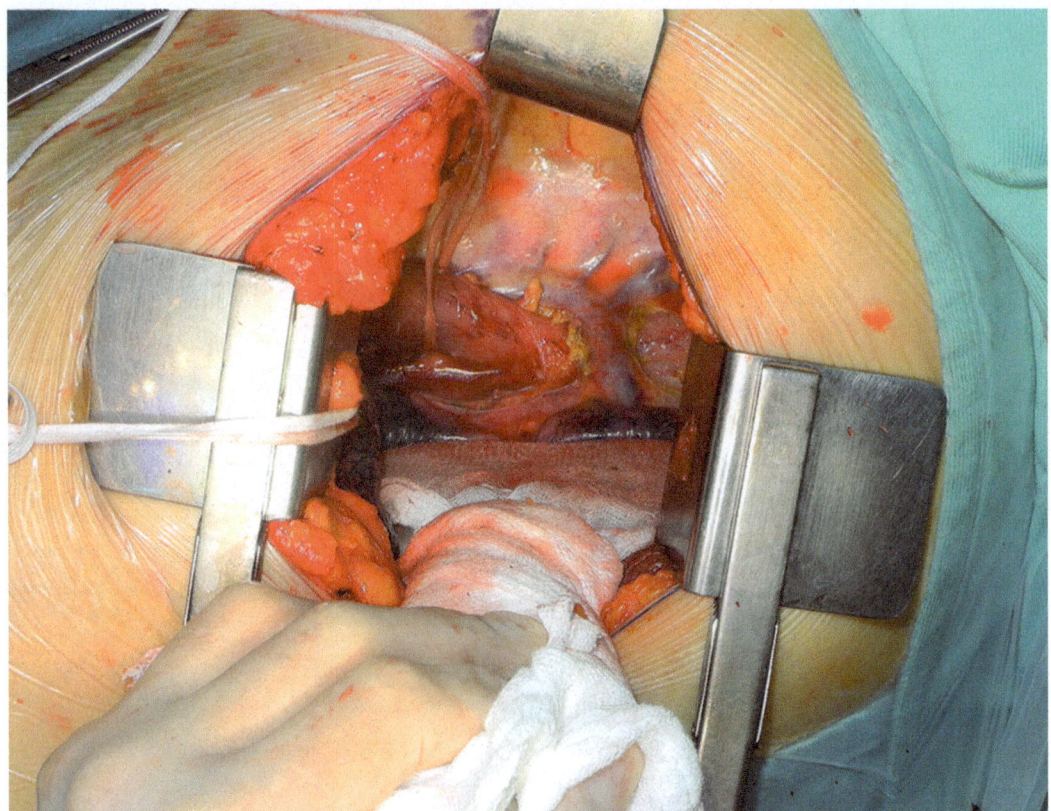

**Fig. 6.40** The esophagus is dissected until the level of the azygos vein which is isolated

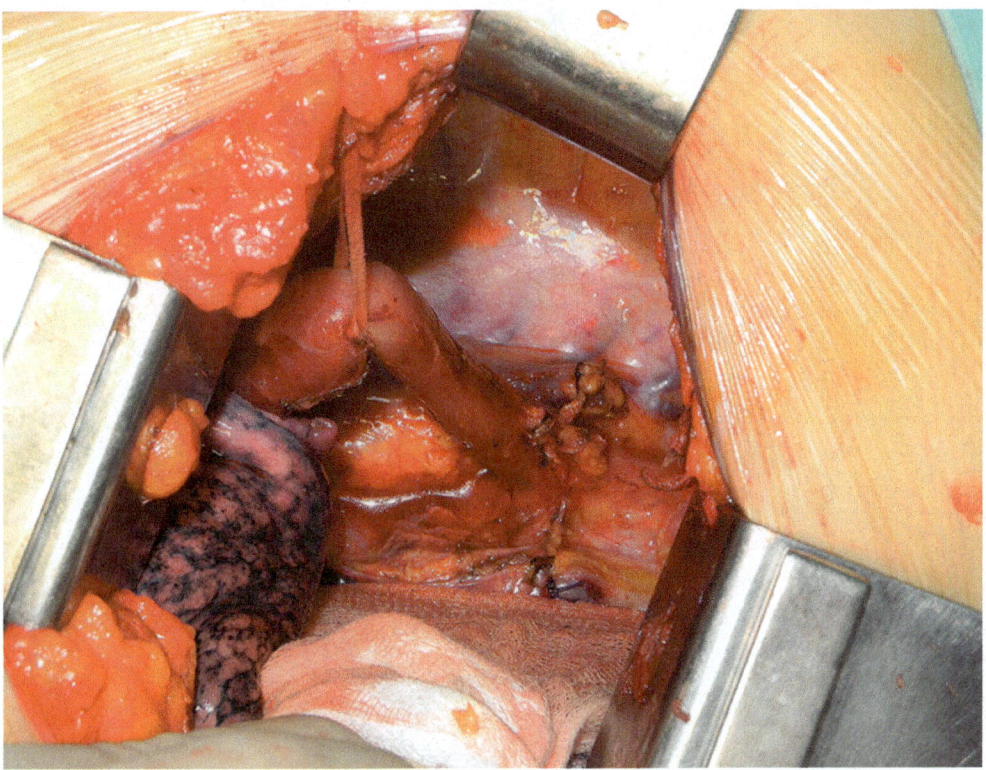

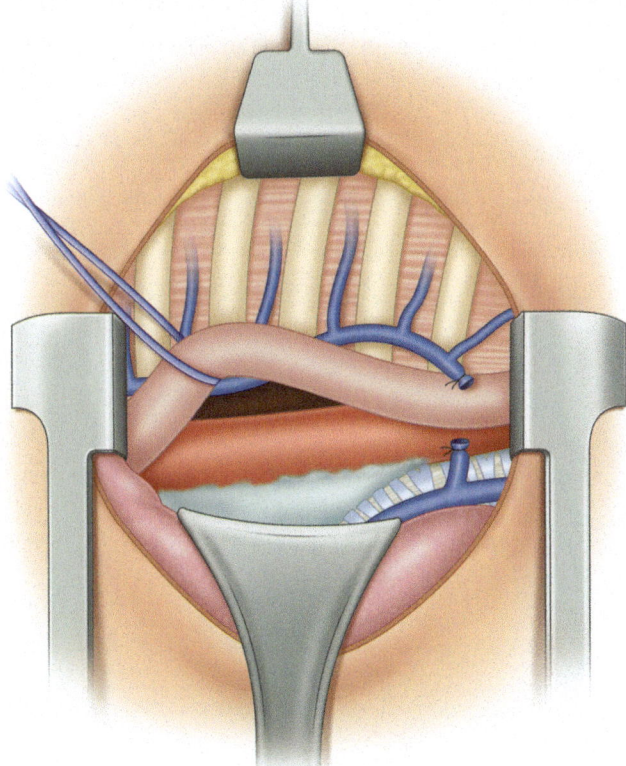

**Figs. 6.41 and 6.42**  The azygos vein is divided

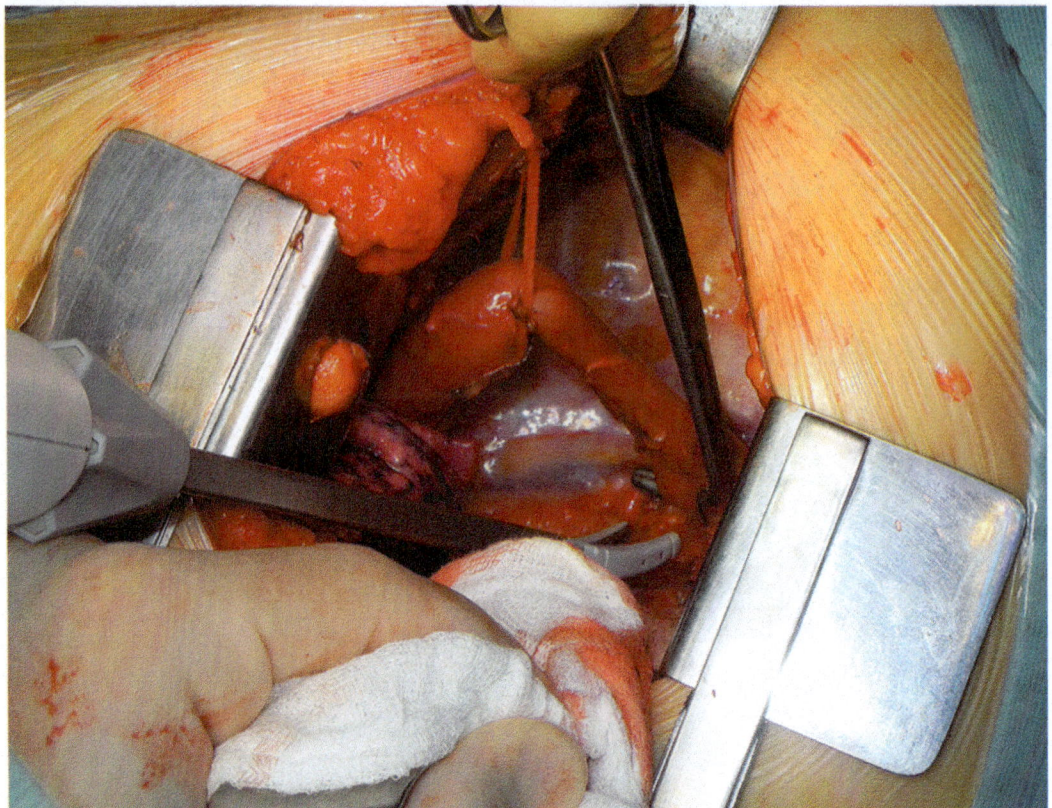

**Fig. 6.43** Dissection is continued toward the upper thoracic esophagus. A two-field extended lymph node dissection is then performed

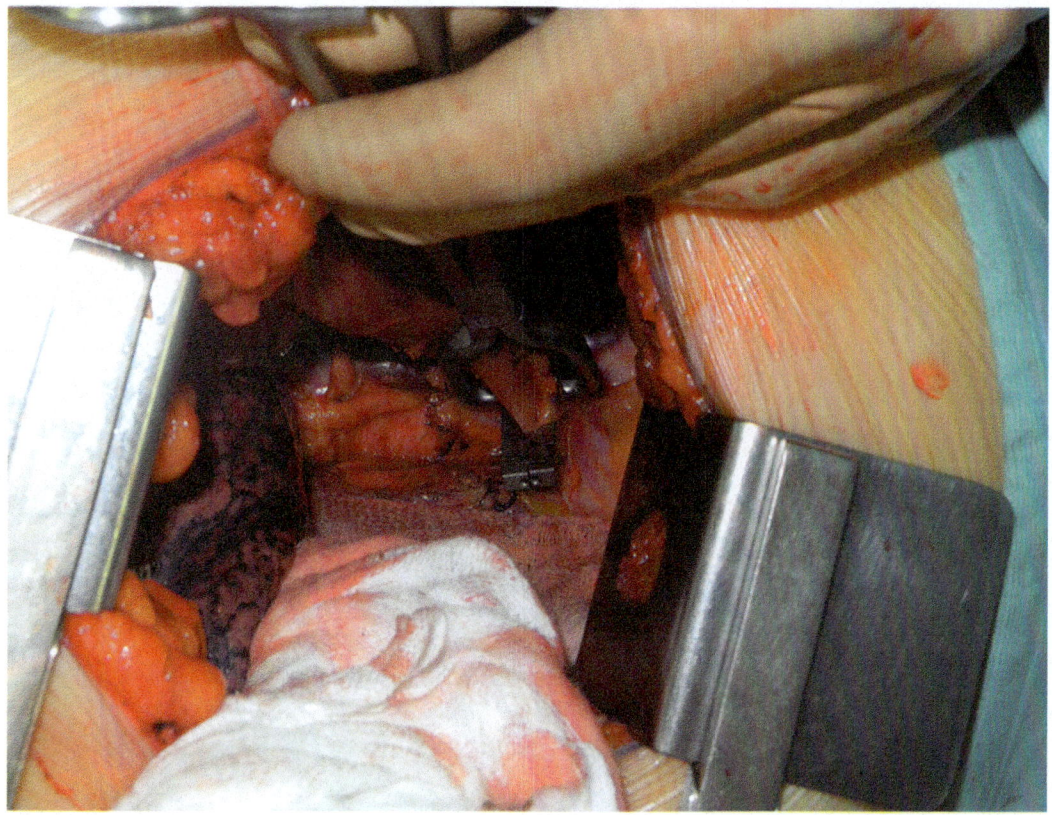

**Fig. 6.44** A rake clamp is placed 2–3 cm above the level of the azygos vein

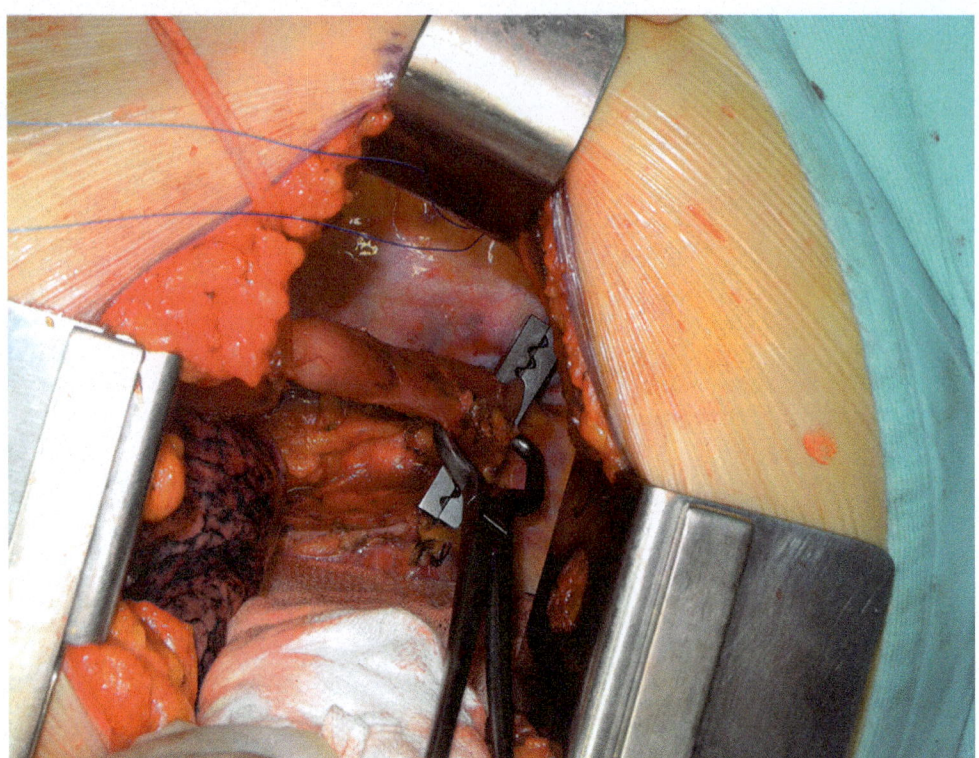

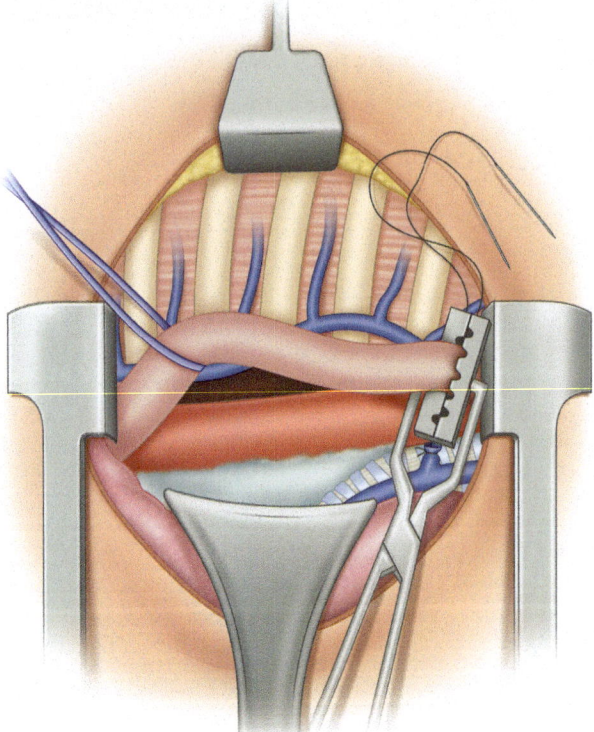

**Figs. 6.45 and 6.46** Two straight needles are inserted through the rake clamp jaws to execute a purse-string suture with 2-0 nonabsorbable monofilament suture

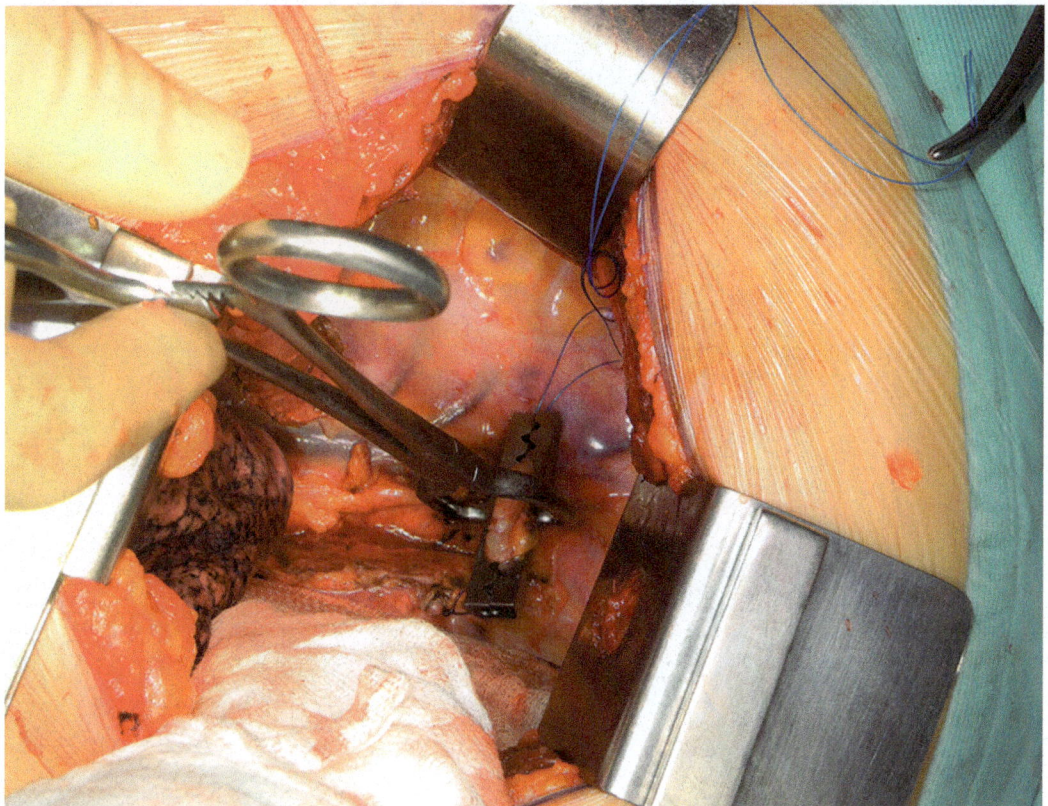

**Fig. 6.47** The esophagus is sectioned and sent for intraoperative histological evaluation of the upper margin

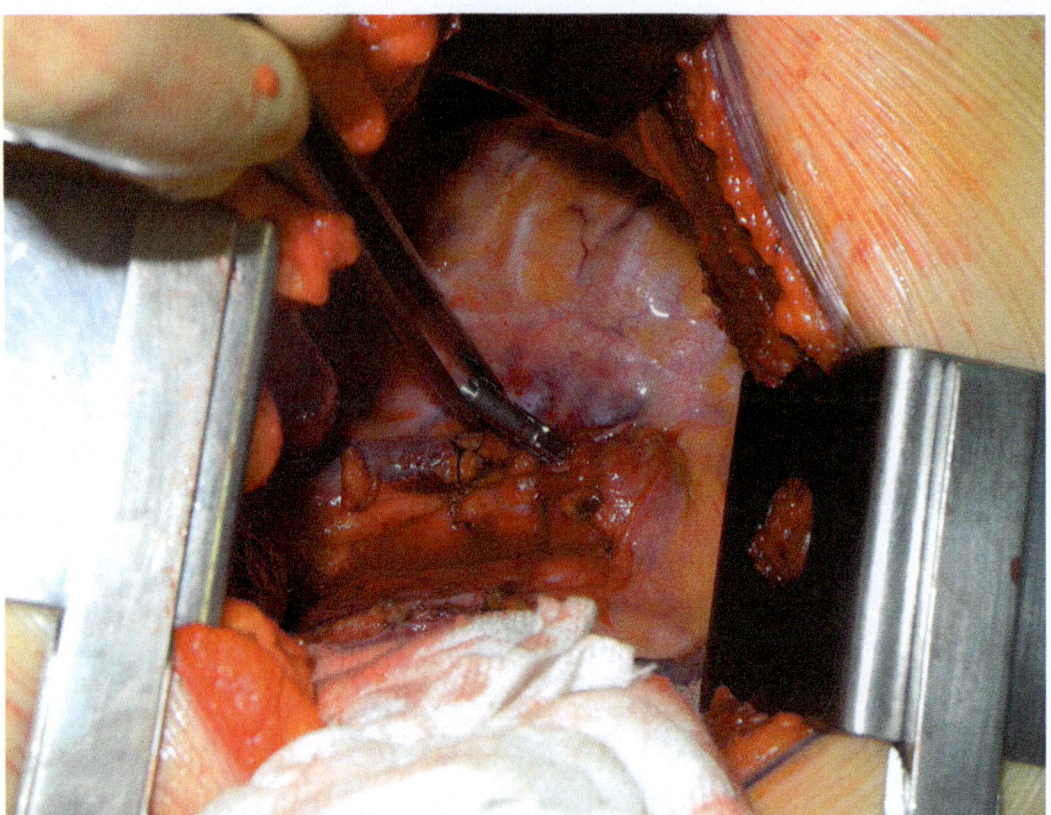

**Fig. 6.48** A 25 mm anvil is inserted in the esophageal stump and blocked with a purse-string suture

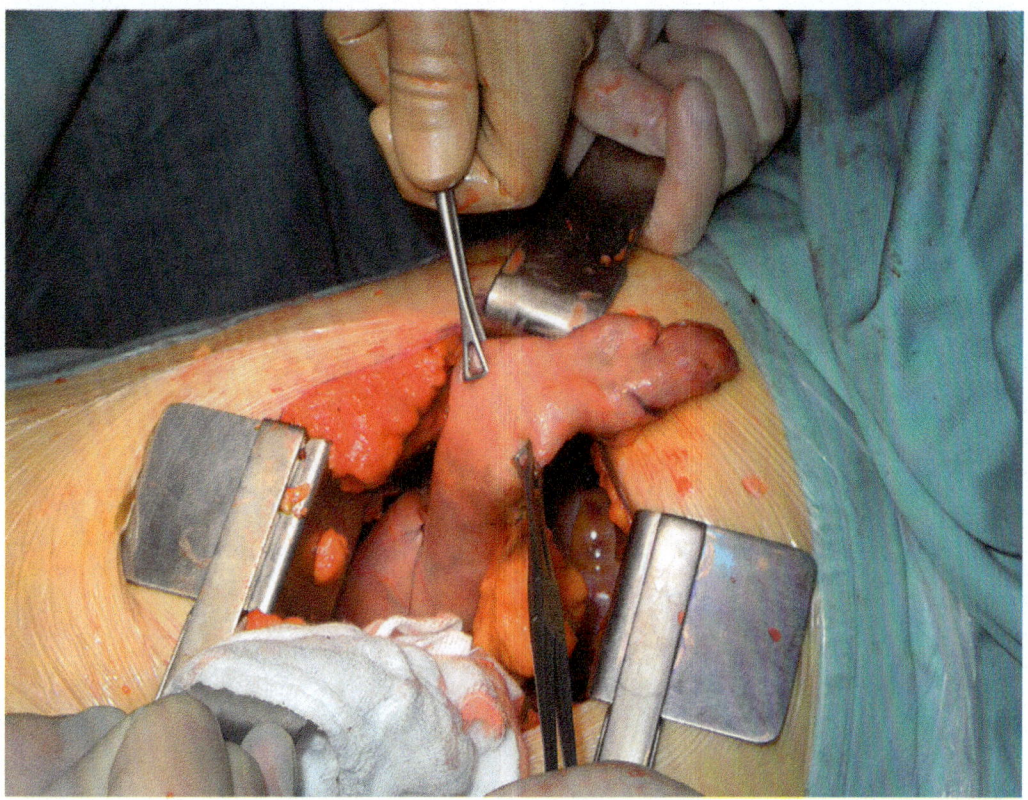

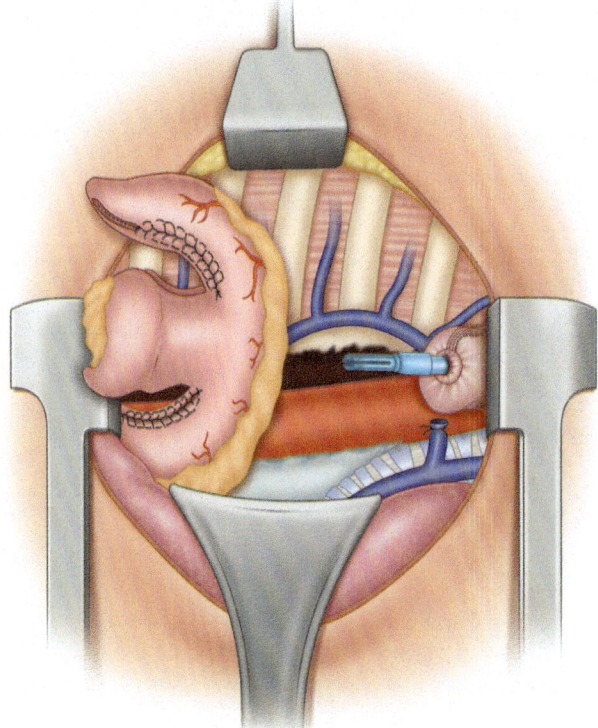

**Figs. 6.49 and 6.50** The gastric conduit is recovered and transposed in the chest cavity

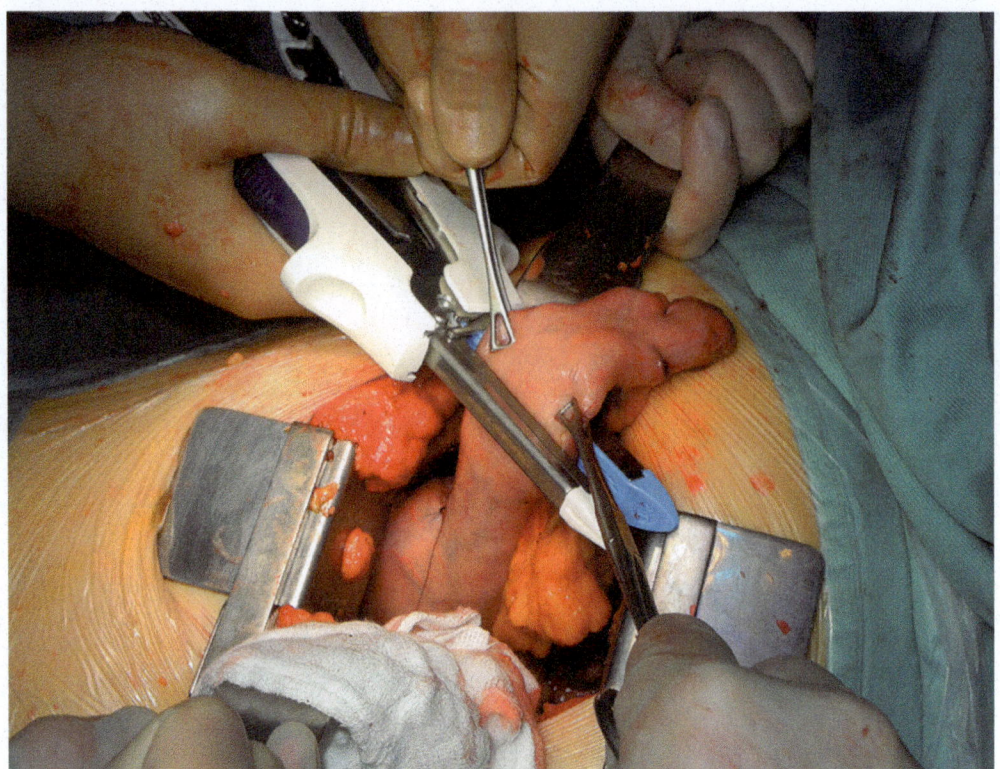

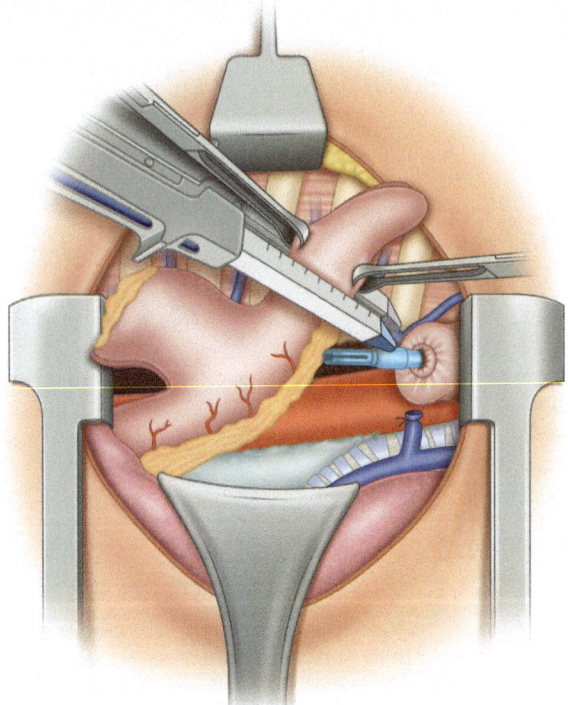

**Figs. 6.51 and 6.52** The length of the gastric tube is calibrated to perform a supple and tension-free anastomosis. At this level the gastric conduit is transected with GIA 60

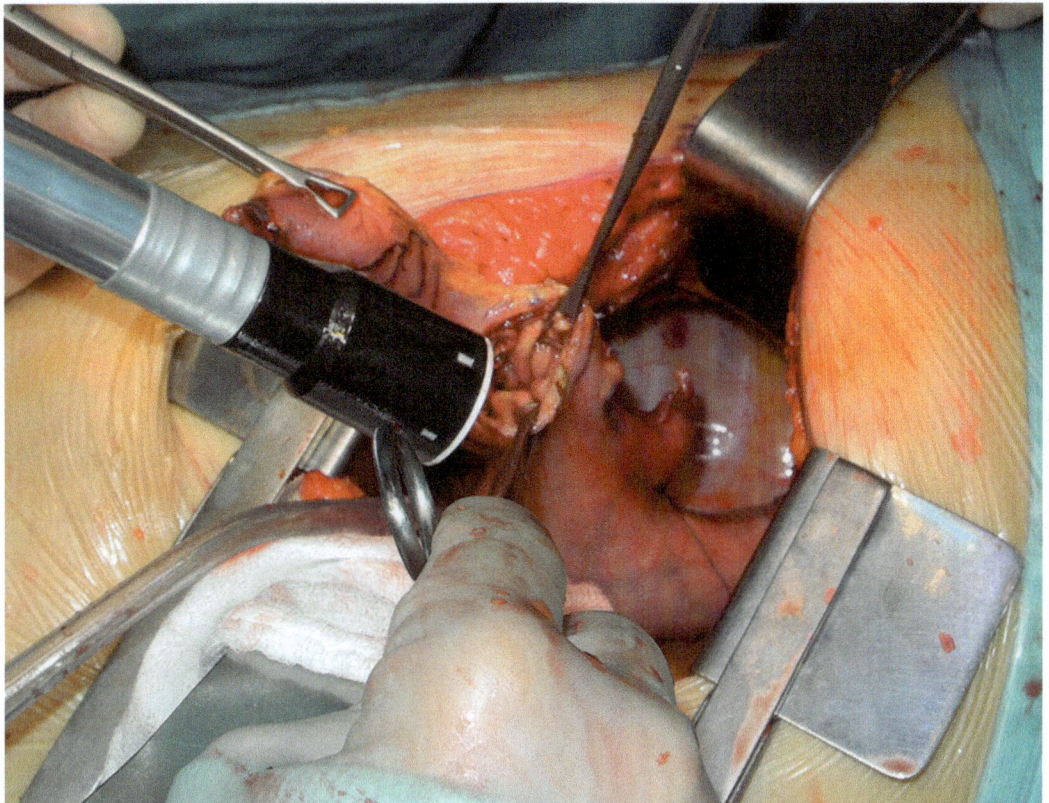

**Fig. 6.53** The circular stapler is inserted through a gastrotomy performed on the access pouch

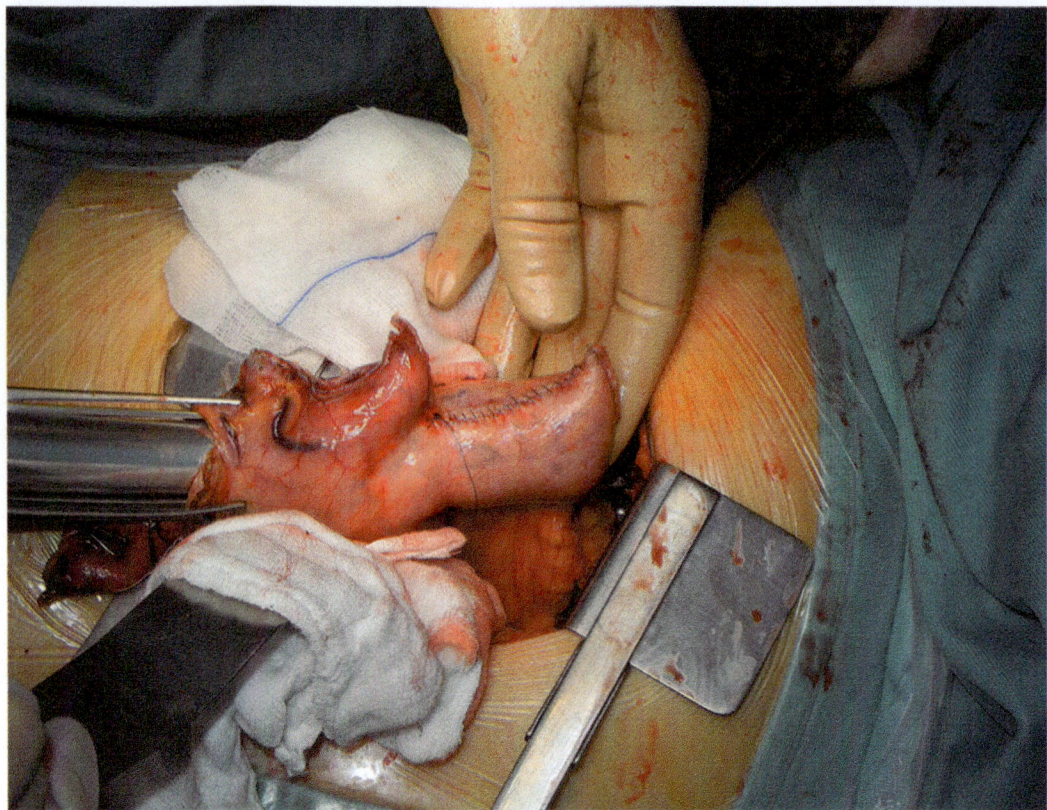

**Fig. 6.54** The stapler is advanced until the top of the transected gastric tube; at this level the gastric conduit is perforated with the spike of the circular stapler

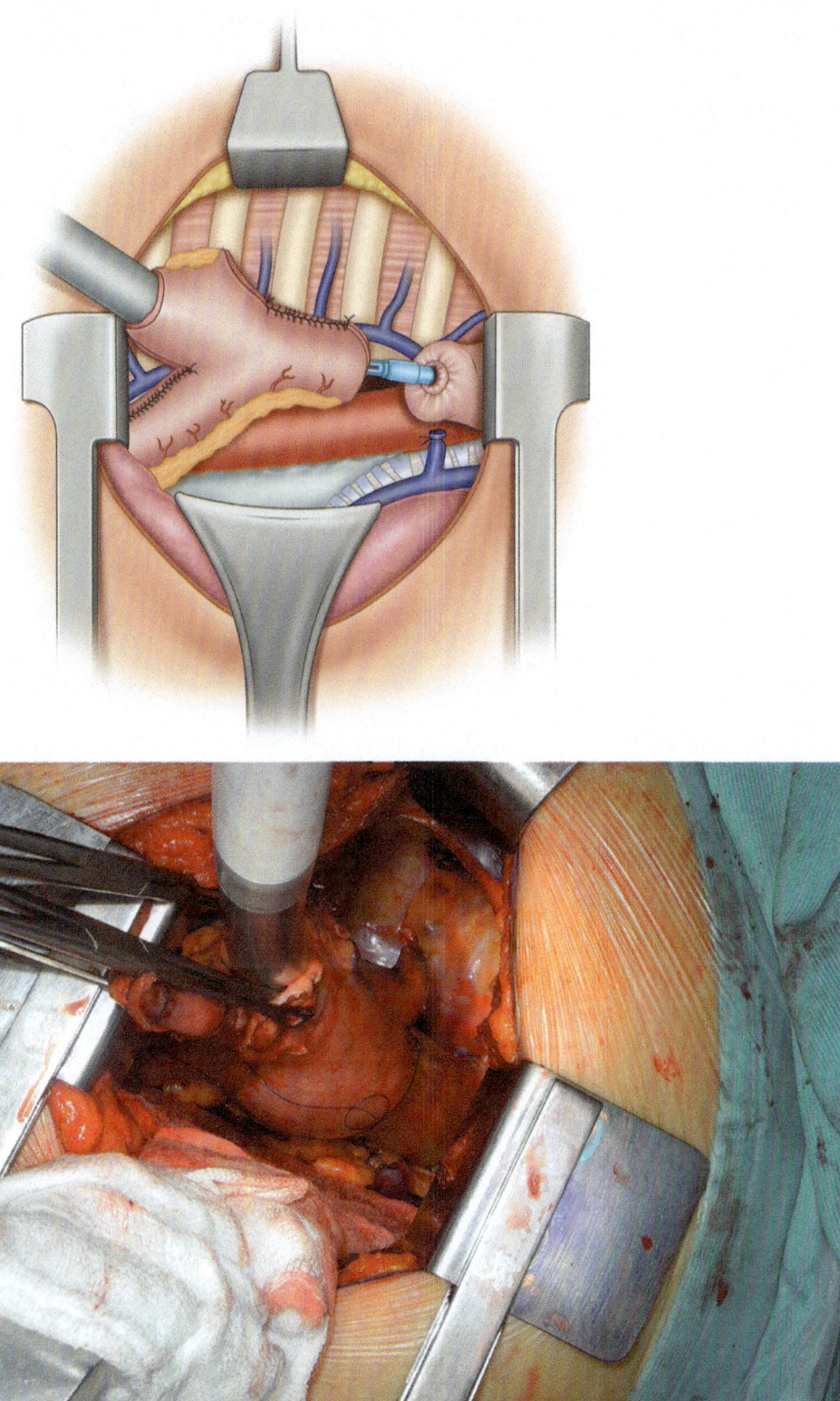

**Figs. 6.55 and 6.56** The cartridge on the circular stapler is joined to the anvil placed in the esophageal stump, and a circular stapled end-to-end anastomosis is performed

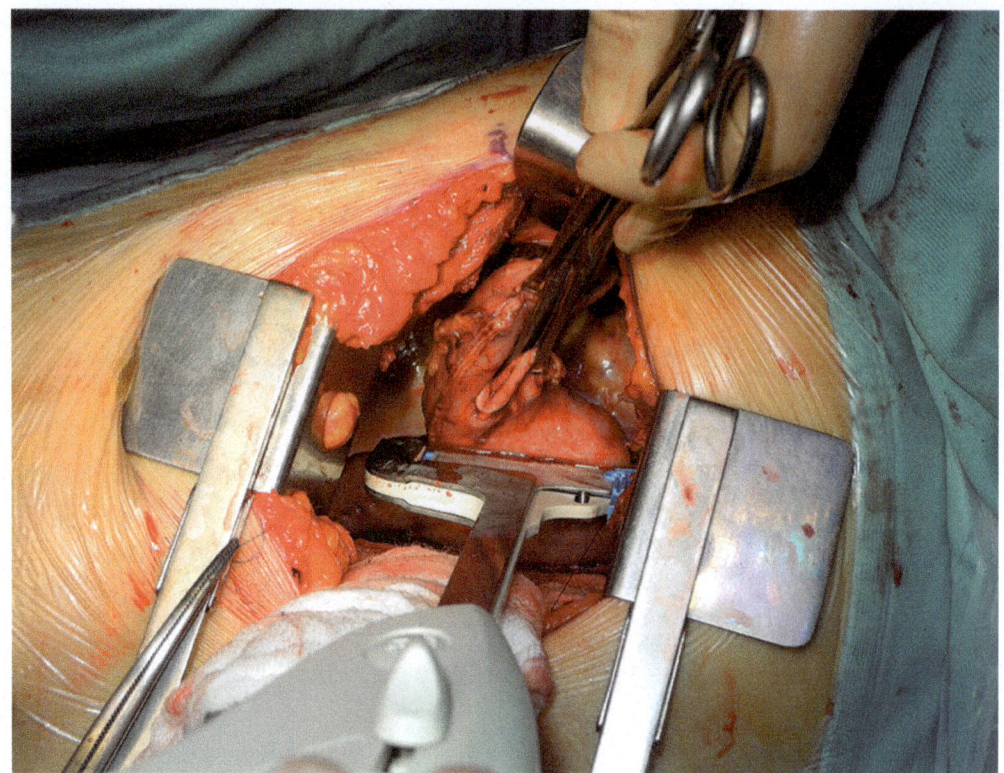

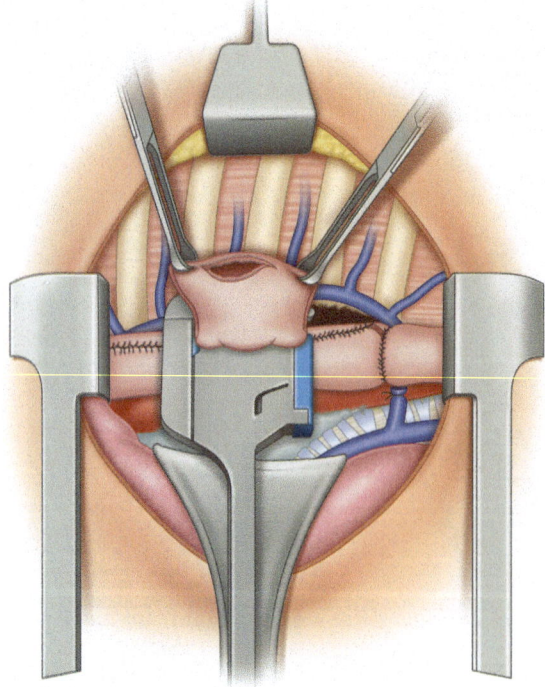

**Figs. 6.57, 6.58, and 6.59** The access pouch is closed with a linear TA 60 stapler and then resected

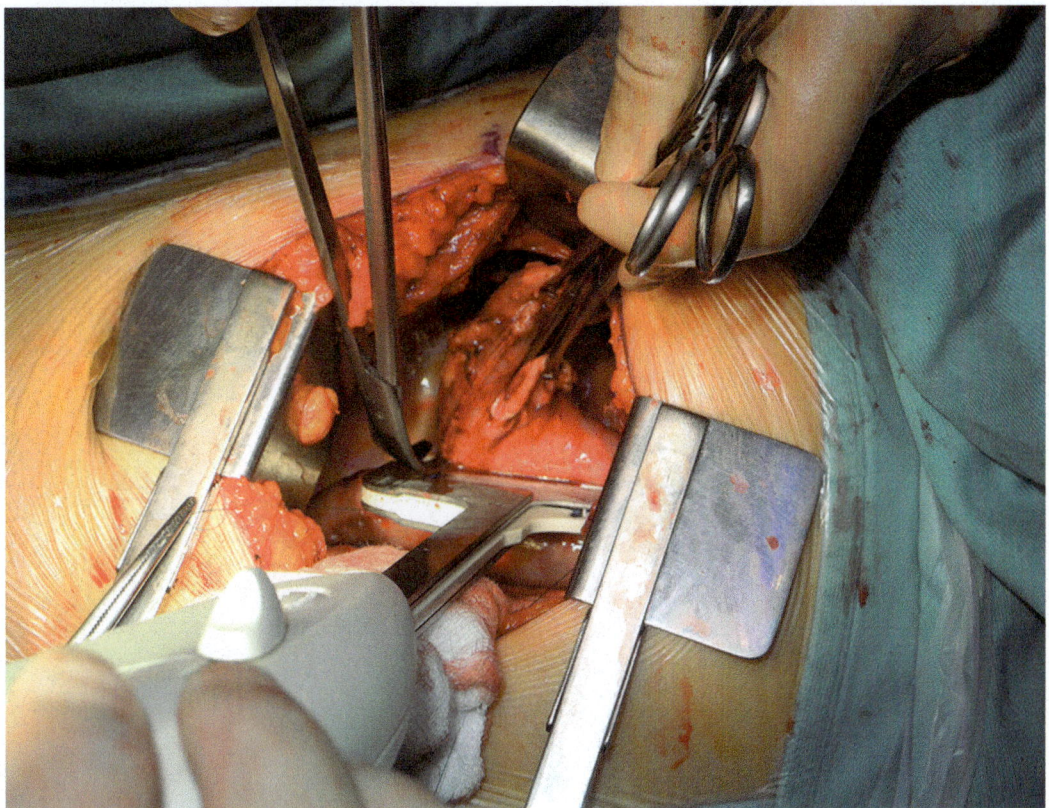

**Figs. 6.57, 6.58, and 6.59** (continued)

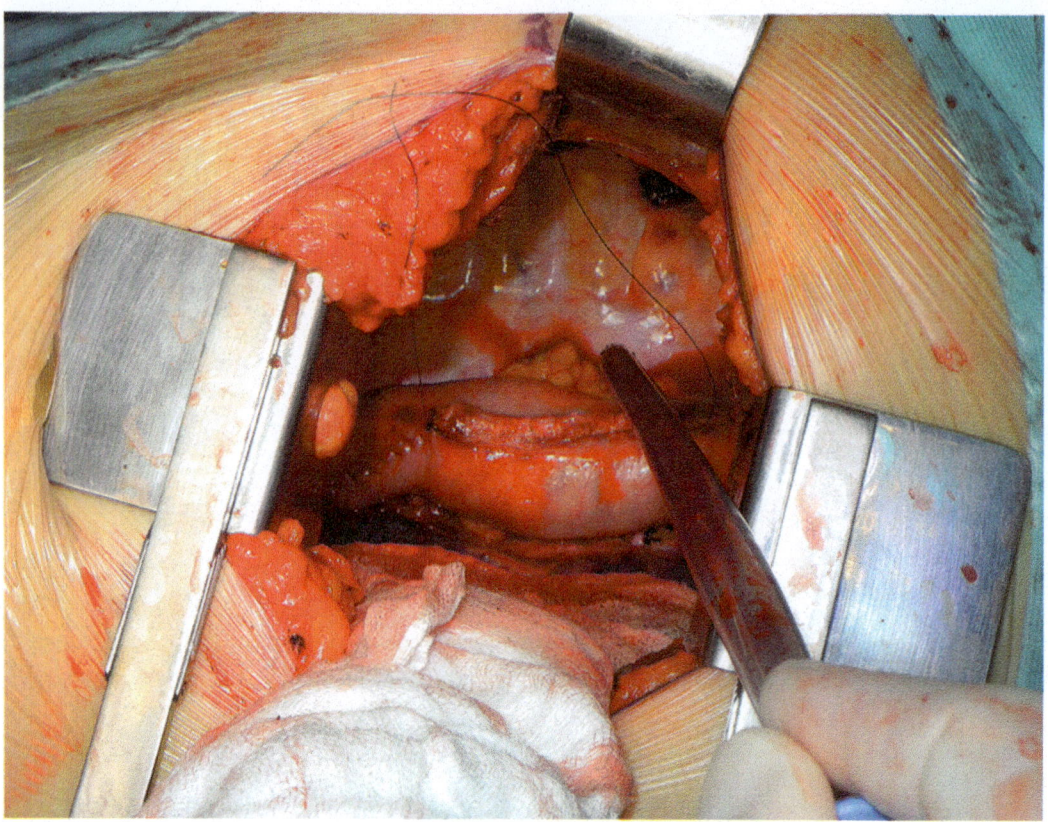

Fig. 6.60 The appearance after gastric access pouch resection

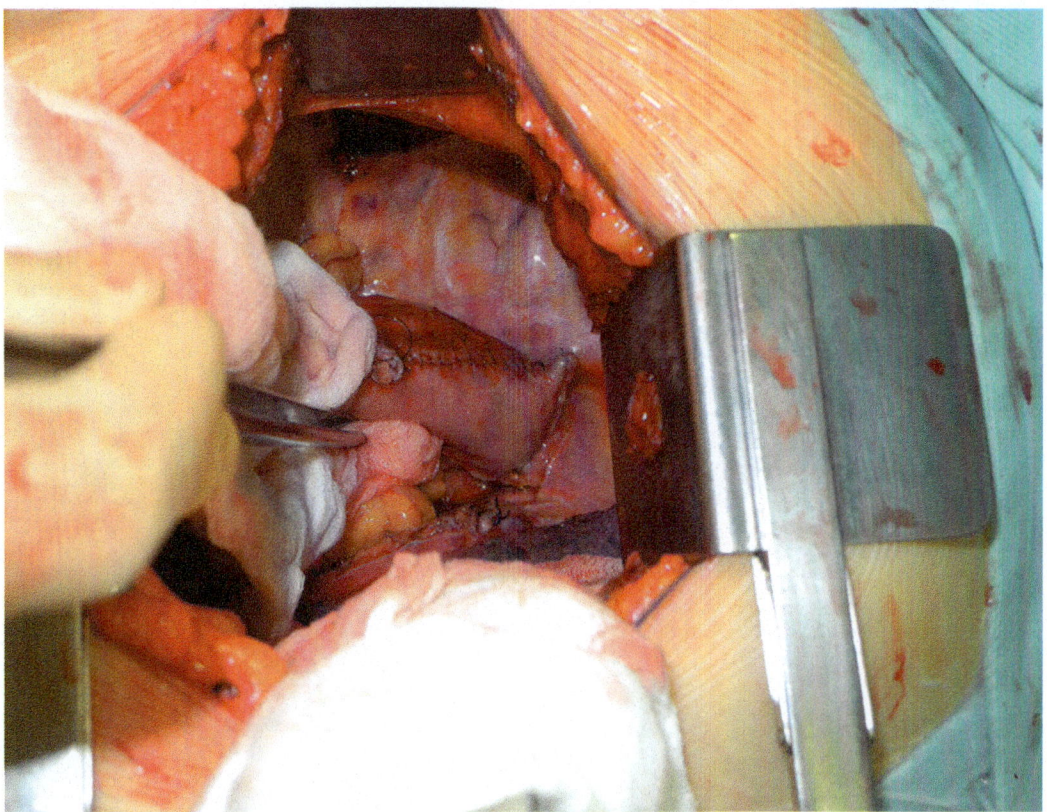

**Fig. 6.61** The appearance of the mechanical esophagogastric tube end-to-end anastomosis

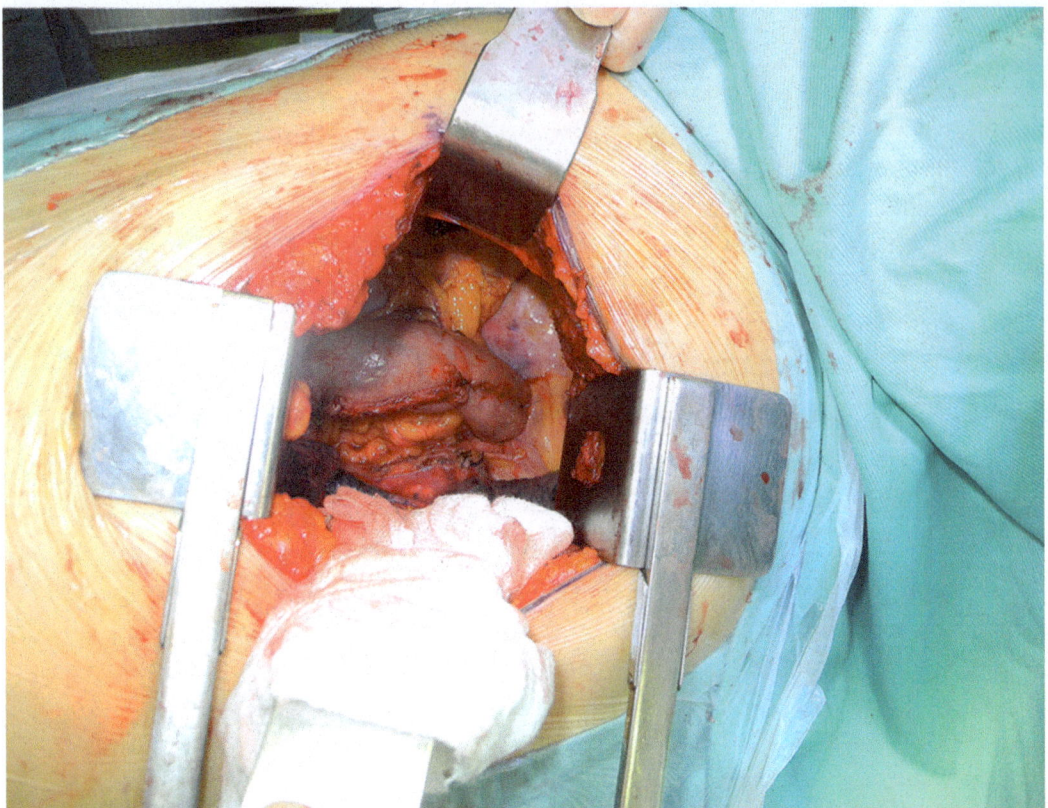

**Fig. 6.62** The anastomosis is very gently oversewn with a PDS 4-0 running suture to avoid staple line tension and reinforce the anastomosis

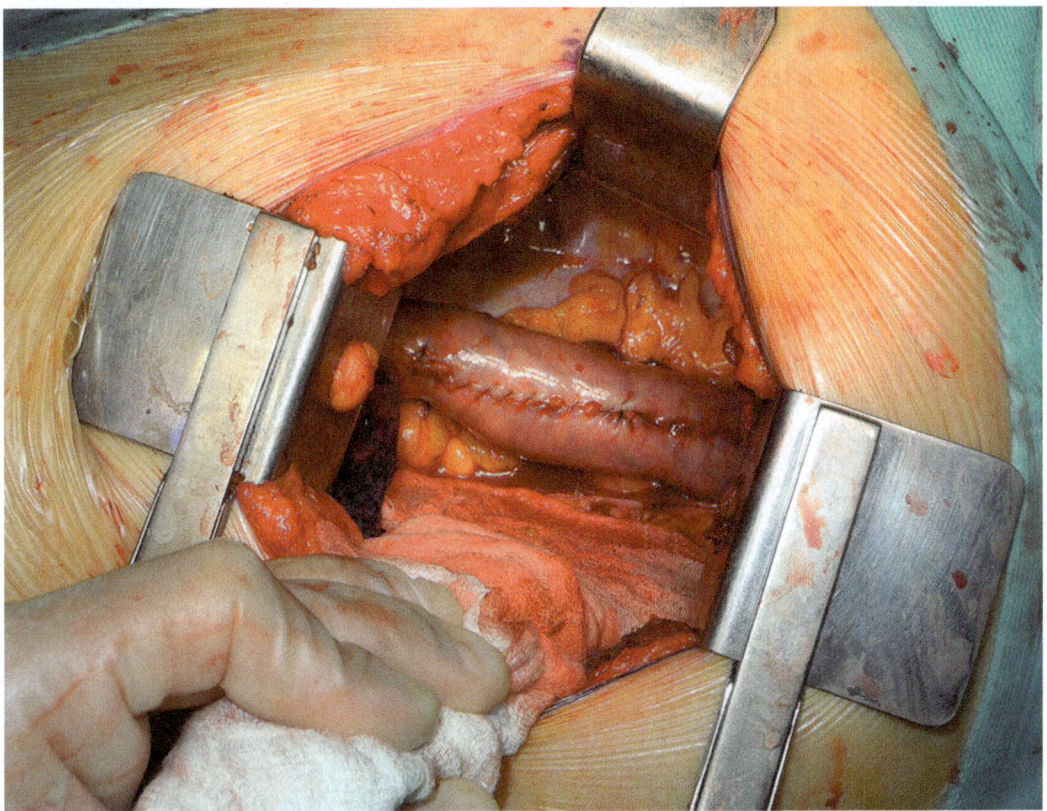

**Fig. 6.63** Even the mechanical suture resulting from access pouch resection is oversewn with a PDS 4-0 running suture. In this way, all the mechanical sutures of the gastric conduit and the anastomosis are reinforced

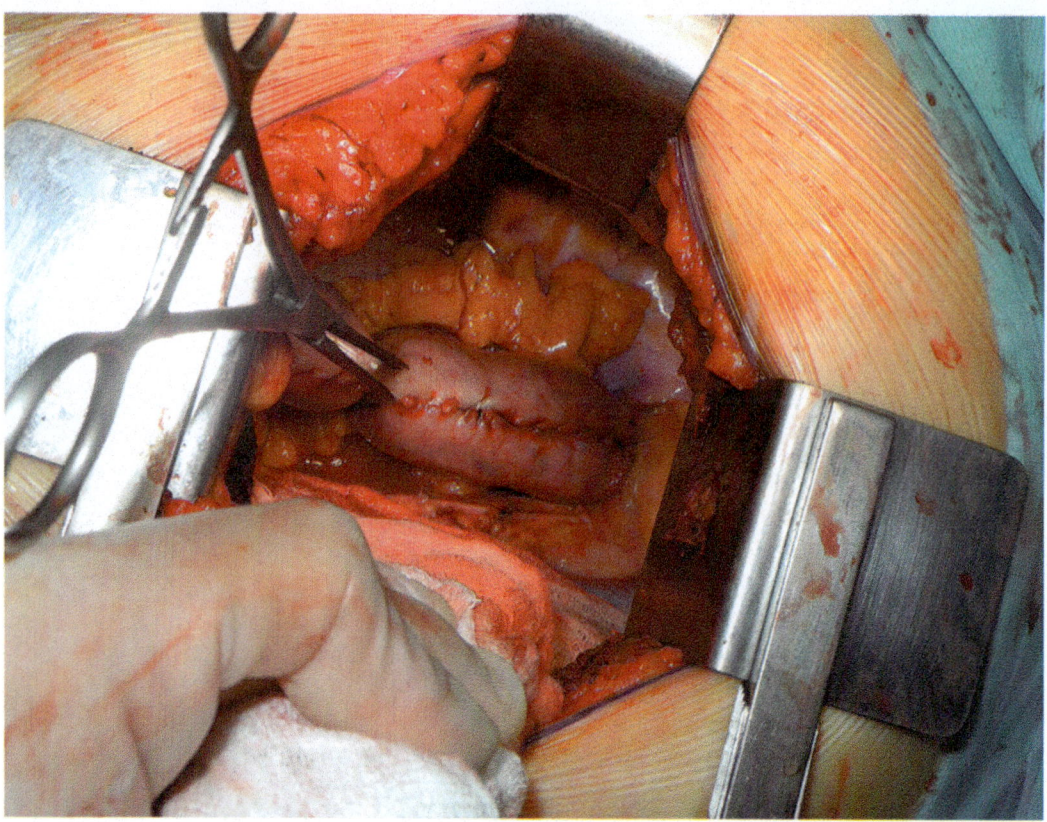

**Fig. 6.64** A non-crushing intestinal clamp is placed on the gastric conduit 10 cm downstream of the anastomosis; the nasogastric tube is then gently advanced ca. 5 cm past the anastomosis and injected with 40–60 ml of saline added with methylene blue for anastomotic and gastric tube suture leak testing. The nasogastric tube is advanced further into the gastric conduit

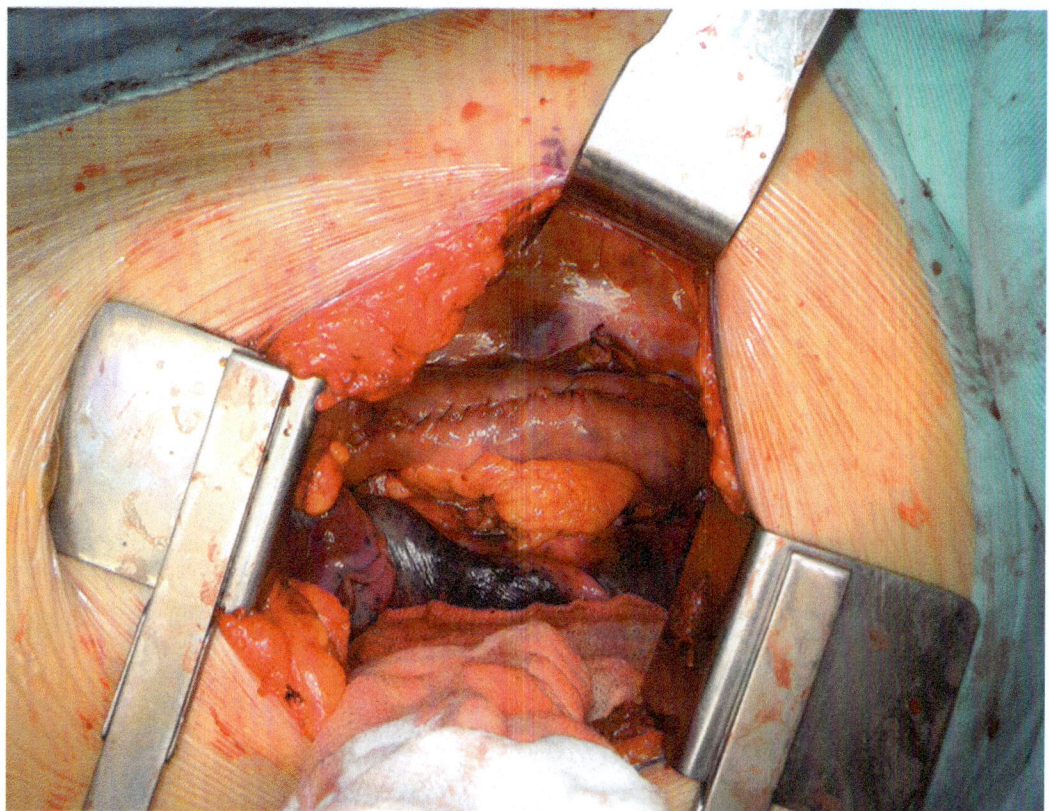

**Fig. 6.65** The gastric tube is repositioned in the posterior mediastinal space and a thoracic tube is placed near the conduit and the anastomosis

# Total and Subtotal D2 Laparoscopic Gastrectomy

**7**

Giorgio Cutini, Francesco Falsetti,
Valerio Caracino, and Pietro Coletta

## 7.1    Introduction

Current gastric cancer treatment is based on gastric resection and regional lymph node dissection.

Even though there is a considerable controversy regarding the appropriate extent of lymph node dissection, in Japan and Europe extended lymph node dissection (D2) is the standard of care for localized gastric cancer and early gastric cancer with a high risk of node metastasis.

The main advantages of this approach are considered to be prolonged survival and improved staging accuracy.

The history of laparoscopic gastrectomies starts in 1991 with the first distal resection with Billroth I reconstruction reported by Kitano, while Goh in 1992 published the first Billroth II for benign ulcer.

The first laparoscopic Billroth II distal gastrectomy for cancer was performed in 1993 by Azagra who also performed the first laparoscopic total gastrectomy.

Laparoscopic distal gastrectomy with D2 lymph node dissection has been recently introduced as a treatment option for distal gastric cancer. Oncologic outcome measures of laparoscopic partial gastrectomy are comparable to those of the conventional open gastrectomy, and the postoperative course is improved in several retrospective and randomized controlled studies.

However, widespread diffusion of this technique is limited by the complexity of D2 lymphadenectomy.

Proximal gastric cancer is treated by total gastrectomy in association with an extended lymph node dissection of splenic, celiac, and paracardial stations. The role of laparoscopic total gastrectomy is still a matter of debate because of technical difficulties (specific node dissection and esophago-jejunal anastomosis) and little evidence on oncologic outcomes of this procedure.

G. Cutini • P. Coletta
Division of General Surgery, "Villa Igea" Private Hospital, Via Maggini, Ancona 60100, Italy
e-mail: giorgiocutini@virgilio.it;
pietro_col@hotmail.com

F. Falsetti (✉)
Division of General Surgery, Jesi Hospital,
Jesi, Italy
e-mail: francesco.falsetti@libero.it

V. Caracino
Division of General Surgery, Pescara Hospital,
Via Fonte Romana, Pescara 65124, Italy
e-mail: valerio.caracino@gmail.com

W. Siquini (ed.), *Total, Subtotal and Proximal Gastrectomy in Cancer: A Color Atlas*,
DOI 10.1007/978-88-470-5749-4_7, © Springer-Verlag Italia 2015

## 7.2    Position of the Patient

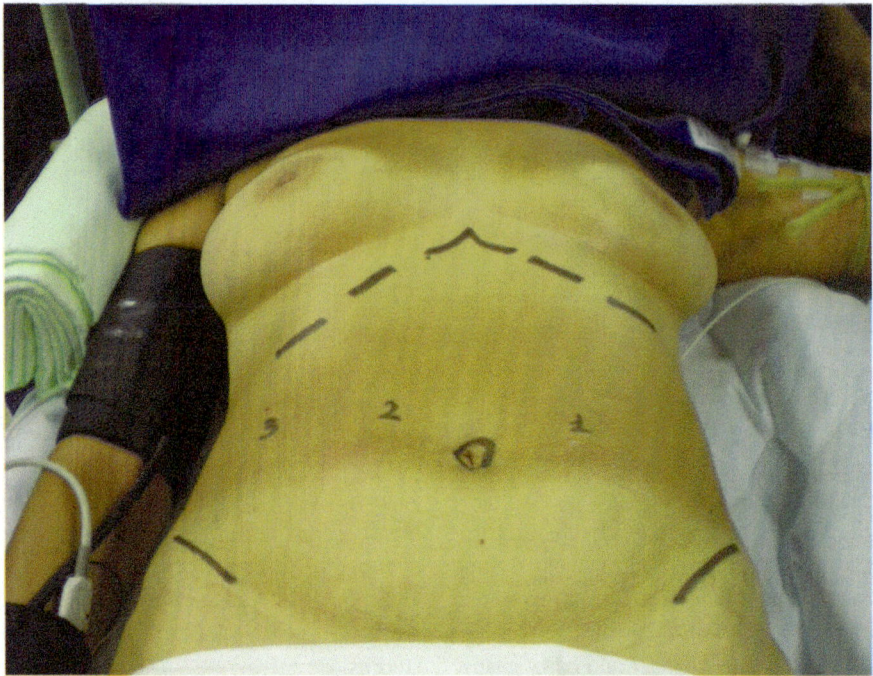

**Fig. 7.1** The patient lies in an articulated table and in the Lloyd-Davies position with the left arm abducted and 20° head-up tilt (reverse Trendelenburg position).

A vesical catheter and a nasogastric tube are applied after induction of anesthesia.

The surgeon works between the legs of the patient with the first assistant (camera assistant) on the right side of the patient. A further assistant is sometimes necessary and stands on the right side too. The scrub nurse and the instrument table are on the left side.

An electrocautery and a bipolar vessel sealing system are placed near the instrument table and main monitor with the laparoscopic instrumentation rack located above the patient's right shoulder. 0,1,2,3 are future trocar positions

**Fig. 7.2** The operative
field is disinfected with
povidone-iodine solution
and protected with
iodine-impregnated drapes.
0,1,2,3 are future trocar
positions

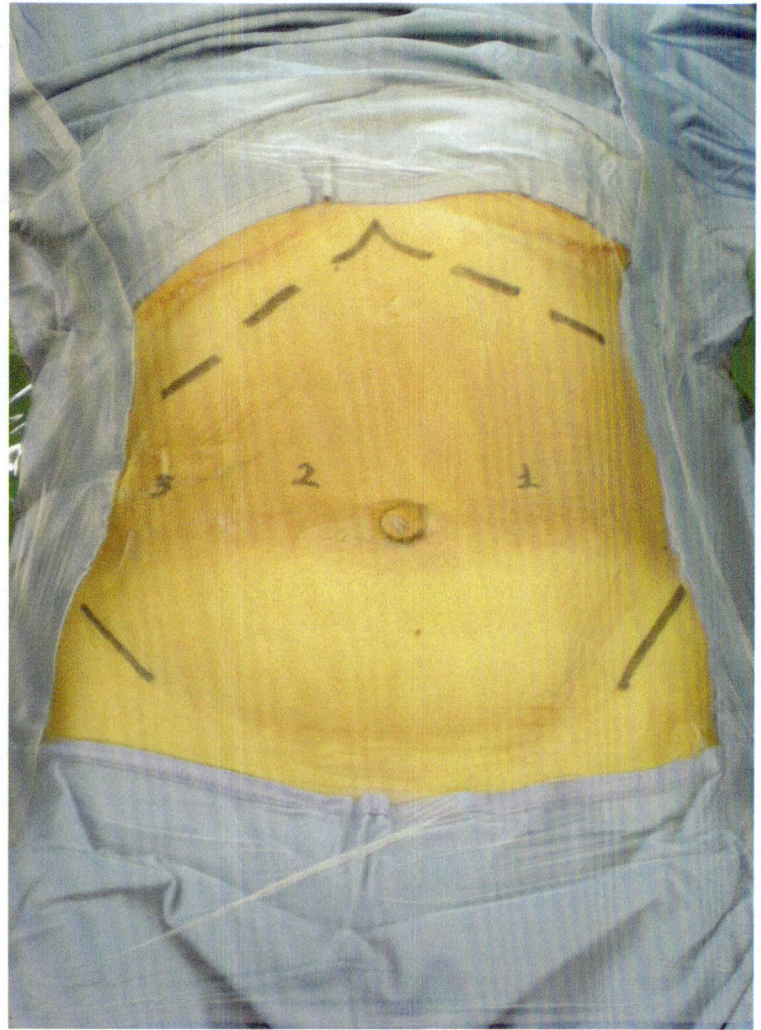

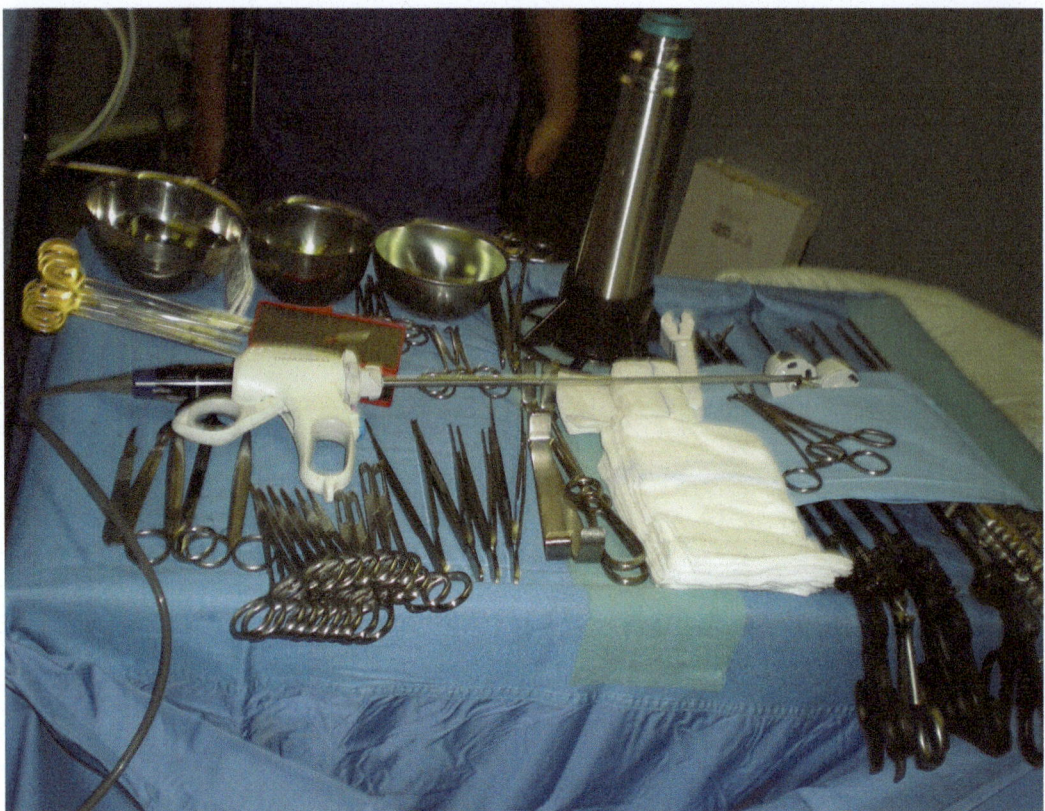

**Fig. 7.3** The surgical procedure is carried up using a harmonic scalpel (Ultracision harmonic scalpel, Ethicon Endo-surgery Inc., Cincinnati, OH) for dissection and vessel sealing. Hemostasis is obtained with the utilization of bipolar forceps and application of titanium clips.

Anastomoses and duodenal and esophageal transection are achieved by the application of a 45 mm cartridge laparoscopic linear stapler (triple-staggered rows of staples). Fenestrated bowel graspers (Johann and Croce-Olmi type) are used for manipulation and traction maneuvers. Curved and angled dissectors are useful for fine dissection, as curved scissors and fixed-tip electrode (J-hook type).

A five-finger fan retractor allows a good exposure of the hepatic hilum and of the esophagogastric junction.

A laparoscopic needle holder is utilized to perform intracorporeal sutures.

A laparoscopic irrigation-suction system and an endo-bag are used for maintaining clean the operative field and for taking out the specimen.

The video camera is connected to a 30° laparoscope and to a wide-screen high-definition monitor

**Fig. 7.4** Four trocars are used. One 12 mm trocar for laparoscope is inserted through the umbilicus (T0). Two 12 mm trocars are placed 2 cm above the umbilicus level in the left (T1) and right (T2) midclavicular line. The fourth 5 or 12 mm trocar (T3) is inserted two centimeters below the right costal margin in the hypochondrium

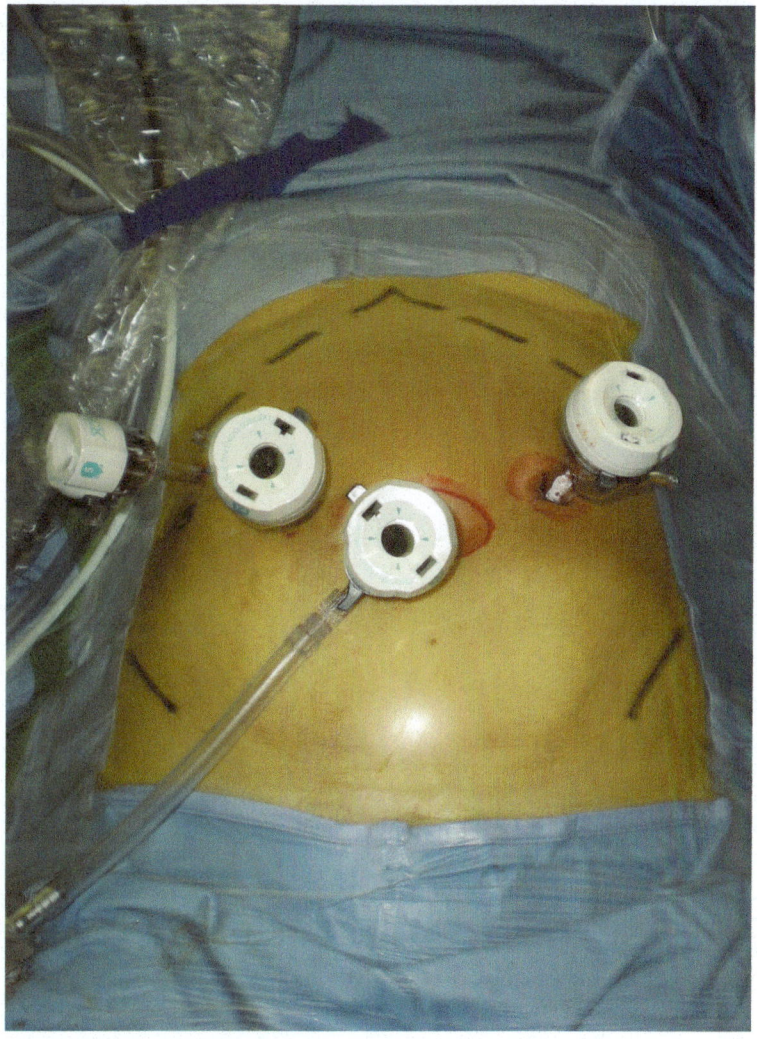

## 7.3 Laparoscopic Total Gastrectomy

### 7.3.1 Preliminary Maneuvers

The liver, diaphragm, serosal surfaces, omentum, bowel, mesentery, and pelvic organs are carefully inspected. Biopsy of suspicious lesions is done and documented pathologically by frozen section. Peritoneal lavage also is obtained and submitted for intraoperative cytology.

At this stage, intraoperative laparoscopic ultrasonography is carried up to scan the liver surface and assess the presence of deep liver metastases.

The identification of hepatic and peritoneal involvement could change the operating strategy.

## 7.3.2   Coloepiploic Detachment and Station 4sb Lymphadenectomy

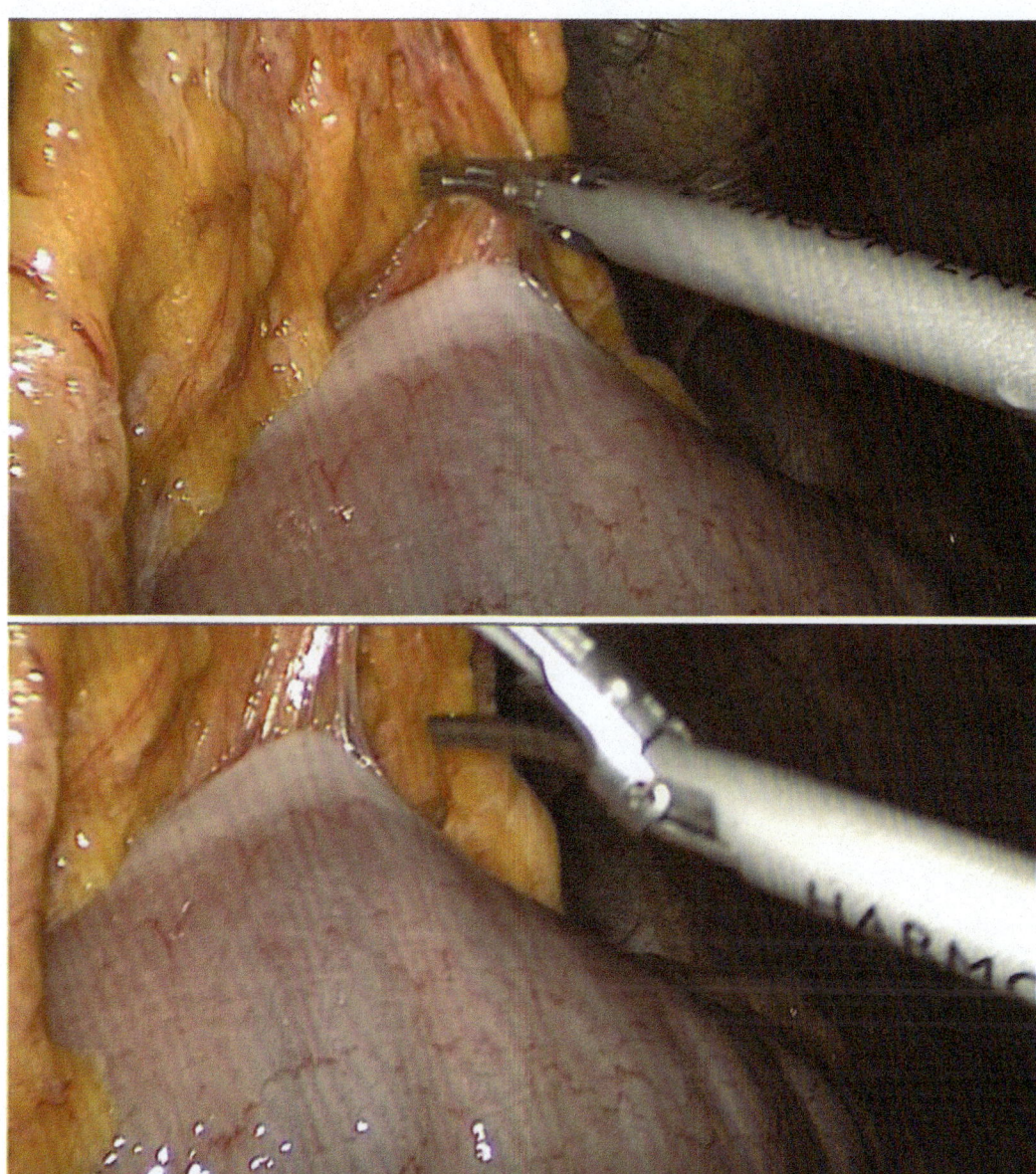

**Figs. 7.5 and 7.6** After exploration of the peritoneal cavity, the greater curvature is mobilized by dissection of the entire greater omentum from the transverse colon. Dissection is extended toward the lower pole of the spleen to ligate left gastroepiploic vessels and short gastric vessels and continued toward the right side to dissect the right gastroepiploic vessels at their roots

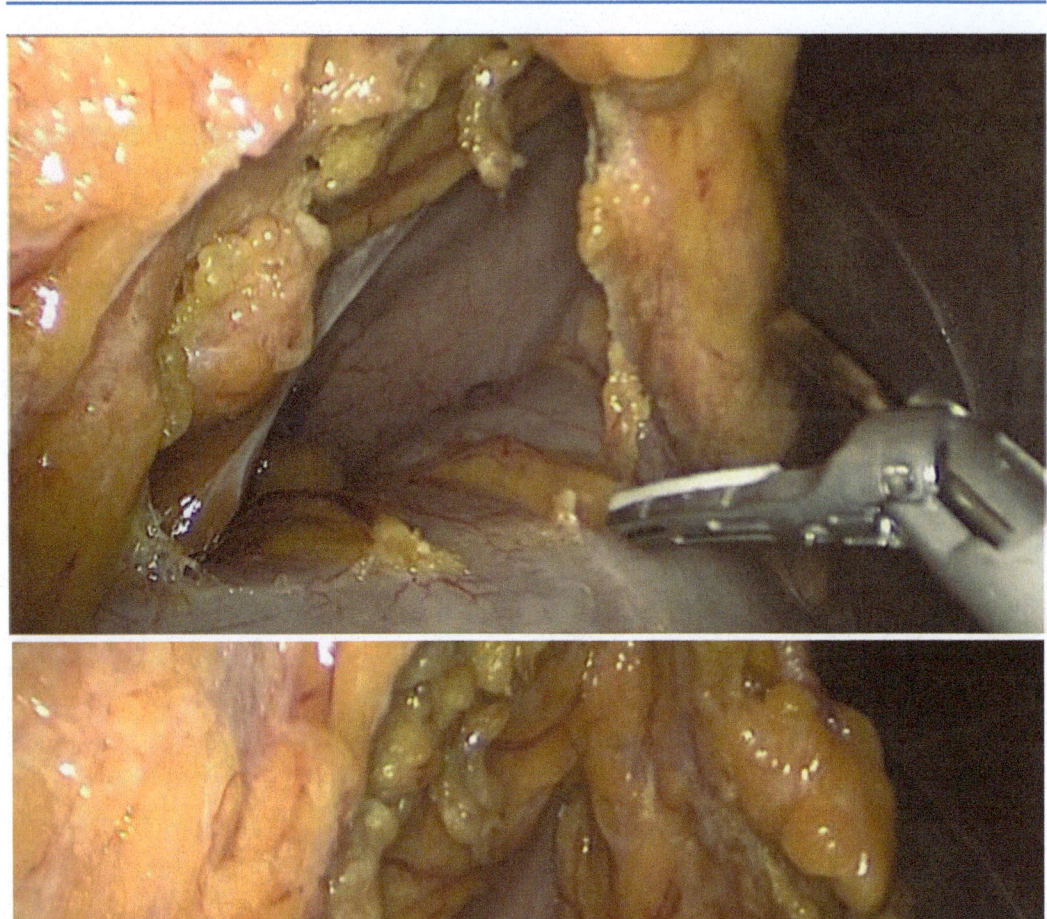

**Figs. 7.7 and 7.8** The assistant inserts through T3 a fenestrated bowel grasper (Johann) in order to lift up the greater omentum and to expose the avascular plane for coloepiploic detachment. The surgeon, using harmonic scalpel and a bowel grasper via T1 and T2, begins the dissection at the middle third of the transverse colon and moves toward the origin of the left gastroepiploic vessels from the splenic artery and vein separating the gastrosplenic ligament and removing the lymph nodes of 4sb station

### 7.3.3 Station 4sa Lymphadenectomy

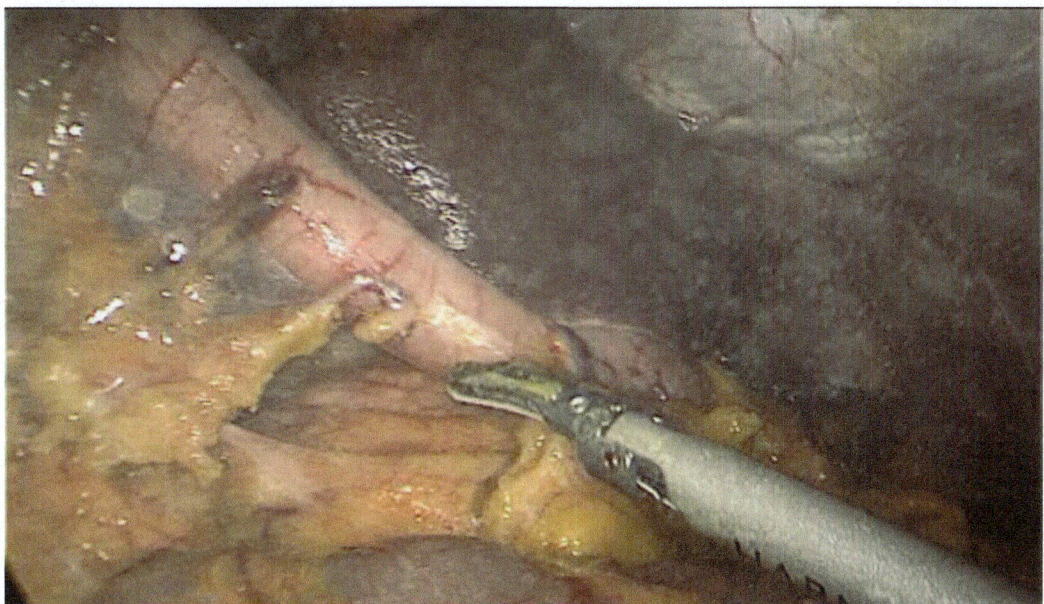

**Fig. 7.9** Left gastroepiploic vessels are divided by a harmonic scalpel or sectioned between titanium clips. For a better exposure of the region, it is useful to dissect the adhesions between the posterior gastric wall and the anterior pancreatic surface opening the lesser peritoneal sac. The identification of the left gastroepiploic vessel roots is facilitated by a gentle mobilization of the pancreatic tail in order to expose the splenic vessels.

Using the same technique the surgeon proceeds cephalad to dissect short gastric vessels. The assistant, by a gentle traction, pulls the gastric fundus down while the surgeon, giving delicate traction on the anterior surface of the spleen, separates by harmonic scalpel the gastrosplenic ligament and the short gastric vessels as near as possible to the spleen to achieve a correct lymphadenectomy of group 4sa nodes

### 7.3.4 Station 2 Lymphadenectomy

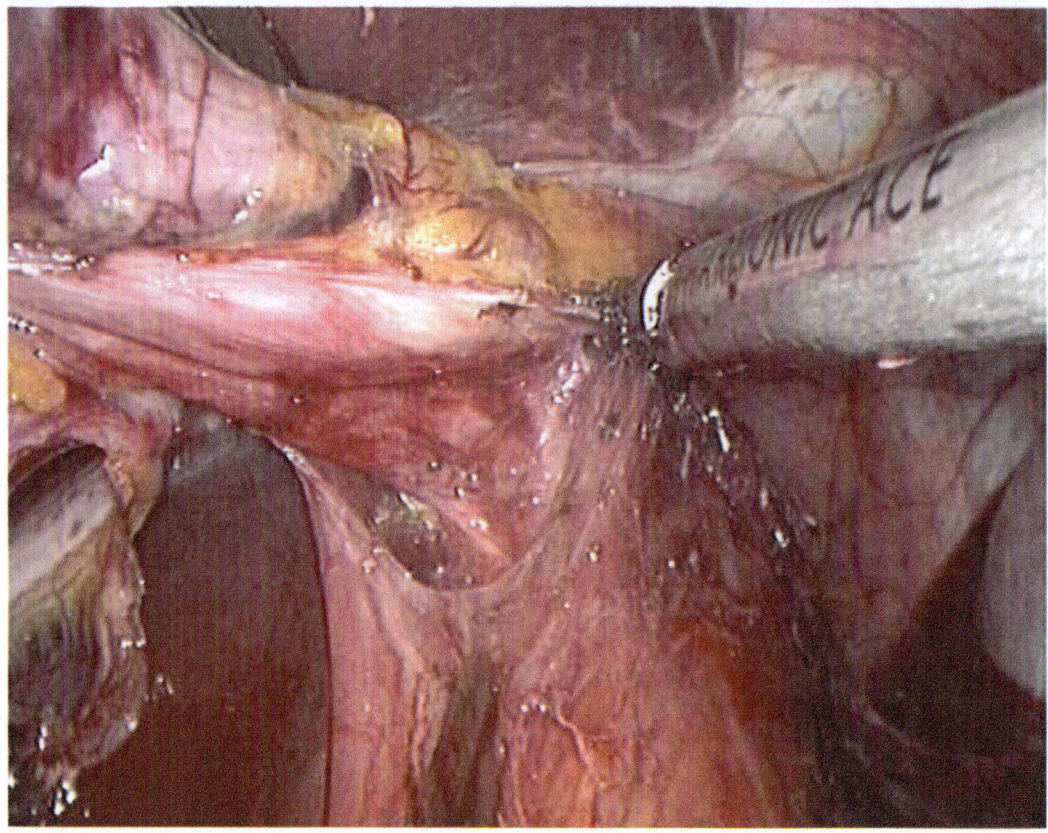

**Fig. 7.10** Now the gastric fundus is free, and the left diaphragmatic crus is exposed. Pulling down the stomach and dissecting the peritoneum over the left diaphragmatic crus, the left paracardial nodes are removed (station n° 2)

## 7.3.5   Station 11p and 7 Lymphadenectomy

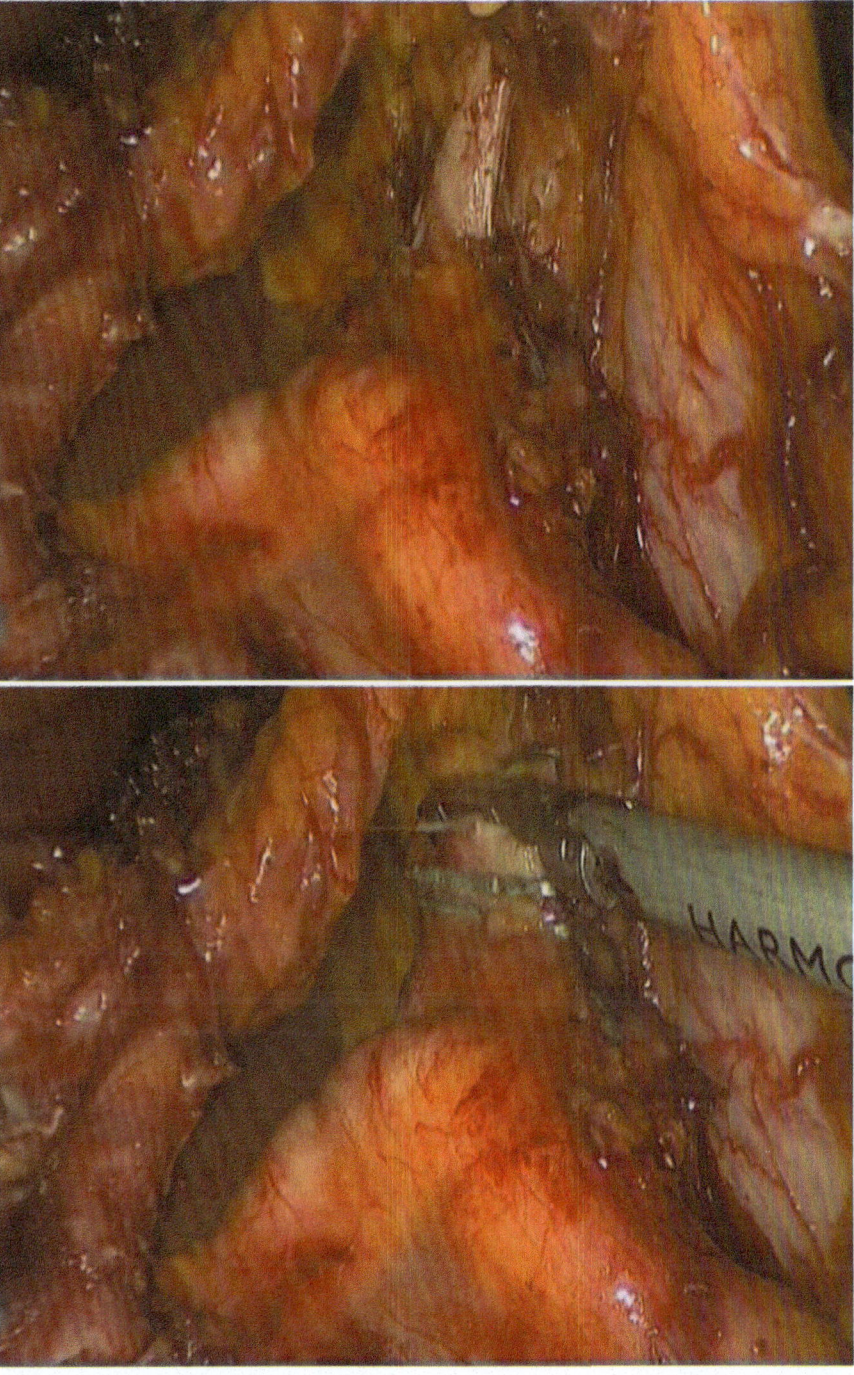

**Figs. 7.11, 7.12, 7.13, 7.14, 7.15, and 7.16** The lymphadenectomy of the 11p station is performed using blunt dissection, and controlling bleeding with bipolar forceps, the splenic artery is dissected by the surgeon while the assistant pulls cephalad the stomach. If present, the posterior gastric artery is clipped and sectioned at the origin from the splenic artery. The dissection moves toward the left gastric vessels. The assistant exposes the posterior gastric wall by a gentle cephalad traction on the stomach with the greater omentum folded up on the anterior aspect of the viscus. This maneuver allows to put the left gastric vessels under tension and enables the surgeon to remove the nodes of station n° 7. The left gastric vessels are isolated using a harmonic scalpel and angled dissector and then clipped and sectioned at their roots. The lymph nodes of the celiac artery are dissected at this time

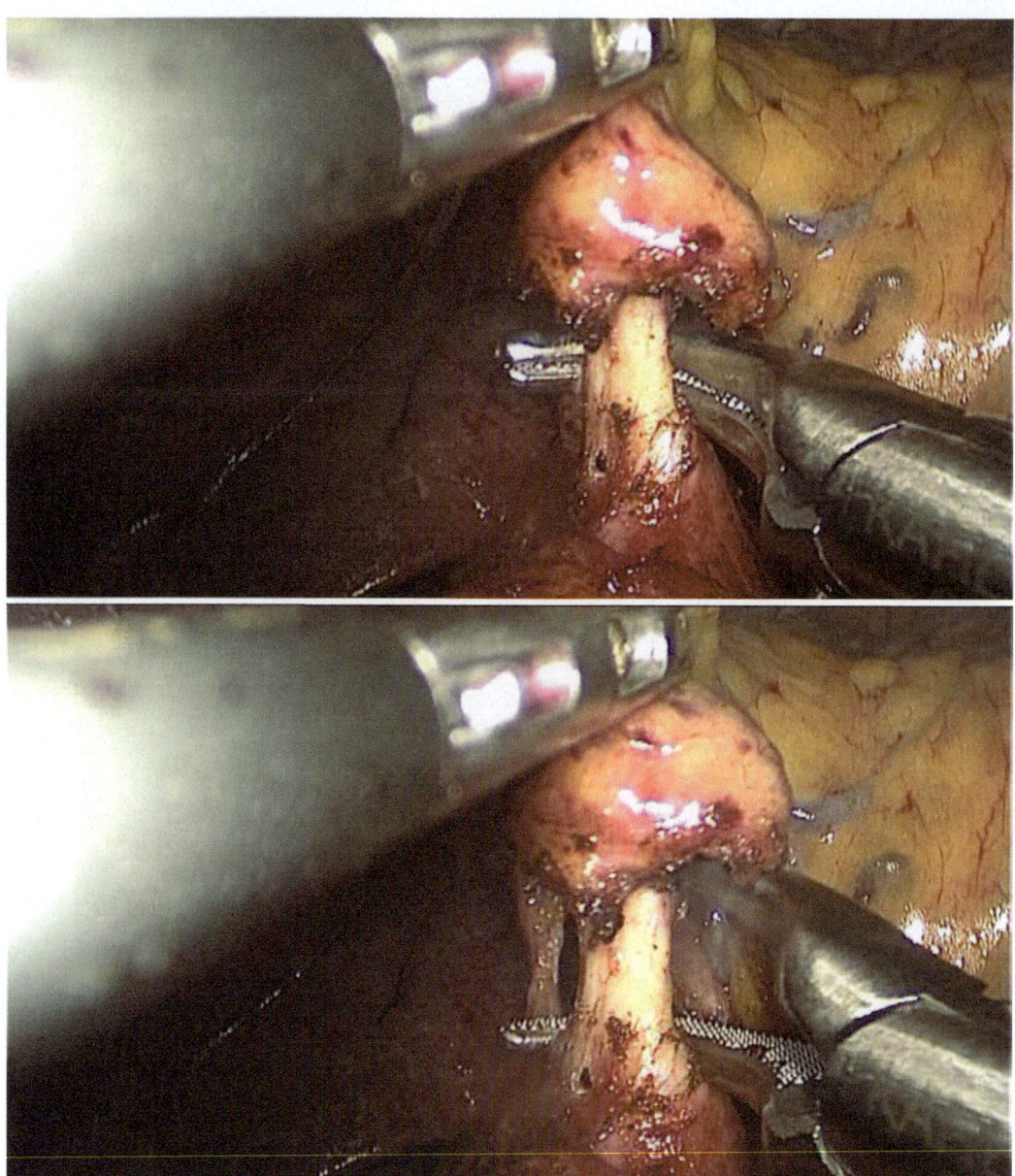

**Figs. 7.11, 7.12, 7.13, 7.14, 7.15, and 7.16** (continued)

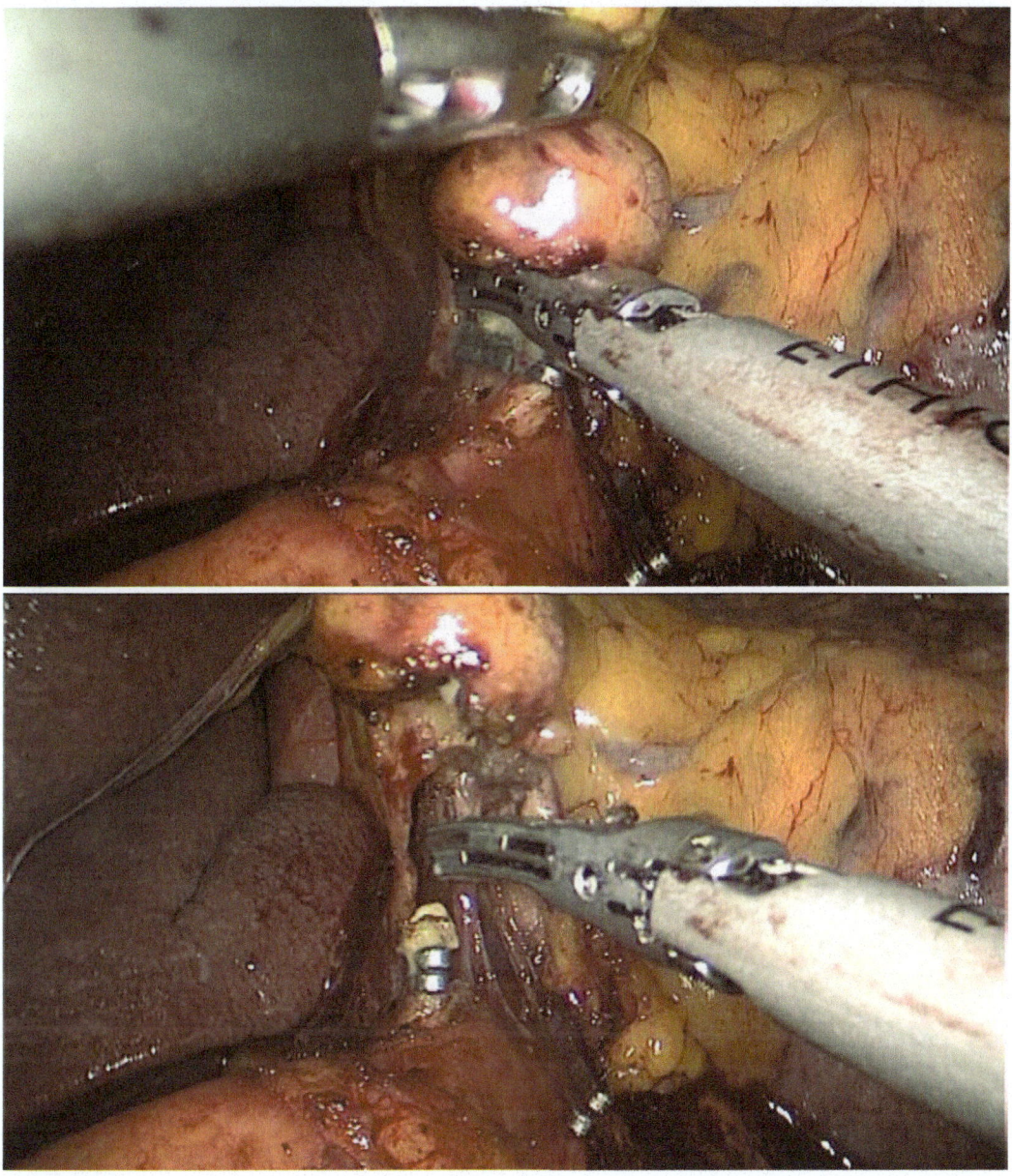

**Figs. 7.11, 7.12, 7.13, 7.14, 7.15, and 7.16**  (continued)

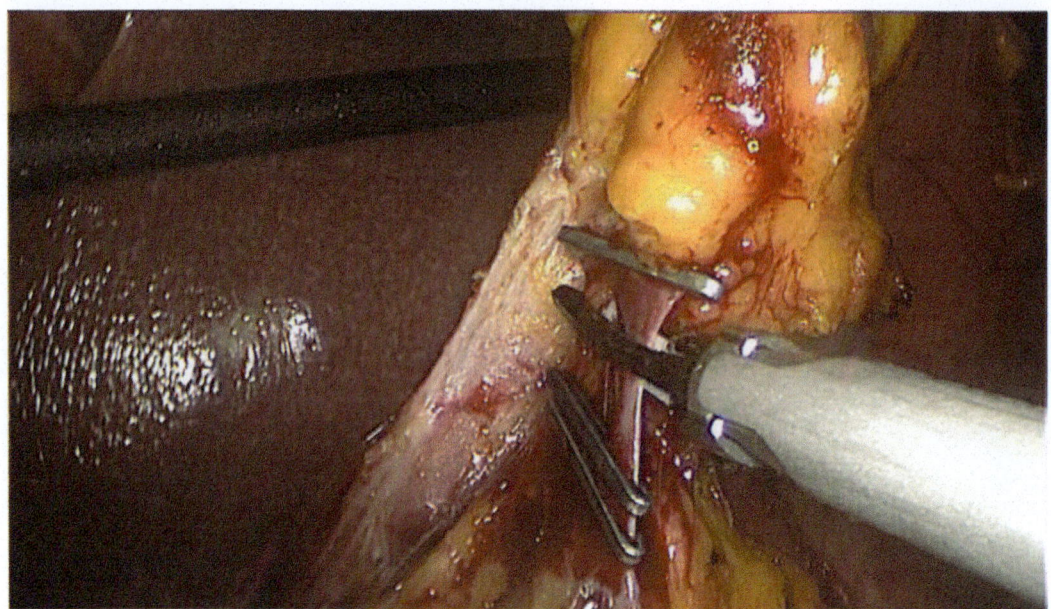

**Fig. 7.17** In the same manner the surgeon completes coloepiploic detachment moving the dissection toward the pylorus and achieving the lymphadenectomy of station 4a. During this maneuver the assistant's grasper pulls up the great curvature of the antropyloric region while the surgeon, dissecting Fredet's area, exposes the superior mesenteric vein. The dissection proceeds in order to identify the right colic vein, the gastroepiploic vein, and Henle's trunk. In this manner the nodes of 14v station are removed, and the right gastroepiploic vein is clipped and sectioned

### 7.3.6   Station 6 Lymphadenectomy

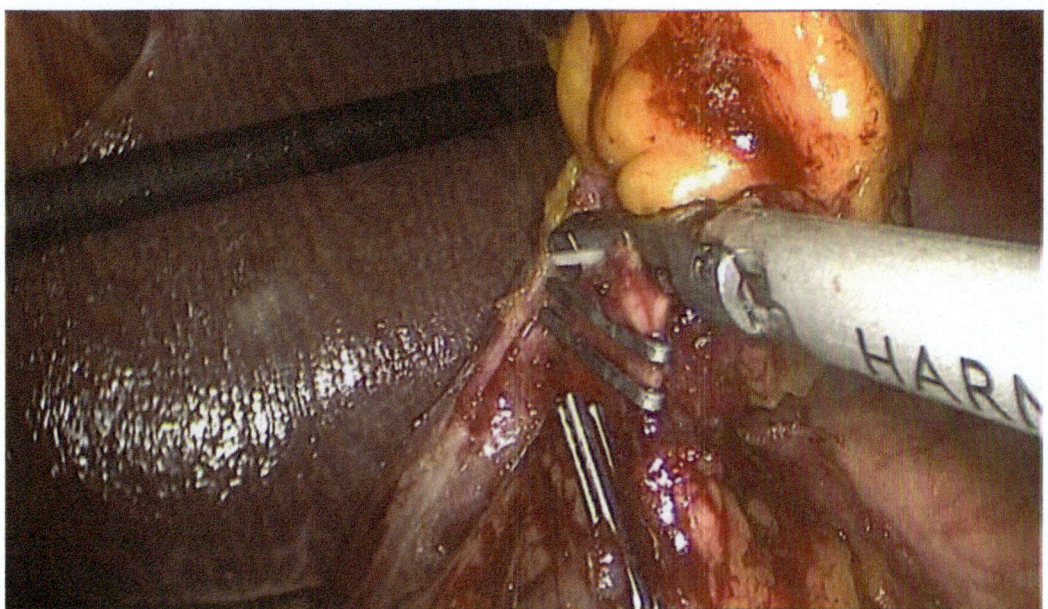

**Fig. 7.18** Using a bipolar forceps and harmonic scalpel, the surgeon removes the infra-pyloric nodes (station n° 6) and, through Fredet's area, exposes the right gastroepiploic artery at her origin from the gastroduodenal artery, just close to the pylorus, along the superior edge of the head of the pancreas. The artery is transected using titanium clips, and the duodenal wall is exposed. Oozing is controlled by bipolar coagulation. The use of a little gauze is useful for maintaining clear the operating field

## 7.3.7 Duodenal Dissection

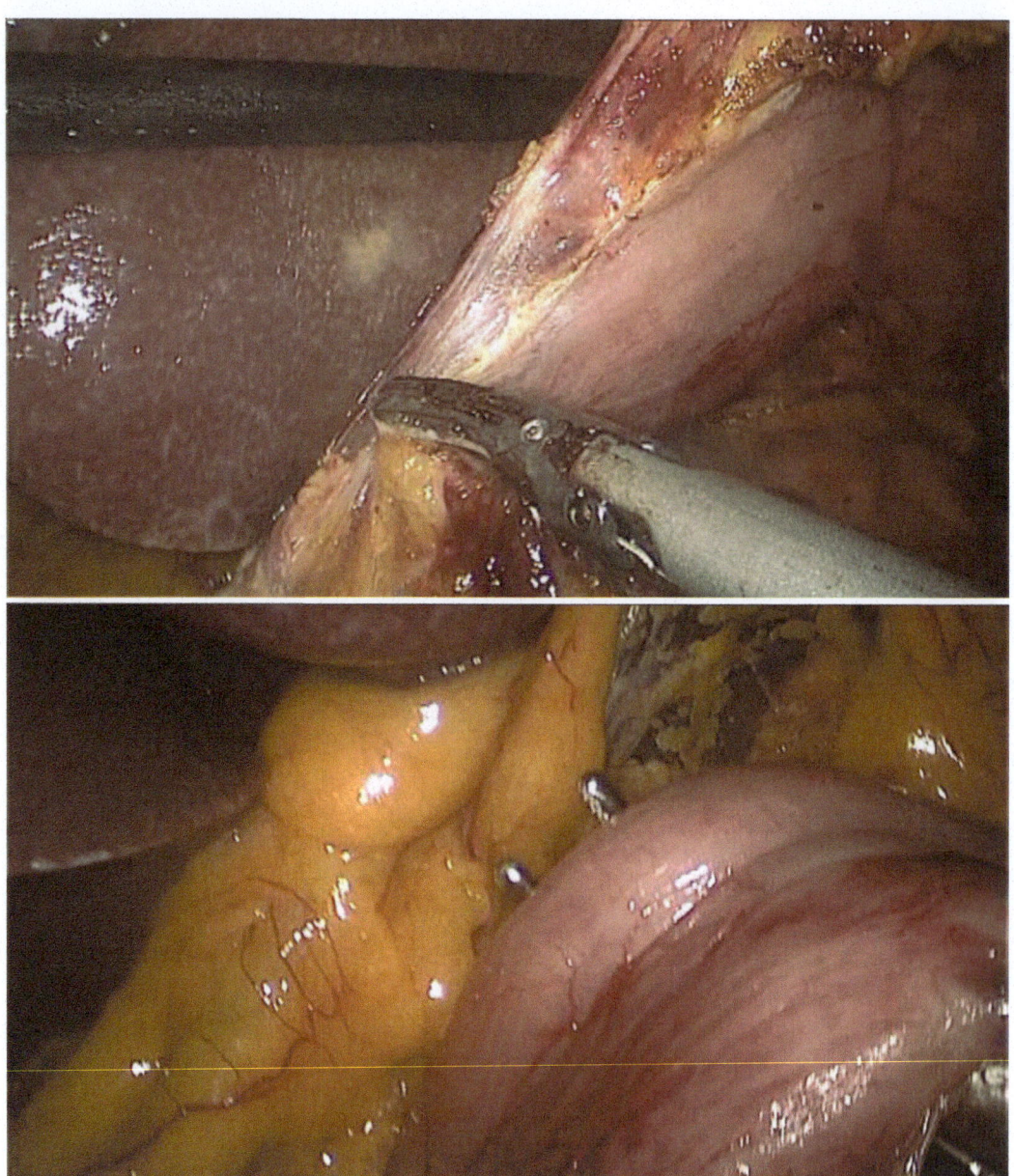

**Figs. 7.19 and 7.20** A gentle traction lifting up the pylorus allows a good exposure of the posterior wall of the first portion of the duodenum. Dissection of the adhe- sions between the duodenum and head of the pancreas and division of the peritoneum over the superior edge of the viscus free completely the first portion of the duodenum

## 7.3.8   Duodenal Transection

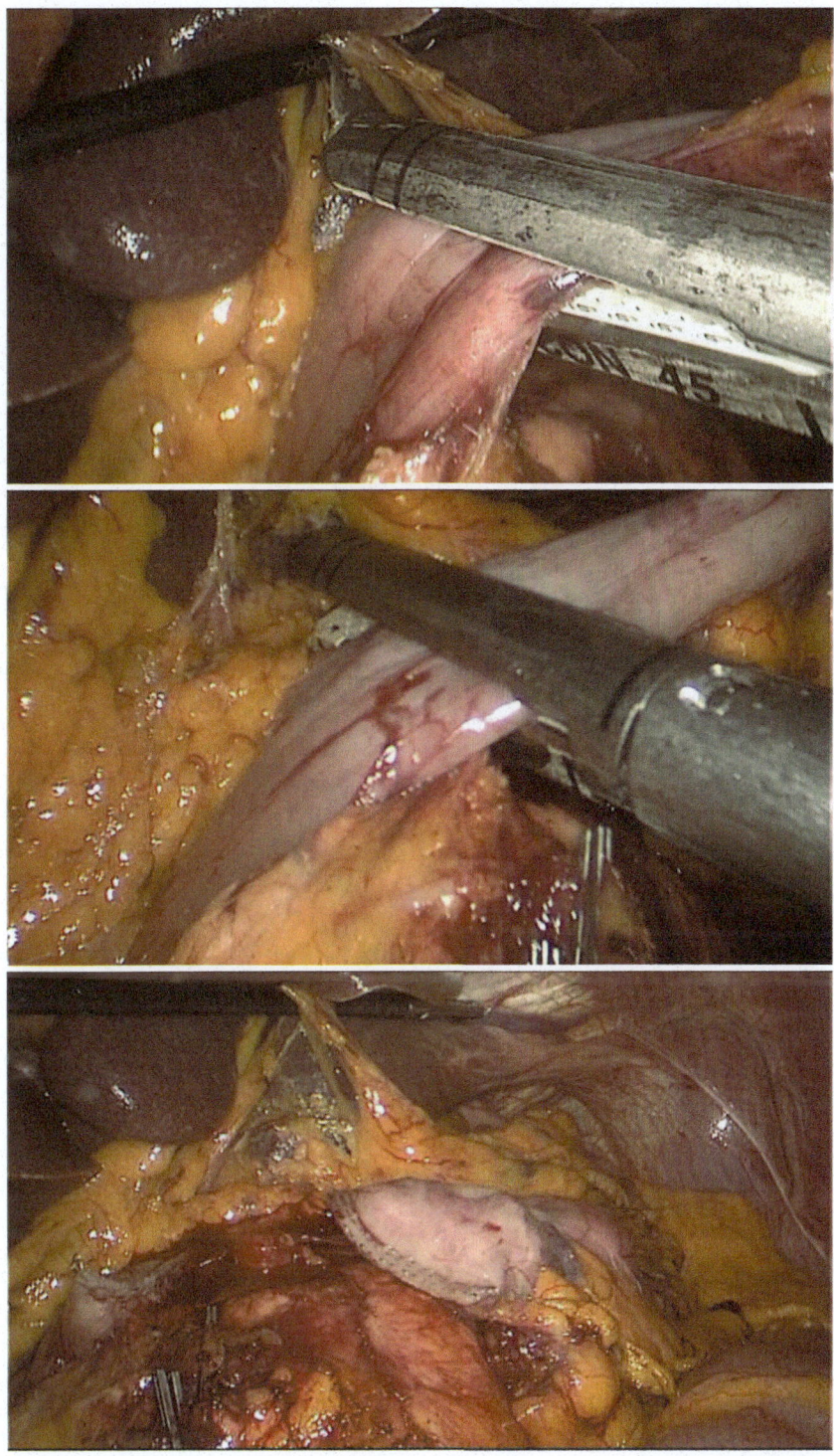

**Figs. 7.21, 7.22, and 7.23** Now is created a window through which is possible to introduce the endoscopic linear stapler (white reloads). The duodenum is tran-sected 2 cm below the pylorus. Straight after duodenal transection the retropancreatic nodes can be removed (station n° 13)

## 7.3.9 Hepatic Hilum Dissection

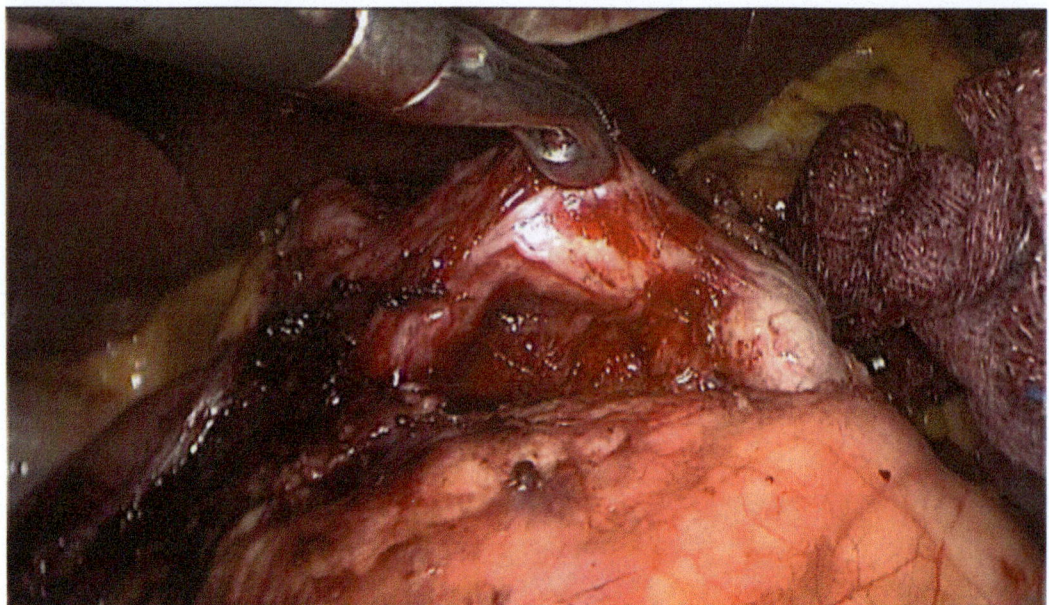

**Fig. 7.24** The introduction via T3 of the hepatic retractor (five-finger fan retractor) allows an excellent exposition of the hepatic hilum. Opening the peritoneum of the lesser omentum with a harmonic scalpel is possible to identify the common hepatic artery and the origin of the right gastric artery. Sectioning of the right gastric artery is done by the application of titanium clips; the removal of the fatty tissue around this vessel allows a correct lymphadenectomy of station n° 5.

Lymphadenectomy continues along the common hepatic artery toward the celiac artery, removing station n° 8 nodes

**Figs. 7.25, 7.26, and 7.27** Dissection of the fatty tissue moves toward the vascular structures of the hepatic hilum to remove the nodes lying on the anterior surface of the right and left hepatic artery clearing the 12a station. Attention must be put in anatomical variations that can be as frequent as 40 % of the cases, in particular when a big posterior gastric artery is found. To accomplish the dis-section, the elements of the hepatic pedicle (left, right, and common hepatic vessels) are carefully isolated and encircled with vascular tapes (in the case presented the left gastric artery comes from the left hepatic artery).

Gentle tractions on these loops facilitate node removal avoiding vascular injuries. Residual oozing after lymph node dissection is best controlled by bipolar coagulation

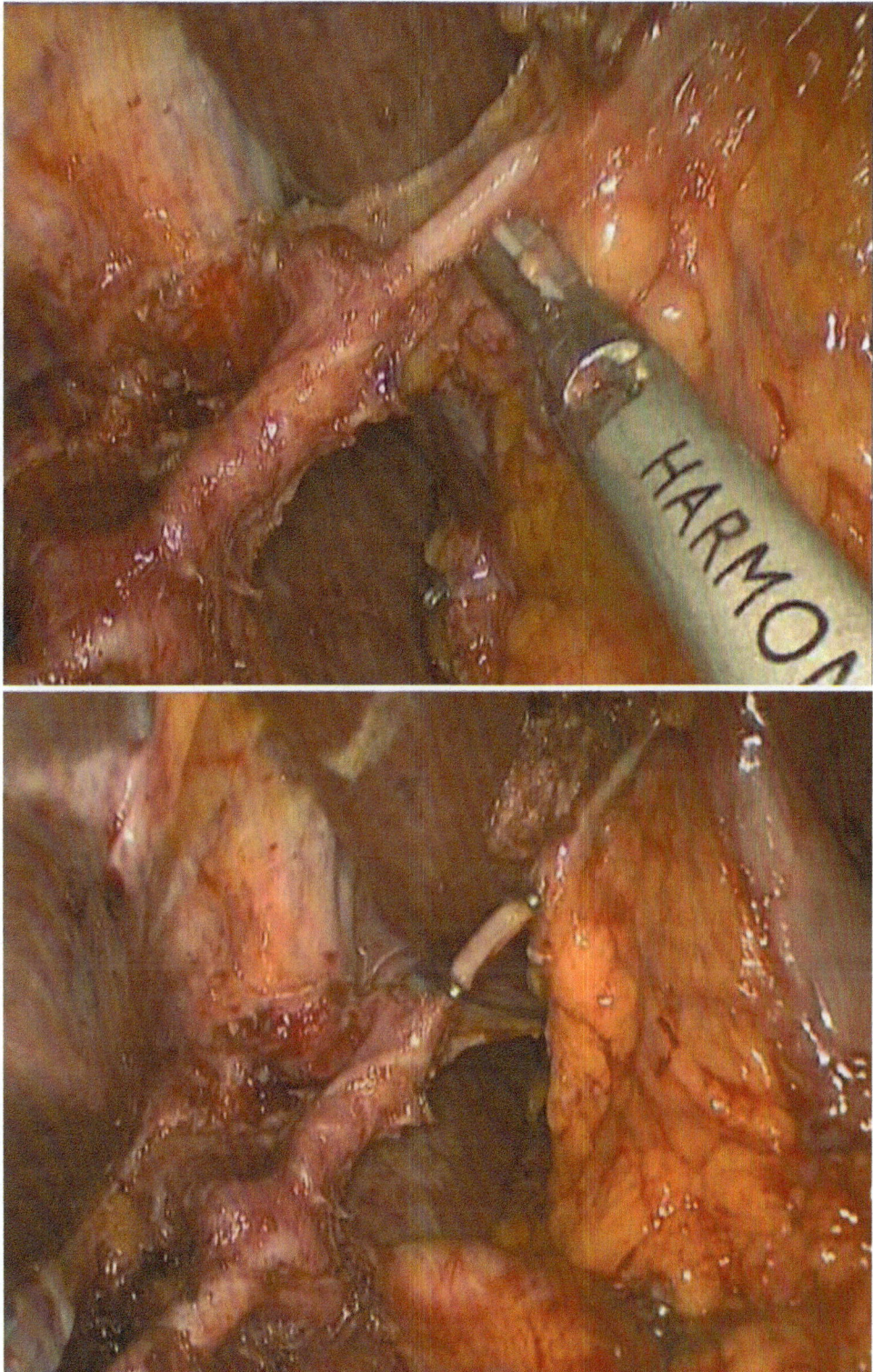

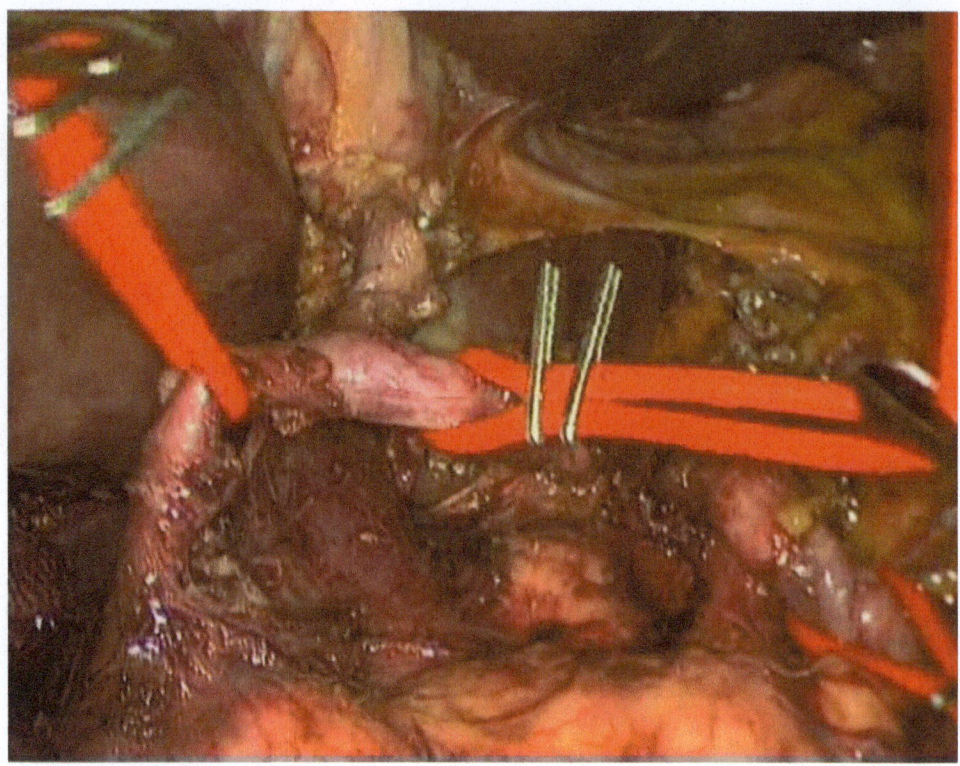

**Figs. 7.25, 7.26, and 7.27** (continued)

### 7.3.10 Station 1 and 3 Lymphadenectomy

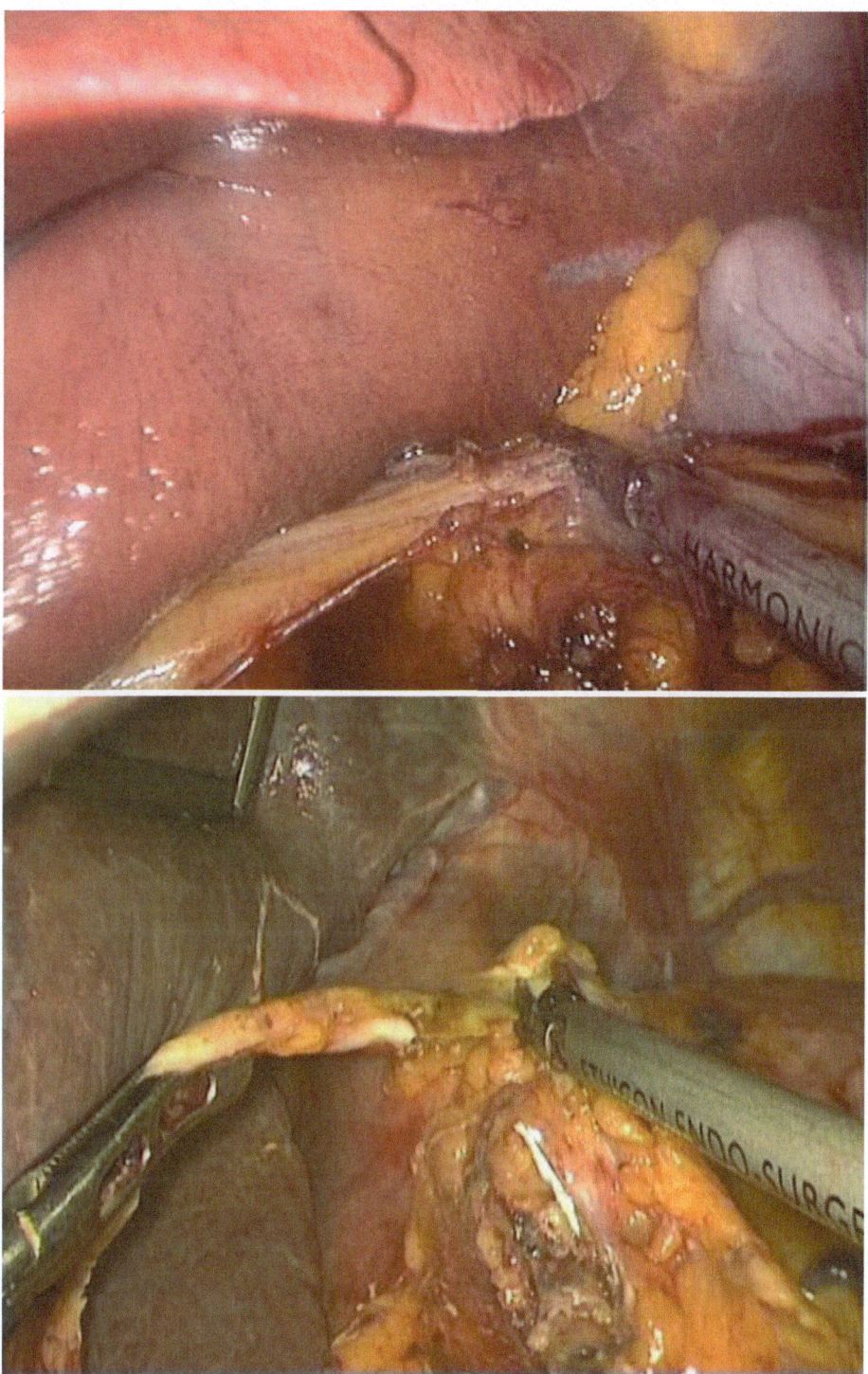

**Figs. 7.28 and 7.29** The surgeon then continues the dissection of the hepatoduodenal ligament toward the esophagogastric junction in order to remove the right paracardial lymph nodes (station n° 1). The dissection of the lesser omentum near the liver using a harmonic scalpel allows a good exposure of the right diaphragmatic crus and facilitates the complete removal of the lymphatic tissue of the paracardial region

## 7.3.11 Dissection of the Hiatus

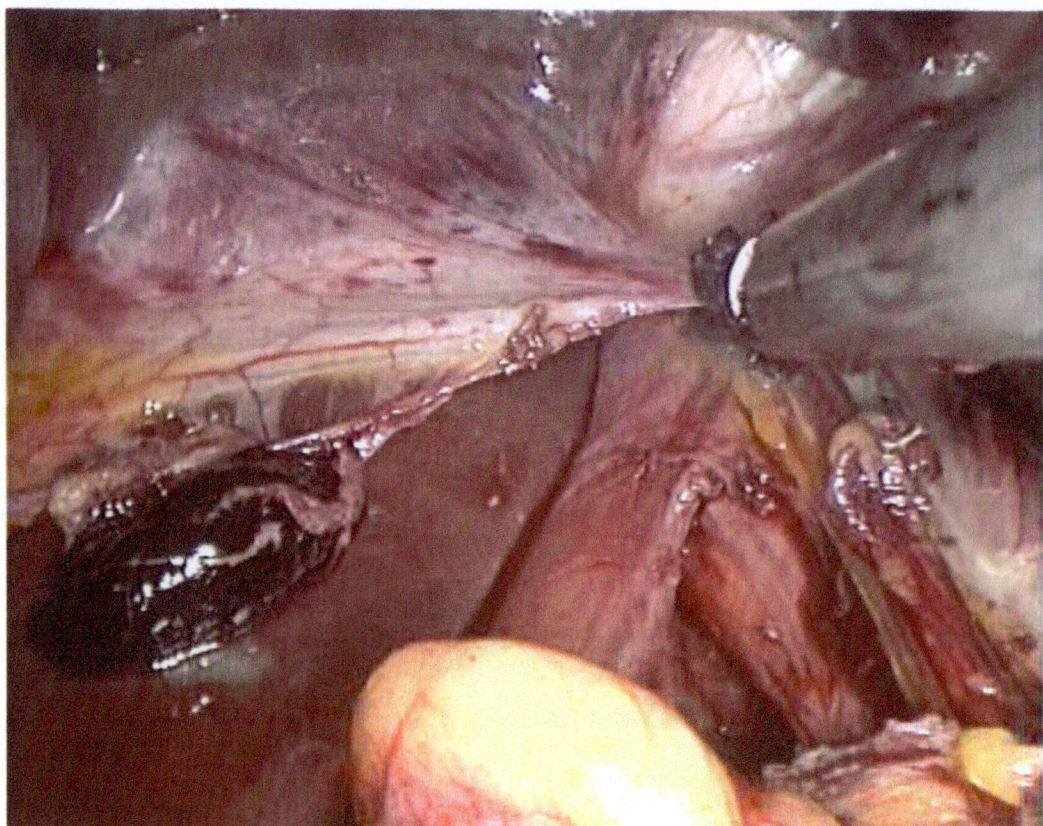

**Fig. 7.30** After the completion of the lymphadenectomy, the fundus and the abdominal esophagus are mobilized by division of the gastrophrenic peritoneal reflection and separation of the gastroesophageal junction from right and left diaphragmatic cruses using a harmonic scalpel and pulling down the stomach. The hiatal canal is entered, and the mediastinal esophagus is dissected and pulled into the peritoneal cavity. The vagal trunks are identified and divided by a harmonic scalpel. The stomach in now completely freed, and the dissection phase is completed

## 7.3.12 Esophago-jejunal Anastomosis

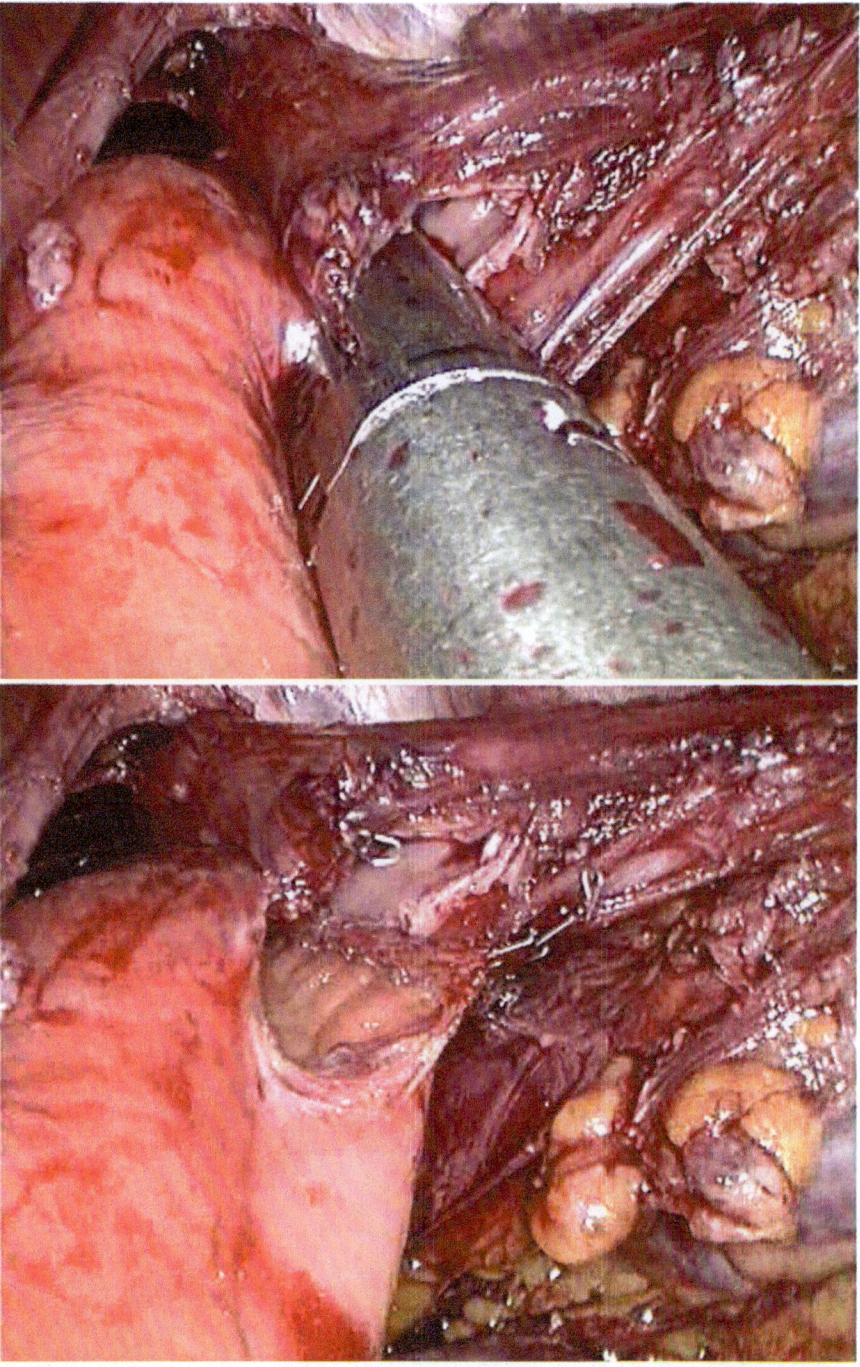

**Fig. 7.31 and 7.32** The second jejunal loop is transected with a linear stapler (45 mm, blue reload) and then transposed through the transverse mesocolon; now the jejunal loop is placed close to the esophagus, just on the right side. No suspension sutures are used between the esophagus and the jejunum, in order to gain freedom of movement. Two small incisions are performed using a harmonic scalpel or a J-hook electrode, one on the antimesenteric side of the jejunum, 5–6 cm from its distal margin, and the other on the posterior wall of the esophagus, 4–5 cm above the esophagogastric junction. The linear stapler (45 mm, blue cartridge) is now introduced through T1 and inserted into the jejunal opening and then into the esophageal hole. Traction and rotation of the stomach are useful maneuvers. A side-to-side esophago-jejunal anastomosis Orringer-like is then fashioned

## 7.3.13  Esophageal Transection

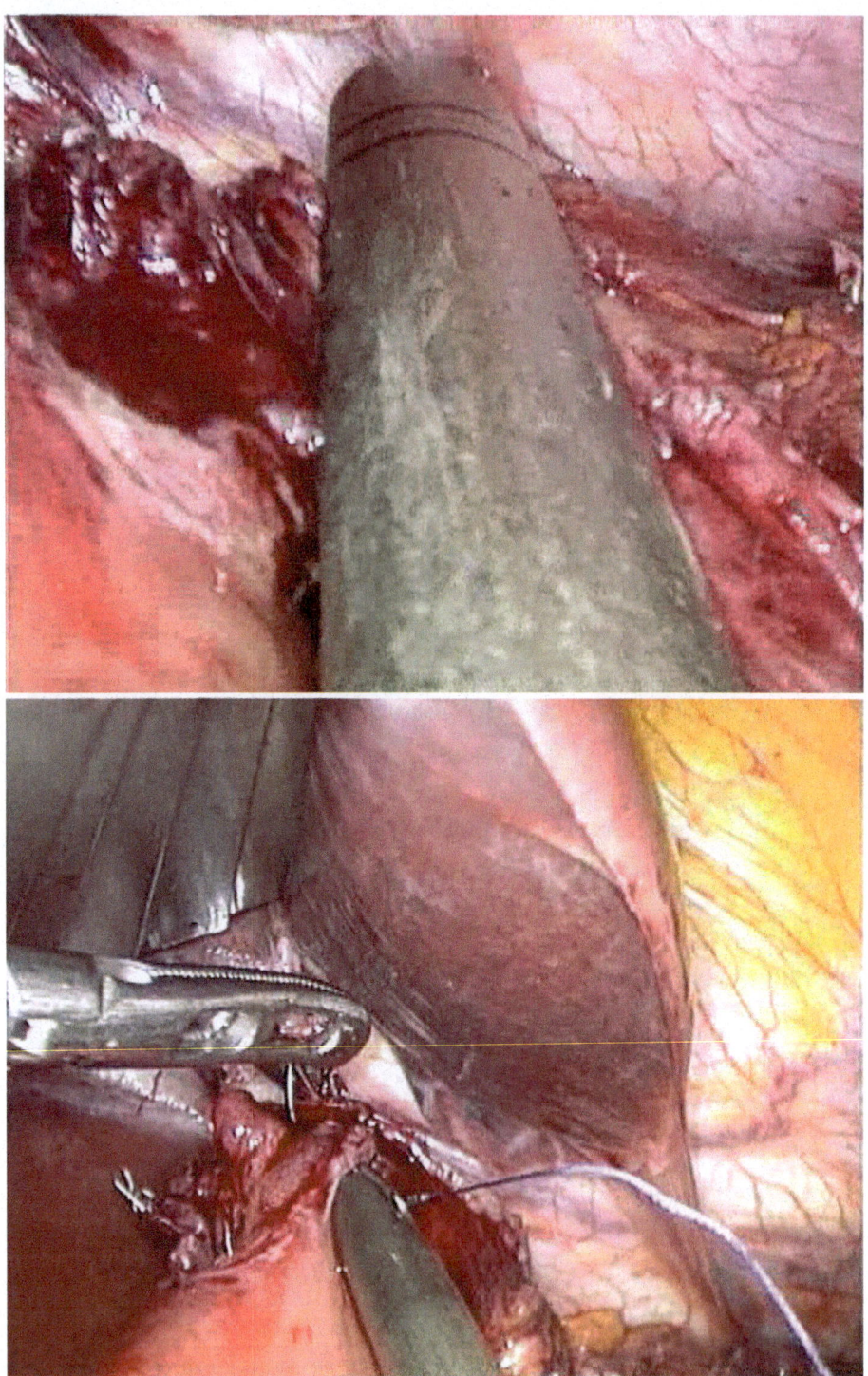

**Figs. 7.33 and 7.34** The esophageal transection is finally done using a linear stapler (45 mm, blue reload), and the residual opening is closed with interrupted stitches of 3-0 reabsorbable suture tied intracorporeally. The resected specimen is placed in a bag and moved toward the right subphrenic space

## 7.3.14 Jejuno-jejunal Anastomosis

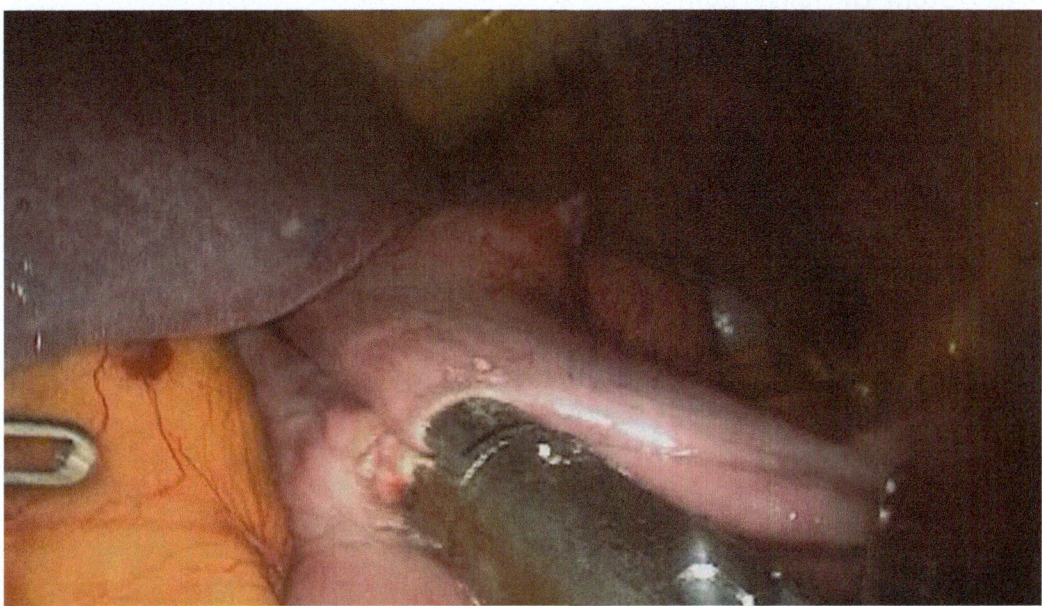

**Fig. 7.35** The side-to-side jejuno-jejunal anastomosis at the foot of the Roux-en-Y loop (about 50–60 cm from the esophago-jejunal anastomosis) is done using an endoscopic linear stapler (45 mm, blue reloads).

For ergonomic reasons, in order to facilitate the completion of the anastomosis, the same is created in the supramesocolic space then transposed through the hole in the transverse mesocolon. The anastomosis is fashioned introducing the stapler through two openings on the antimesenteric jejunal limbs. The access opening is hand sutured with interrupted stitches (3-0 reabsorbable).

A check of esophago-jejunal anastomosis is done by methylene blue test, and two drains are placed, one in Morrison's pouch near the duodenal stump and the other in the left subphrenic space close to the anastomosis.

The operative specimen is removed through a minimal enlargement of the umbilical incision (about 3–4 cm)

## 7.4 Laparoscopic Subtotal Gastrectomy

### 7.4.1 Stomach Transection

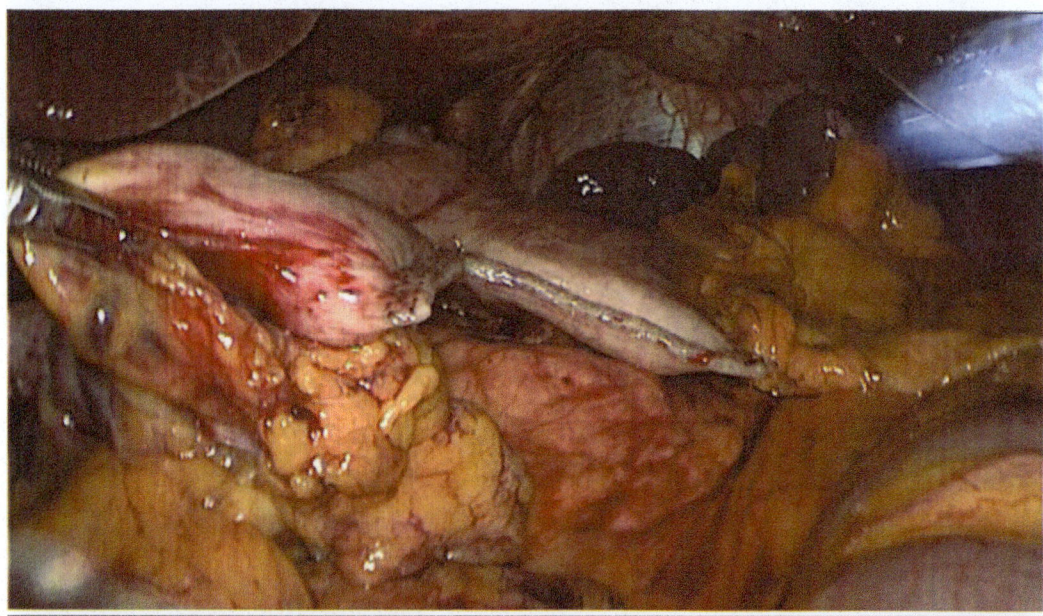

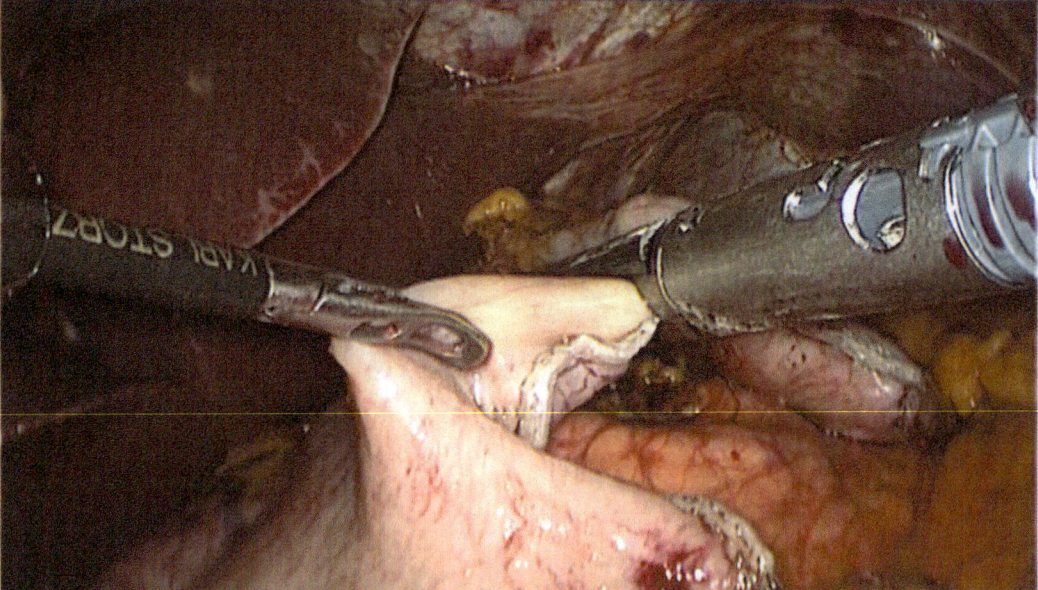

**Figs. 7.36 and 7.37** Coloepiploic detachment moves from the middle third of the transverse colon toward the short gastric vessels with the same technique as for the total gastrectomy; the left gastroepiploic artery is divided between titanium clips; only the first two short gastric vessels are divided. Gastric stump vascularization is best preserved if two or more short gastric vessels and the posterior gastric artery are carefully respected.

After the nodes of the right paracardial station are freed and D2 lymphadenectomy is completed, the stomach is transected with multiple endostapler applications (45 mm, blue cartridge), moving from the greater curve, just below the second short gastric vessel, to the right side, 3–4 cm below the esophagogastric junction

## 7.4.2    Side-to-Side Vertical Gastrojejunal Anastomosis

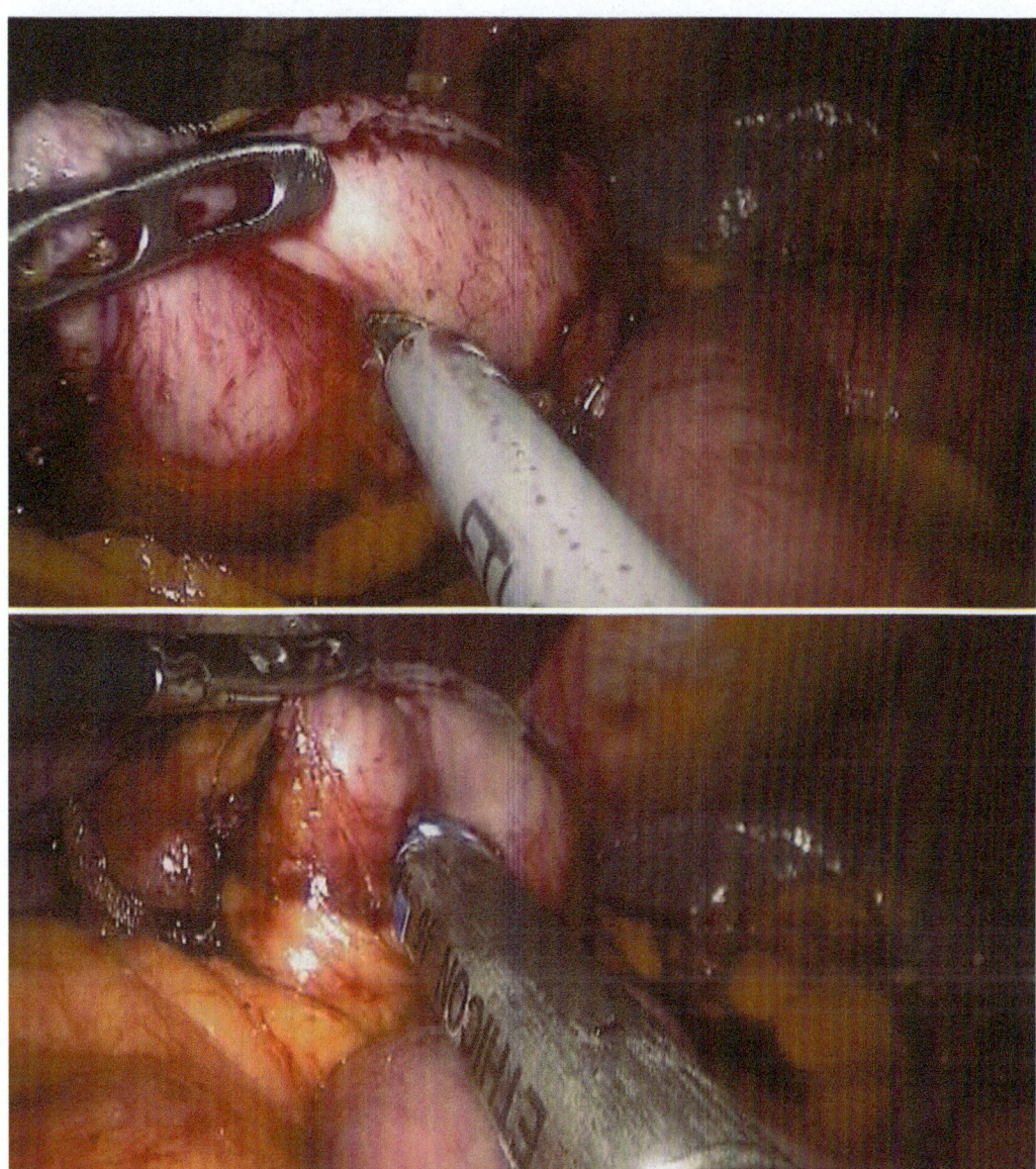

**Figs. 7.38, 7.39, 7.40, and 7.41** The gastric remnant is now free, and the second jejunal loop is transposed in the upper abdomen in order to prepare a Roux-en-Y transmesocolic loop. Straight after the transection of the jejunal loop with an endostapler (45 mm, blue reloads), we fashion a side-to-side gastrojejunal anastomosis by inserting the branches of a 45 mm blue cartridge linear stapler through two openings, one on the antimesenteric edge of the jejunum and the other on the posterior wall of the gastric stump

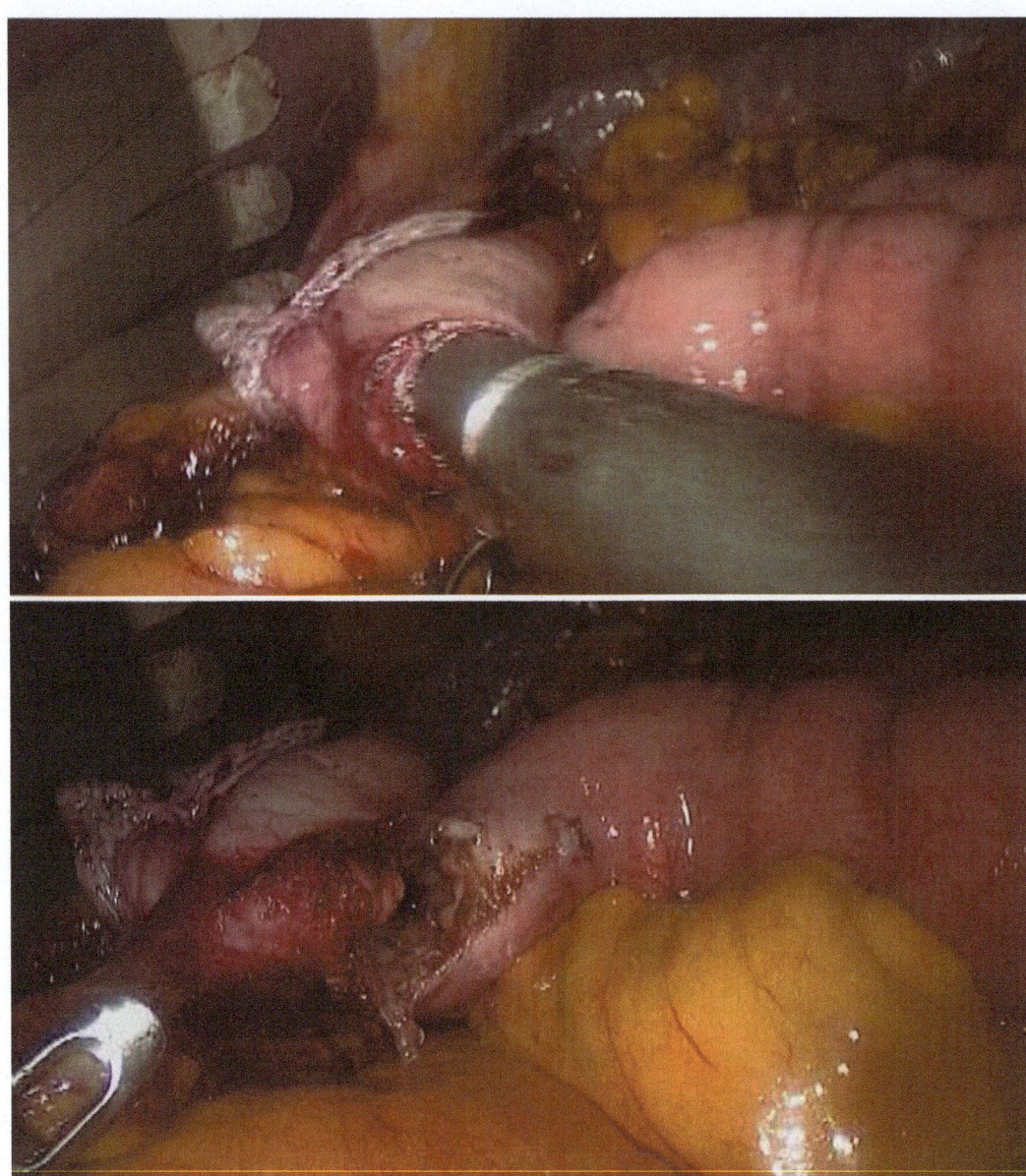

**Figs. 7.38, 7.39, 7.40, and 7.41** (continued)

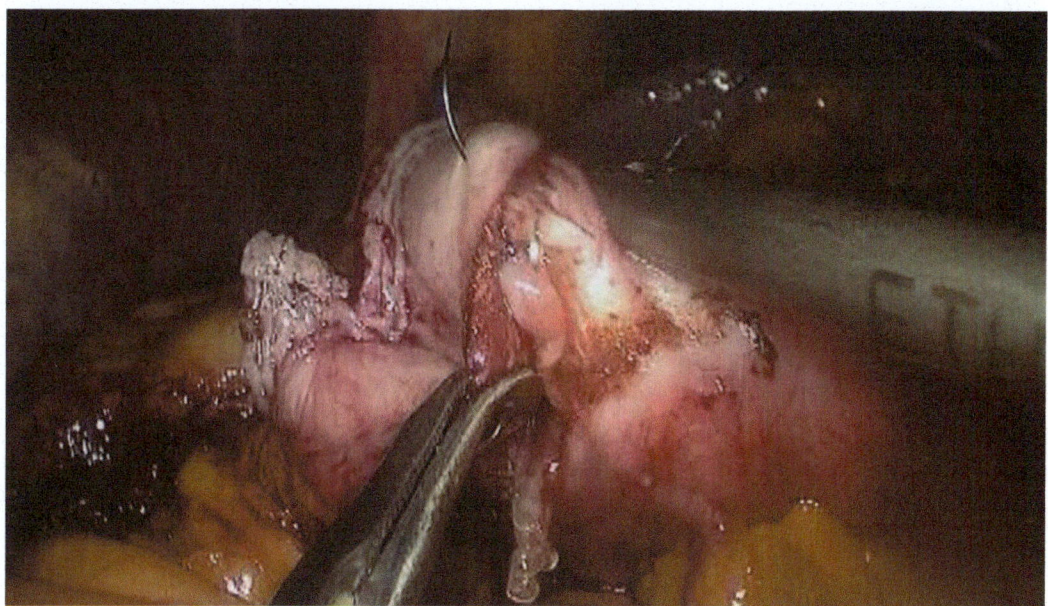

**Fig. 7.42** The closure of the incisions is performed by interrupted stitches of 3-0 reabsorbable suture intracorporeally. A nasogastric tube is collocated through the anastomosis. Finally we carry out the side-to-side jejuno-jejunal anastomosis at the foot of the Roux-en-Y loop, about 50–60 cm from the gastro-jejunal anastomosis, in the same manner as the procedure for total gastrectomy

# Lymphadenectomy

**8**

Emilio Feliciotti, Pierpaolo Stortoni, Raffaella Ridolfo, and Walter Siquini

Radical total or subtotal gastrectomy with lymph node dissection is the only potentially curative therapy for gastric cancer, and local control of lymph node metastases through extended node dissection appears essential in order to cure the disease.

The lymph nodes of the stomach have been arranged into a very useful classification by the Japanese Gastric Cancer Association (JGCA). According to this classification, lymph nodes surrounding stomach are divided into 20 stations (Fig. 8.1 and Table 8.1), and these are classified into three groups depending on the anatomical position of the station in relation to the location of the primary tumor (Figs. 8.2, 8.3, and 8.4). This grouping system is based on the results of studies of lymphatic flow at various tumor sites, together with the observed survival associated with metas-

tasis to each nodal station. In this grouping system, most perigastric LNs (stations 1–6) are defined as group 1, whereas the nodes along the left gastric artery (station 7), common hepatic artery (station 8), celiac axis (station 9), splenic artery (station 11), and proper hepatic artery (station 12) are defined as group 2, and nodes at the base of superior mesenteric artery (station 14), on the posterior surface of the pancreatic head (station 13), and para-aortic nodes (station 16) are designated as group 3. Lymph node dissection may be classified as D0, D1, or D2 depending on the extent of lymph nodes removed. D0 refers to incomplete resection of group 1 lymph nodes. D1 gastrectomy is defined as dissection of all the group 1 nodes, and D2 is defined as dissection of all the group 1 and group 2 nodes, and D3 is defined as dissection of all the group 1, 2, and 3 nodes. Recently, the new Japanese Classification of Gastric Carcinoma and guideline for Diagnosis and Treatment of Carcinoma of the Stomach edited by the Japanese Gastric Cancer Society were published in May and October 2010 to match to the standard of TNM classification of UICC. In this guideline the definition of lymphadenectomy has been remarkably simplified: the lymph node stations to be dissected in D1, D1+, and D2 are defined for total and subtotal gastrectomy regardless of the tumor location (Figs. 8.5 and 8.6). It should be noted that the lymph nodes along the left gastric artery (N° 7), which used to be classified as N2 for tumors in any location, are now included in D1 for any type of gastrectomy.

E. Feliciotti (✉)
Department of Surgery, "Ospedali Riuniti" University Hospital, Ancona, Italy
e-mail: feliciotti@live.it

P. Stortoni
Division of General Surgery, "A. Murri" Hospital, Fermo, Italy
e-mail: pierpaolostortoni@libero.it

R. Ridolfo
Division of General Surgery, Senigallia General Hospital, Senigallia, Italy
e-mail: raffaella.ridolfo@email.it

W. Siquini
Division of General Surgery,
"Madonna del Soccorso" Hospital,
San Benedetto del Tronto, Italy
e-mail: walter.siquini@sanita.marche.it

W. Siquini (ed.), *Total, Subtotal and Proximal Gastrectomy in Cancer: A Color Atlas*,
DOI 10.1007/978-88-470-5749-4_8, © Springer-Verlag Italia 2015

In the new Japanese Gastric Cancer Treatment Guidelines, D3 is no longer defined because the rationale to recommend this super-extended surgery was lost by the negative results of the Japanese randomized controlled trial (RCT) JCOG 9501.

The appropriate extent of lymph node dissection accompanied by gastrectomy for cancer remains controversial. In East Asian countries, especially in Japan and Korea, D2 lymph node dissection has been regularly performed as a standard procedure since the 1960s, and D1 dissection is considered unethical today. In Western countries, surgeons perform gastrectomy with D1 dissection only because D2, in two randomized trials, is associated with high mortality and morbidity compared to those associated with D1 alone but does not improve the 5-year survival rate. However, more recent studies have demonstrated that Western surgeons can be trained to perform D2 lymphadenectomies on Western patients with a lower morbidity and mortality.

D2 dissection is now recommended as standard surgical treatment by the major surgical and oncological scientific society guidelines worldwide [3–6].

D2 lymphadenectomy, originally developed by Eastern surgeons, is now becoming the procedure of choice also in the West. Recently the latest edition of the American National Comprehensive Cancer Network (NCCN) guidelines, published on March 2015, included for the first time, the D2 dissection as surgical standard of treatment for gastric cancer [6]. The current consensus view in the West is that for patients deemed to be medically fit, D2 dissection with spleen and pancreas preservation should be the standard procedure carried out in specialized, high-volume centers with appropriate surgical expertise and postoperative care. The current UICC/AJCC TNM classification recommendations (7th edition) include excision of a minimum of 15 lymph nodes to allow reliable staging, but D2 lymphadenectomy with a minimum of 25 or more nodes removed should be considered the best treatment for patients undergoing gastrectomy.

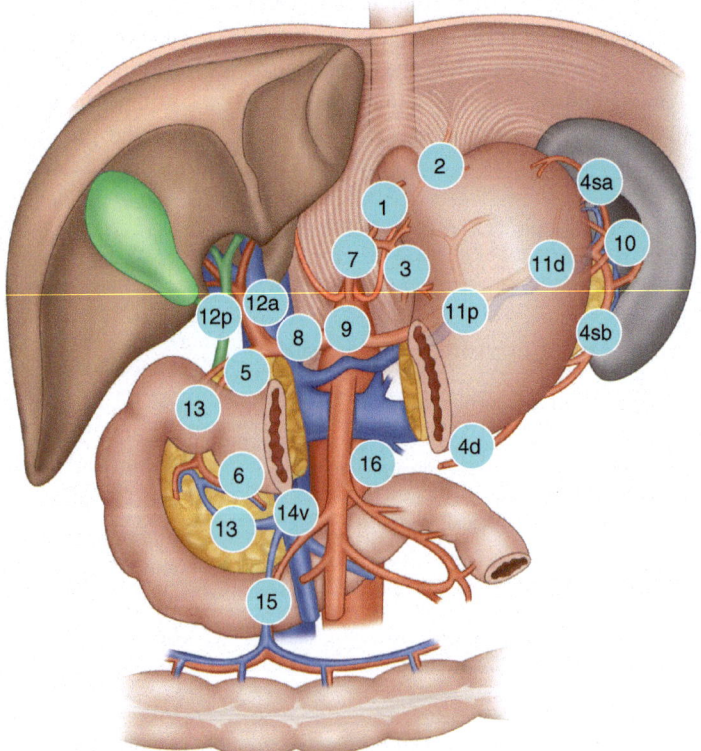

**Fig. 8.1** Regional lymphatic stations of the stomach according to the Japanese Gastric Cancer Association

**Table 8.1** Regional gastric lymph nodes

| No. 1 | Right paracardial LN |
|---|---|
| No. 2 | Left paracardial LN |
| No. 3 | LN along the lesser curvature |
| No. 4sa | LN along the short gastric vessels |
| No. 4sb | LN along the left gastroepiploic vessels |
| No. 4d | LN along the right gastroepiploic vessels |
| No. 5 | Suprapyloric LN |
| No. 6 | Infrapyloric LN |
| No. 7 | LN along the left gastric artery |
| No. 8a | LN along the common hepatic artery (anterosuperior group) |
| No. 8p | LN along the common hepatic artery (posterior group) |
| No. 9 | LN around the celiac artery |
| No. 10 | LN at the splenic hilum |
| No. 11p | LN along the proximal splenic artery |
| No. 11d | LN along the distal splenic artery |
| No. 12a | LN in the hepatoduodenal ligament (along the hepatic artery) |
| No. 12b | LN in the hepatoduodenal ligament (along the bile duct) |
| No. 12p | LN in the hepatoduodenal ligament (behind the portal vein) |
| No. 13 | LN on the posterior surface of the pancreatic head |
| No. 14v | LN along the superior mesenteric vein |
| No. 14a | LN along the superior mesenteric artery |
| No. 15 | LN along the middle colic vessels |
| No. 16a1 | LN in the aortic hiatus |
| No. 16a2 | LN around the abdominal aorta (from the upper margin of the celiac trunk to the lower margin of the left renal vein) |
| No. 16b1 | LN around the abdominal aorta (from the lower margin of the left renal vein to the upper margin of the inferior mesenteric artery) |
| No. 16b2 | LN around the abdominal aorta (from the upper margin of the inferior mesenteric artery to the aortic bifurcation) |
| No. 17 | LN on the anterior surface of the pancreatic head |
| No. 18 | LN along the inferior margin of the pancreas |
| No. 19 | Infradiaphragmatic LN |
| No. 20 | LN in the esophageal hiatus of the diaphragm |
| No. 110 | Paraesophageal LN in the lower thorax |
| No. 111 | Supradiaphragmatic LN |
| No. 112 | Posterior mediastinal LN |

**Figs. 8.2, 8.3, and 8.4**
Extent of lymphadenectomy
(D1, D2, D3) according to the
site of the gastric tumor as
defined in the first edition
(2001) of the treatment
guidelines by the Japanese
Gastric Cancer Association [1]
    Gastric antrum: Pic.1
    Body: Pic.2
    Gastric fundus: Pic.3
    D1 lymphadenectomy:
    *Yellow circles*
    D2 lymphadenectomy:
    *Red circles*
    D3 lymphadenectomy:
    *Blue circles*

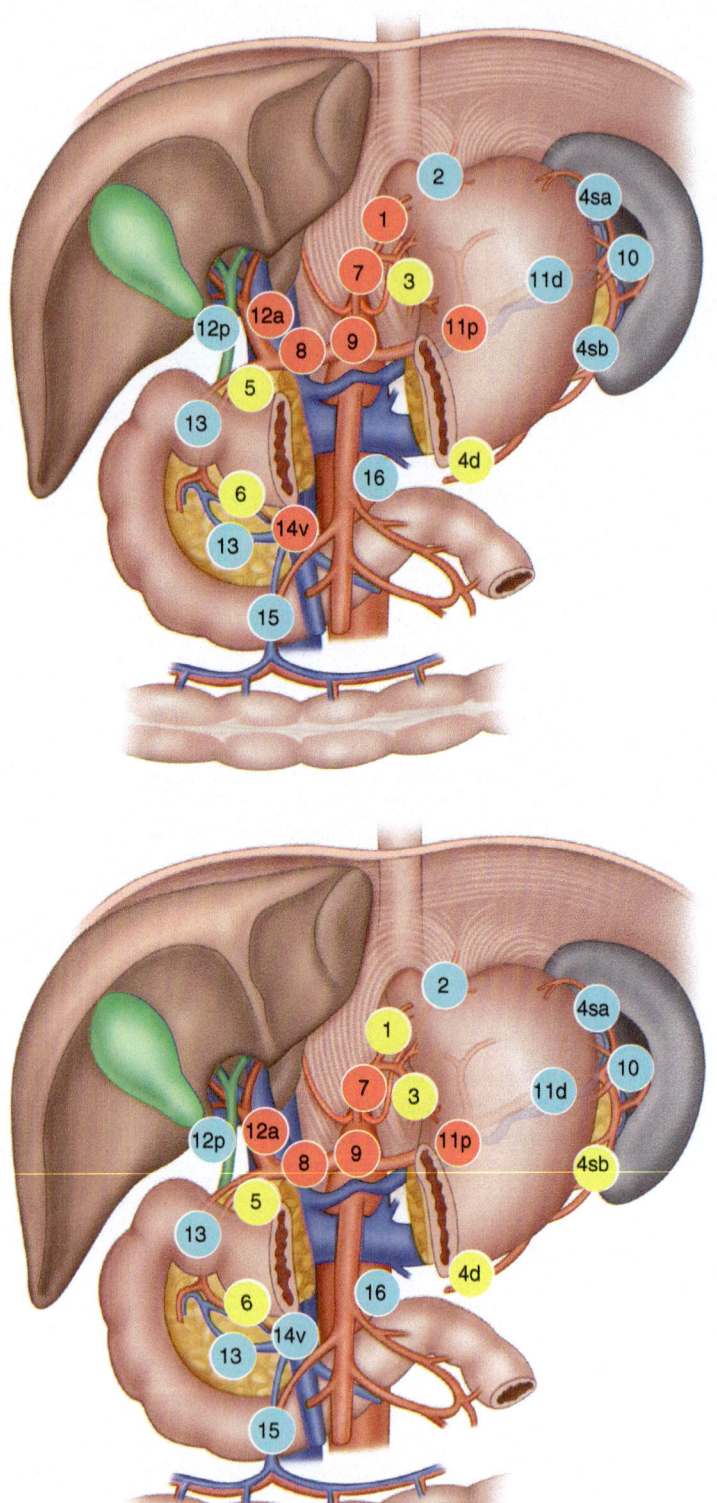

**Figs. 8.2, 8.3, and 8.4** (continued)

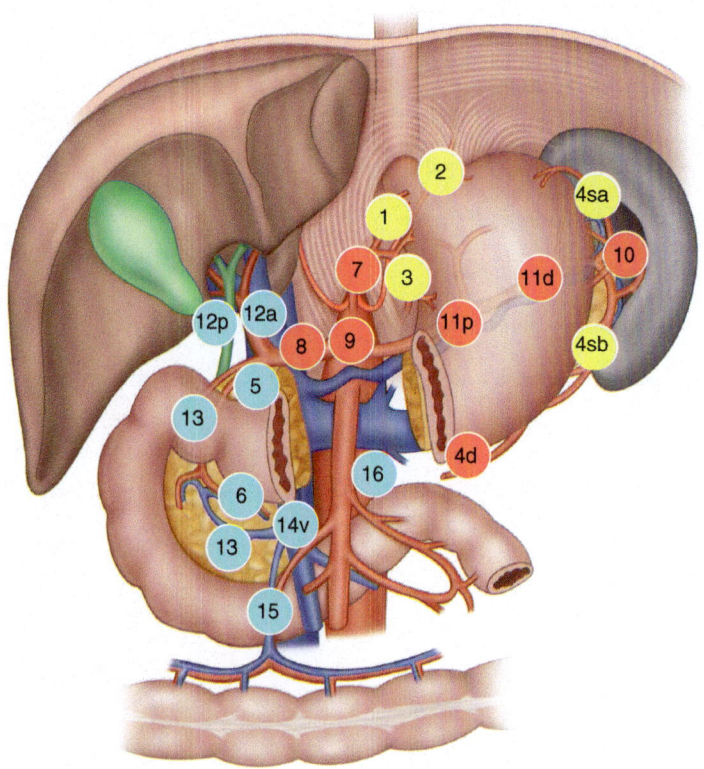

**Figs. 8.5 and 8.6** In the new Japanese Gastric Cancer Treatment Guidelines (2010), the definition of lymphadenectomy has been remarkably simplified: the lymph node stations to be dissected in D1, D1+, and D2 are defined for total (Pic.1) and subtotal (Pic.2) gastrectomy regardless of the tumor location [2, 3]

    D1 lymphadenectomy: *Blue circles*

    D1+ lymphadenectomy: *Yellow circles*

    D2 lymphadenectomy: *Red circles*

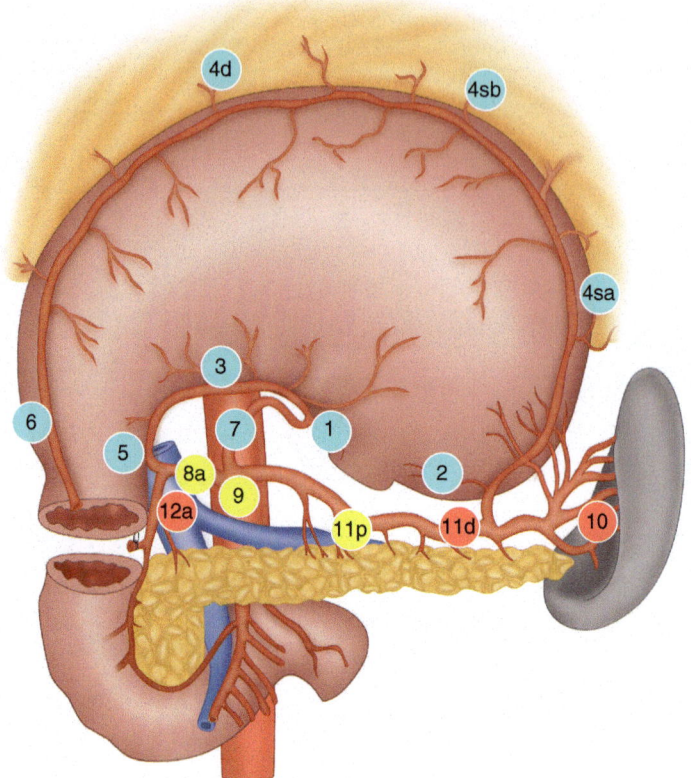

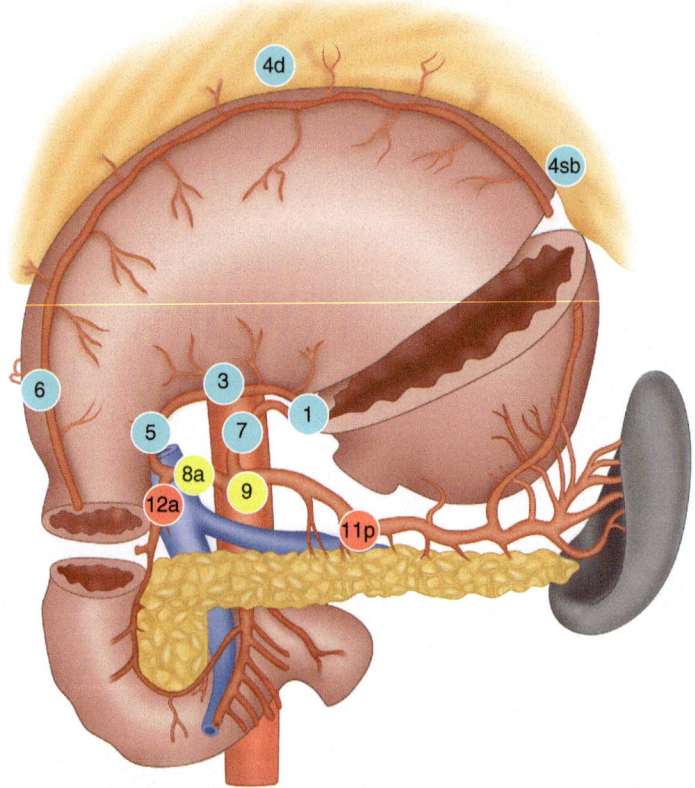

**Figs. 8.7 and 8.8**
Accurate examination of the contrast-enhanced abdominal CT scans allows preoperative identification of any enlarged nodes (*arrows*) in the 16 node stations defined by the JGCA, minimizing the risk of missing or neglecting any involved nodes

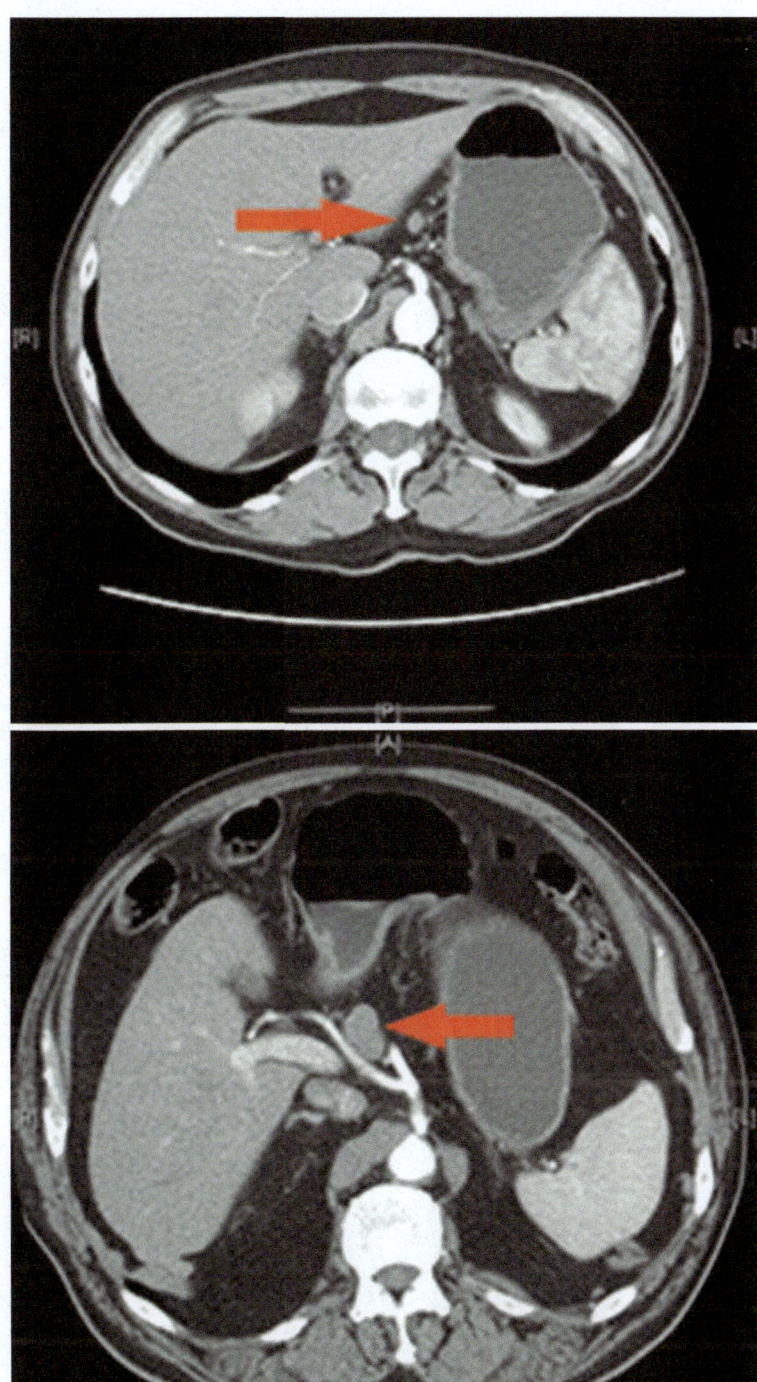

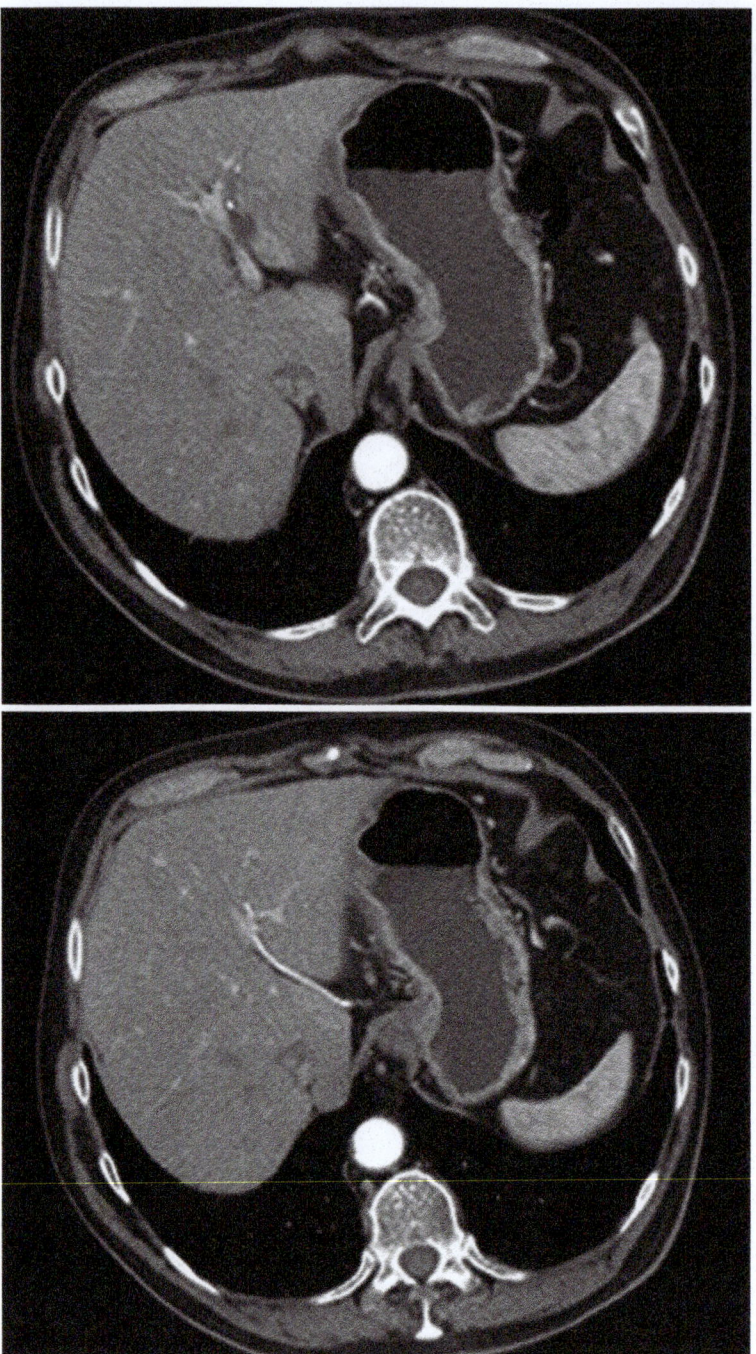

**Figs. 8.9, 8.10, 8.11, and 8.12** The arterial phase CT scans show the course of the arterial branches of the celiac trunk and any anatomical variation, which need to be identified to avoid possible errors. Recognition of any abnormalities prior to the operation provides for safe and correct execution of D2 lymphadenectomy

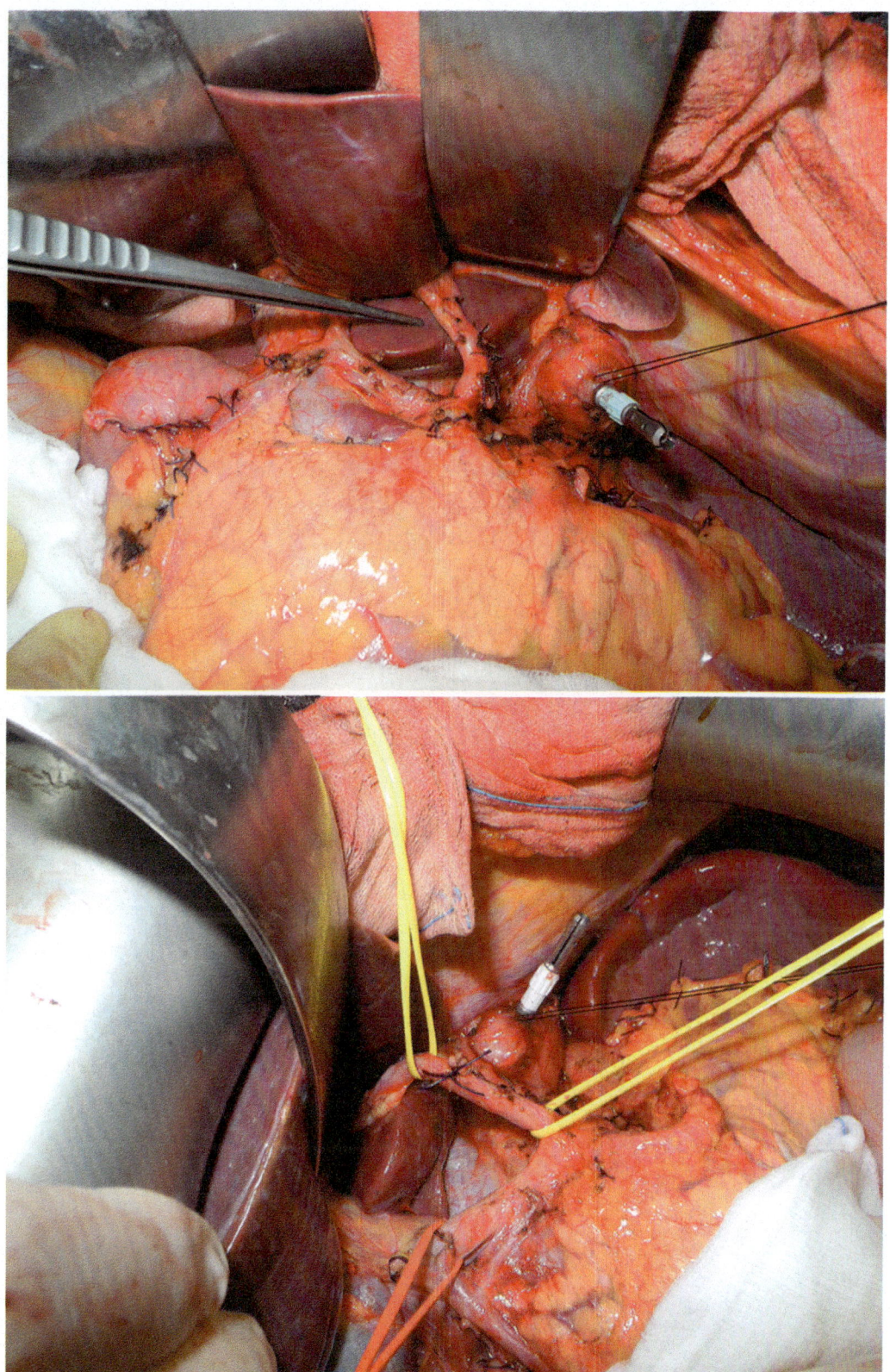

**Figs. 8.9, 8.10, 8.11, and 8.12**  (continued)

**Figs. 8.13 and 8.14**
Infrapyloric and left gastric
artery nodes

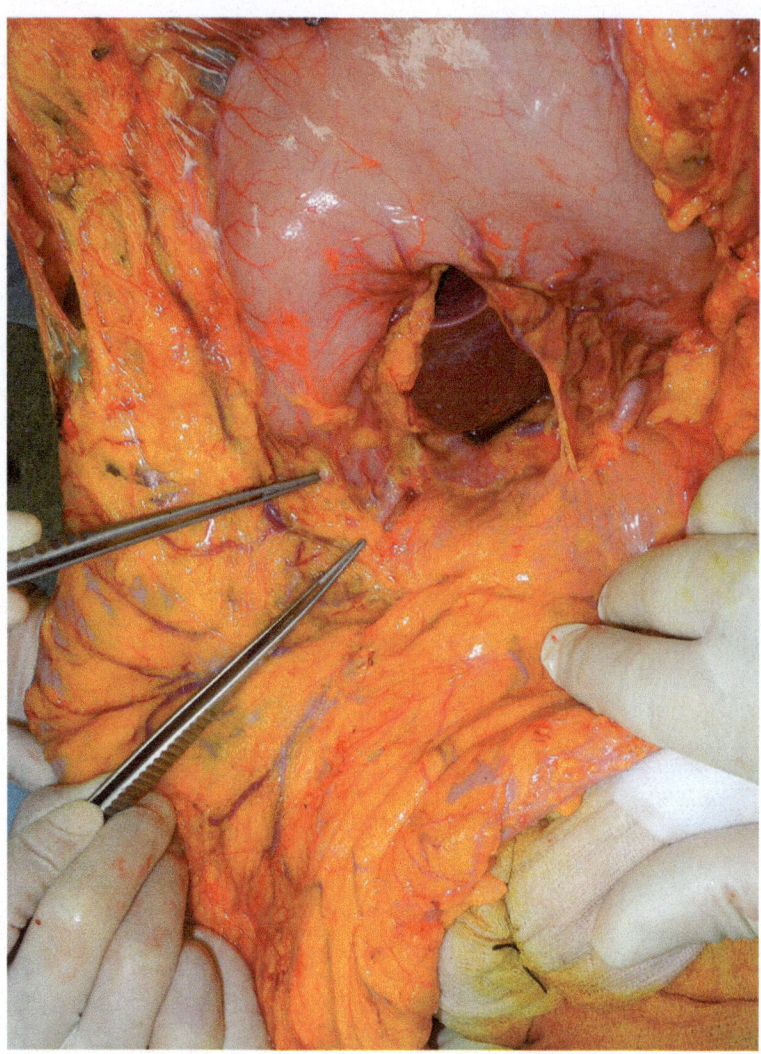

**Figs. 8.13 and 8.14**
(continued)

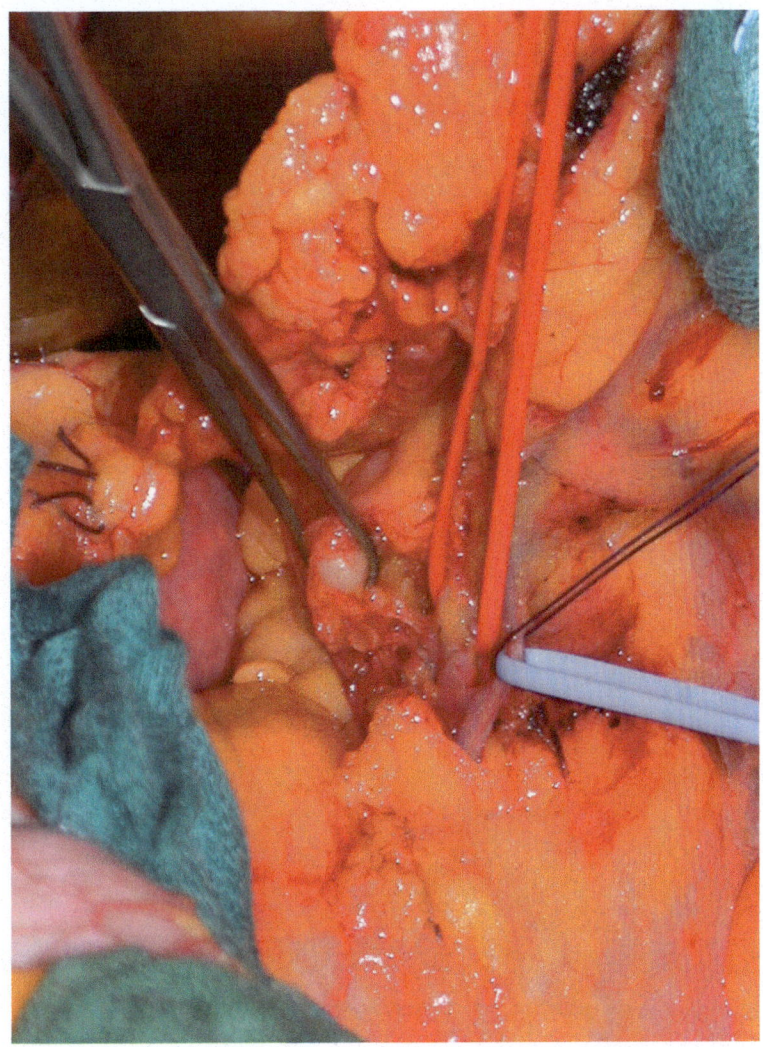

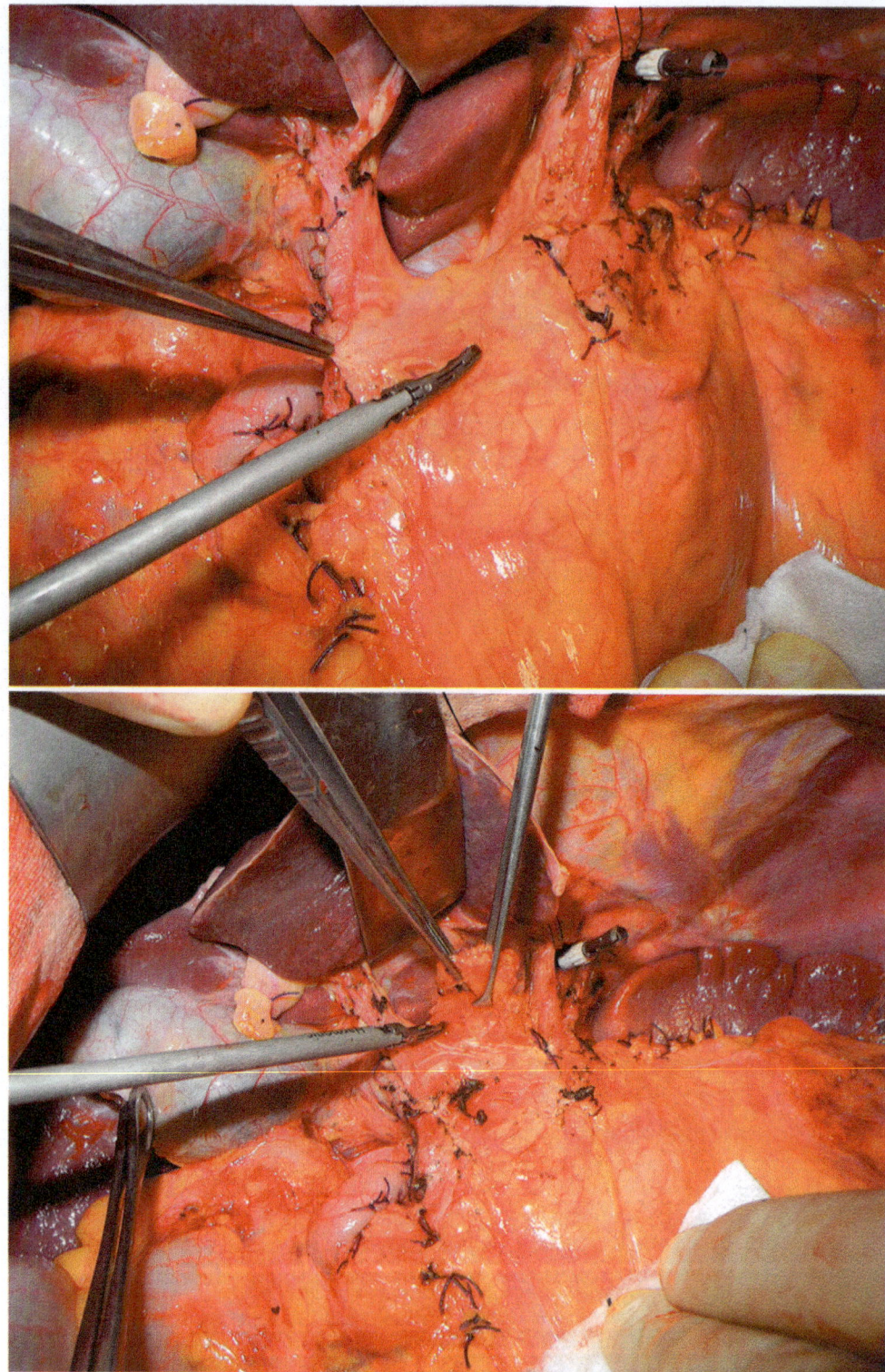

**Figs. 8.15, 8.16, and 8.17** After removal of the stomach and prior to reconstruction, D2 lymphadenectomy is performed.

We prefer to begin the lymph node dissection by identifying, medial to the duodenal stump, the gastroduodenal artery, which is dissected backward until its origin in the common hepatic artery

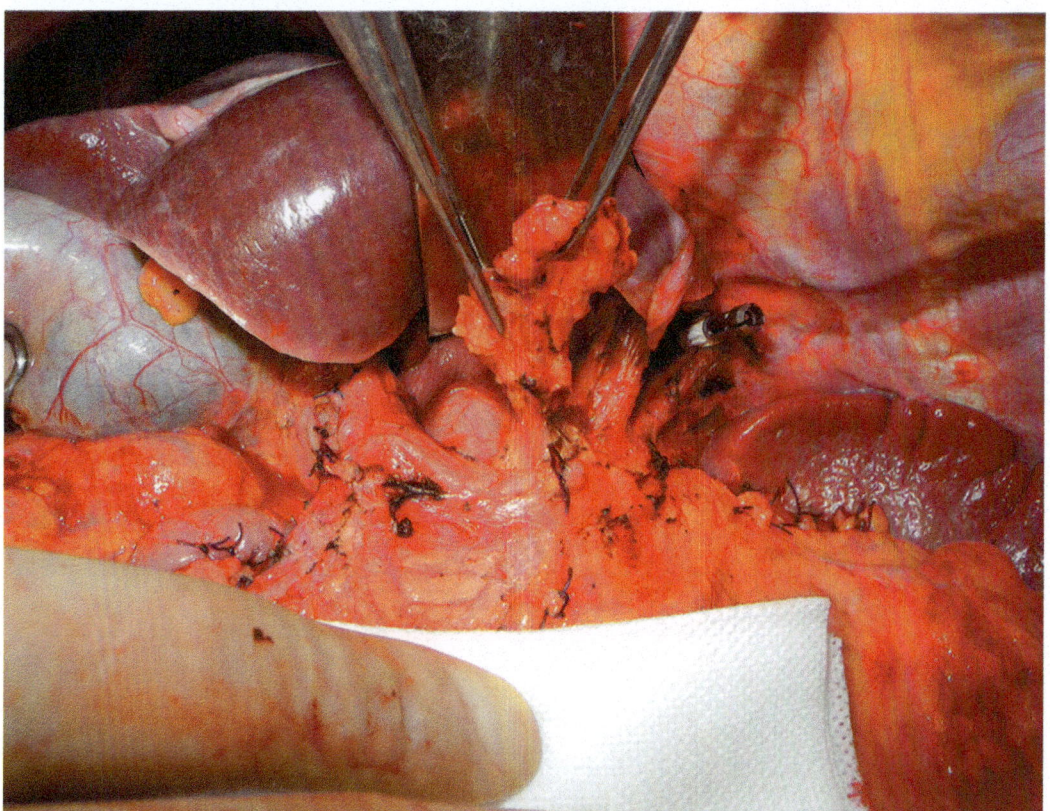

**Figs. 8.15, 8.16, and 8.17** (continued)

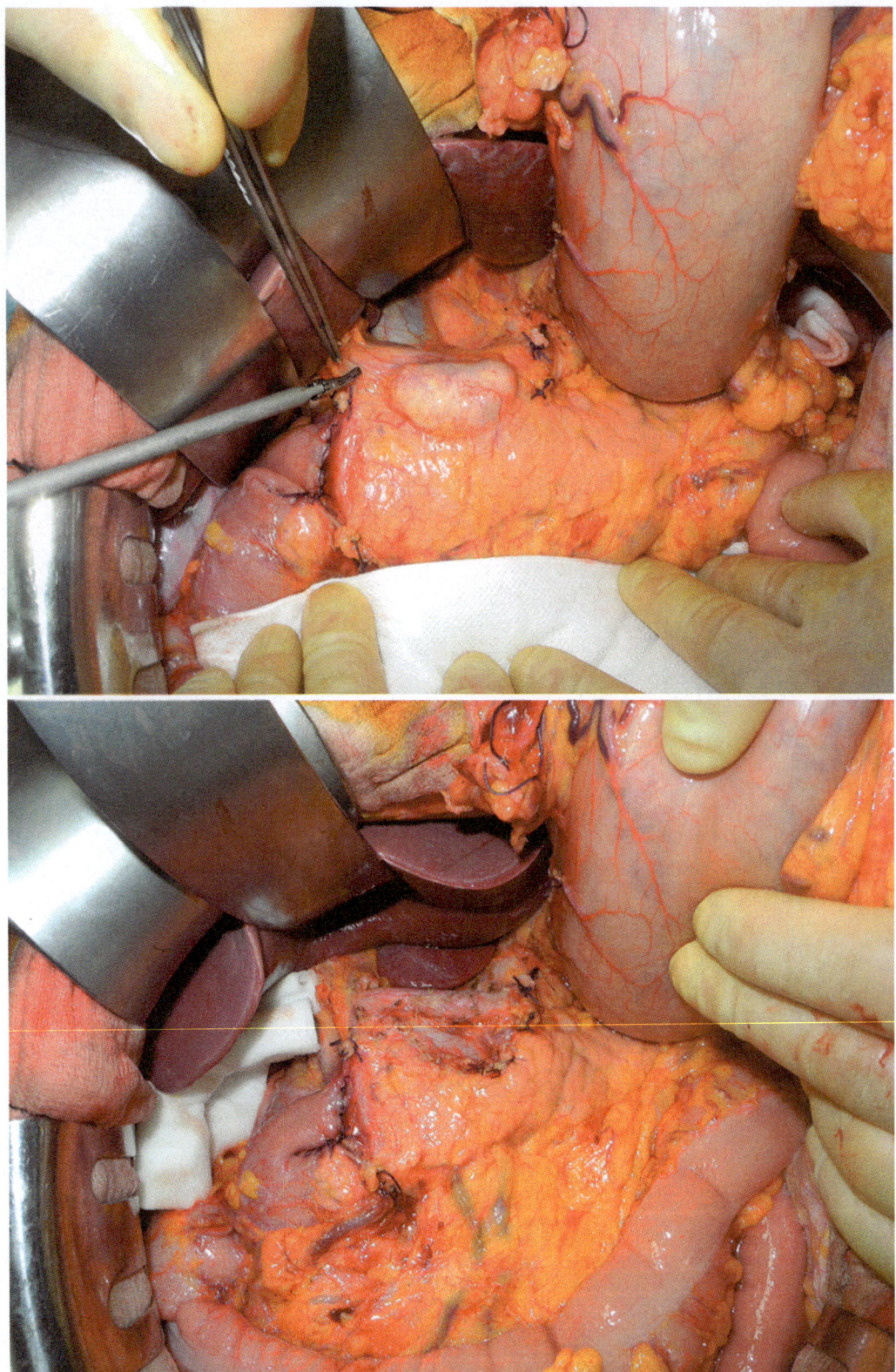

**Figs. 8.18 and 8.19** A large metastatic node on the common hepatic artery in contact with the portal vein

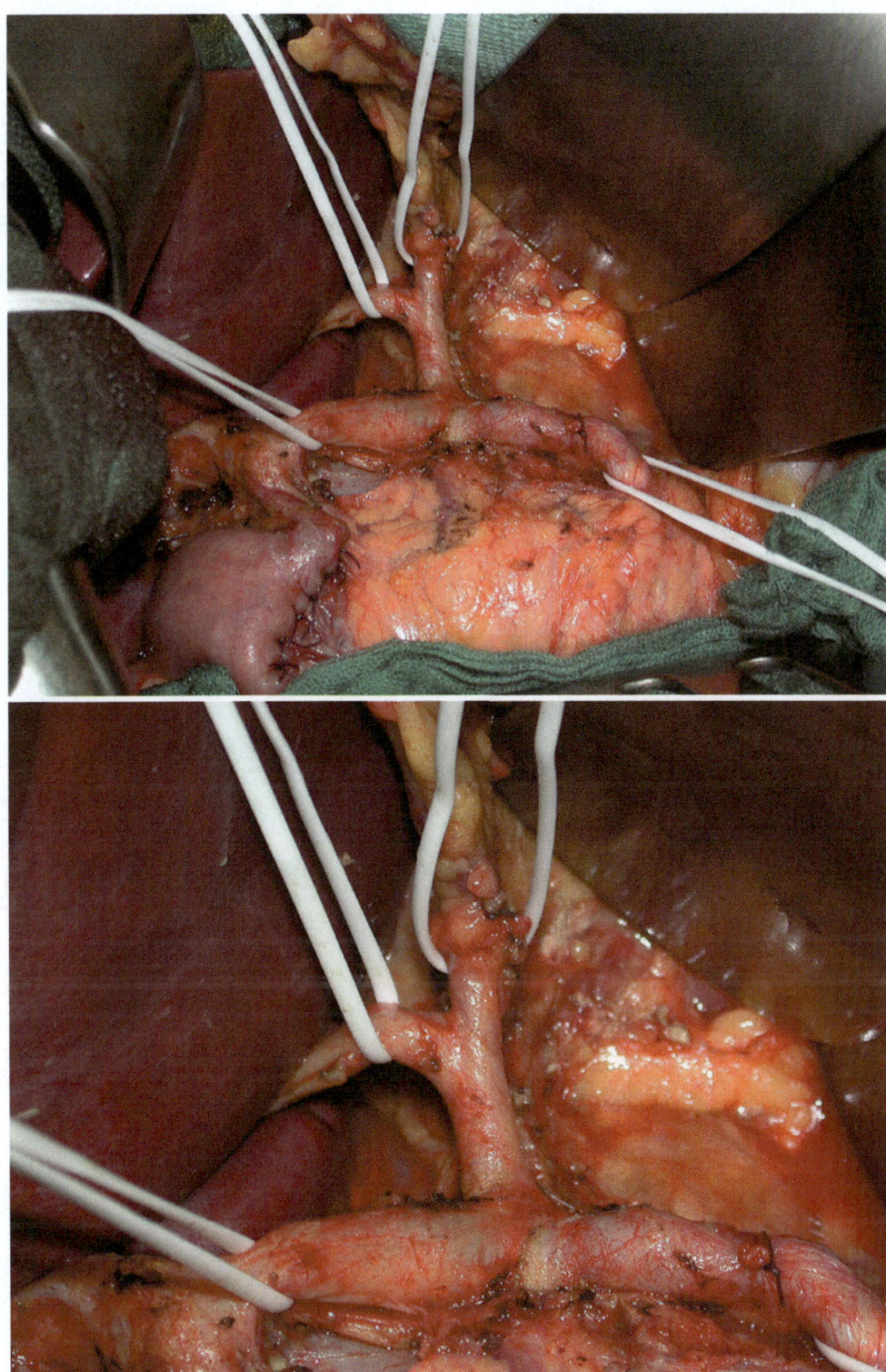

**Figs. 8.20 and 8.21** The common hepatic pedicle is dissected in the direction of the celiac trunk, which is now completely exposed. Complete lymphadenectomy involving the left gastric artery (station 7), the common hepatic artery (station 8), and the celiac trunk (station 9) is then performed. This patient had an anatomical variant, the left hepatic artery originating from the left gastric artery

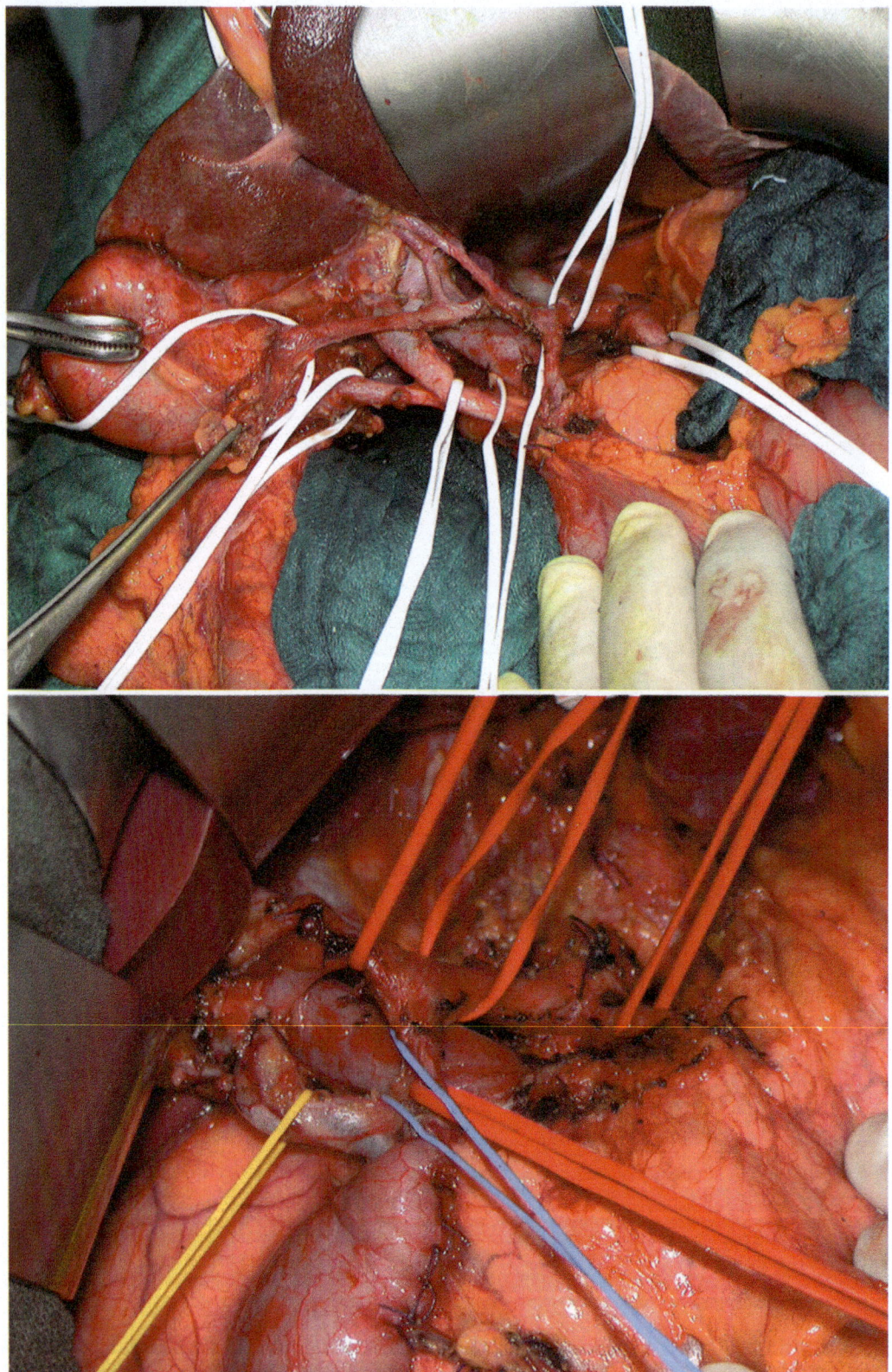

**Figs. 8.22 and 8.23** Lymphadenectomy of the arterial (12a), common bile duct (12c), and portal (12p) portions of the hepatoduodenal ligament is performed after preparing and placing these structures in a vascular tape

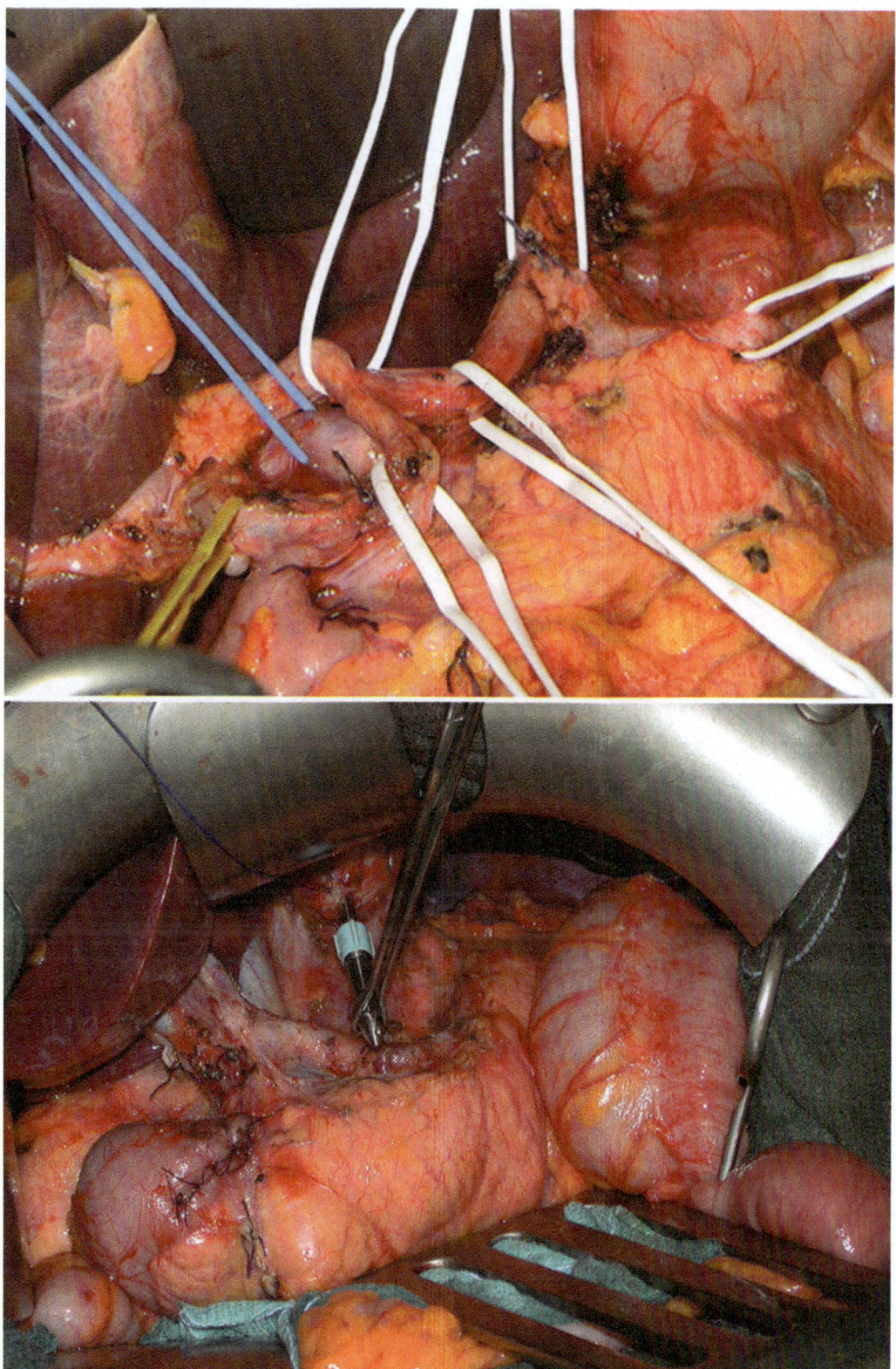

**Figs. 8.24, 8.25, and 8.26** View of the operating field after D2 lymphadenectomy with removal of the node stations of the splenic artery and splenic hilum (stations 11 and 10)

**Figs. 8.24, 8.25, and 8.26** (continued)

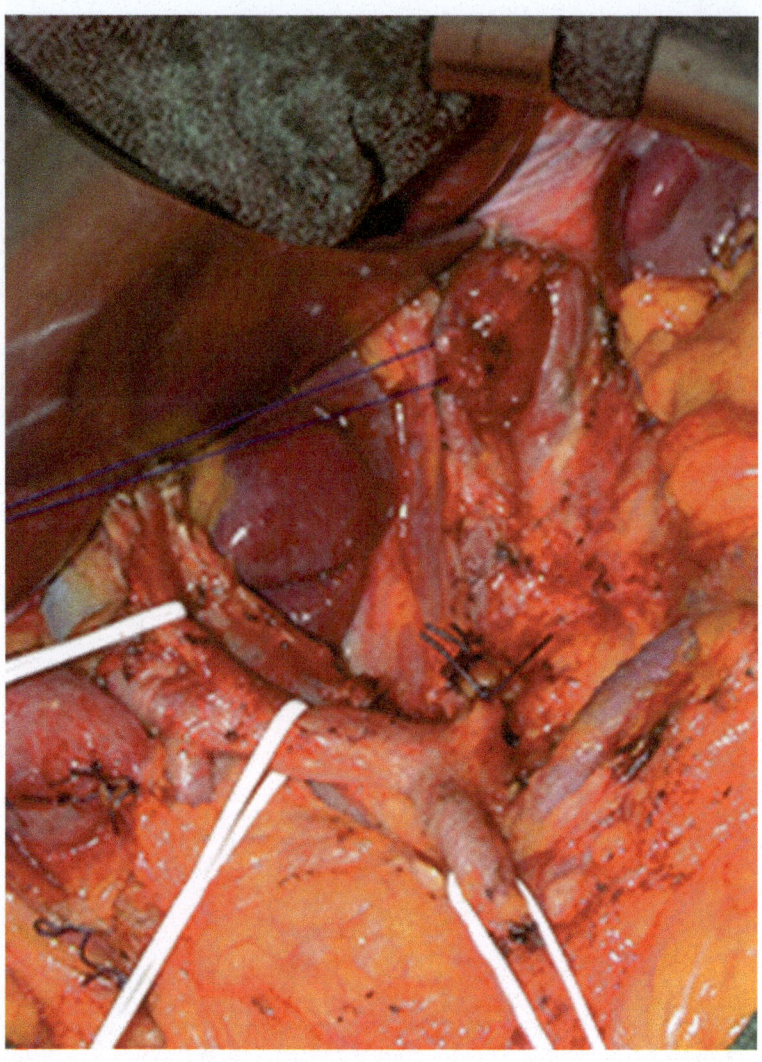

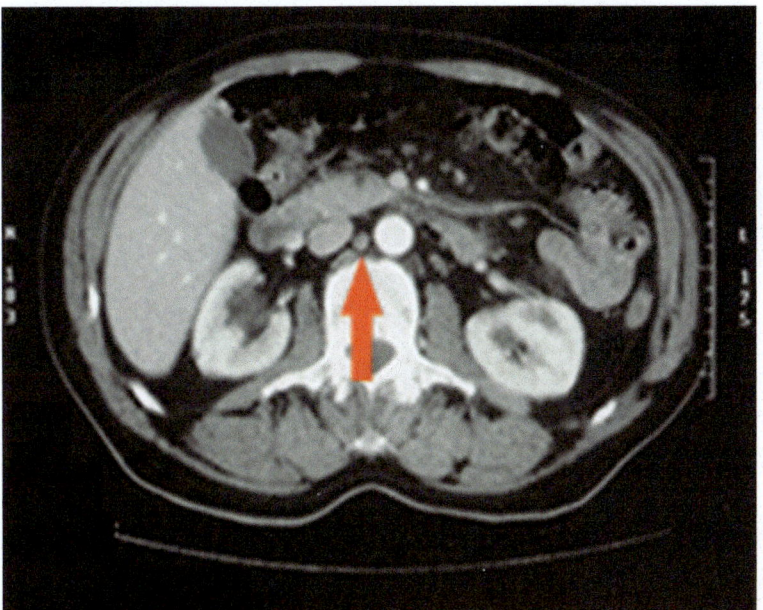

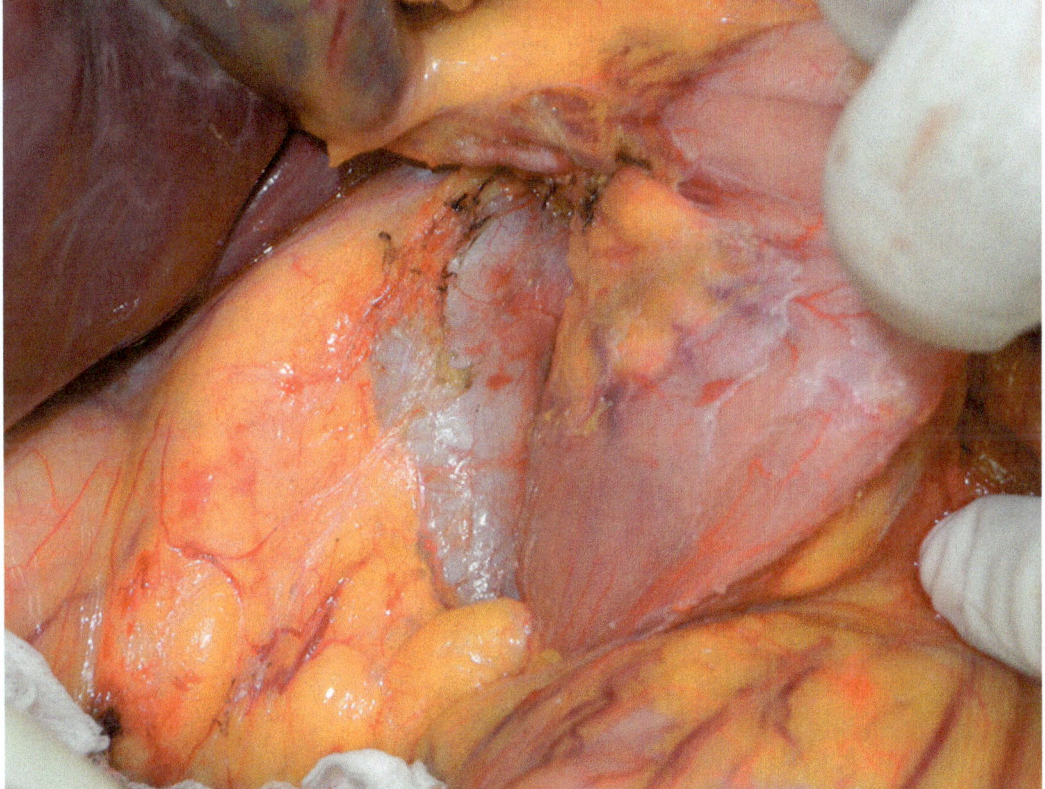

**Fig. 8.27, 8.28, 8.29, and 8.30** If the para-aortic lymph nodes are enlarged on preoperative CT (*arrow*), these node stations should be removed before the duodenal resection. Kocher's maneuver is executed with gentle duodenopancreatic mobilization and exposure of the inferior vena cava and aorta. The para-aortic lymphatic and adipose tissue between the left renal vein and the origin of the inferior mesenteric artery is removed

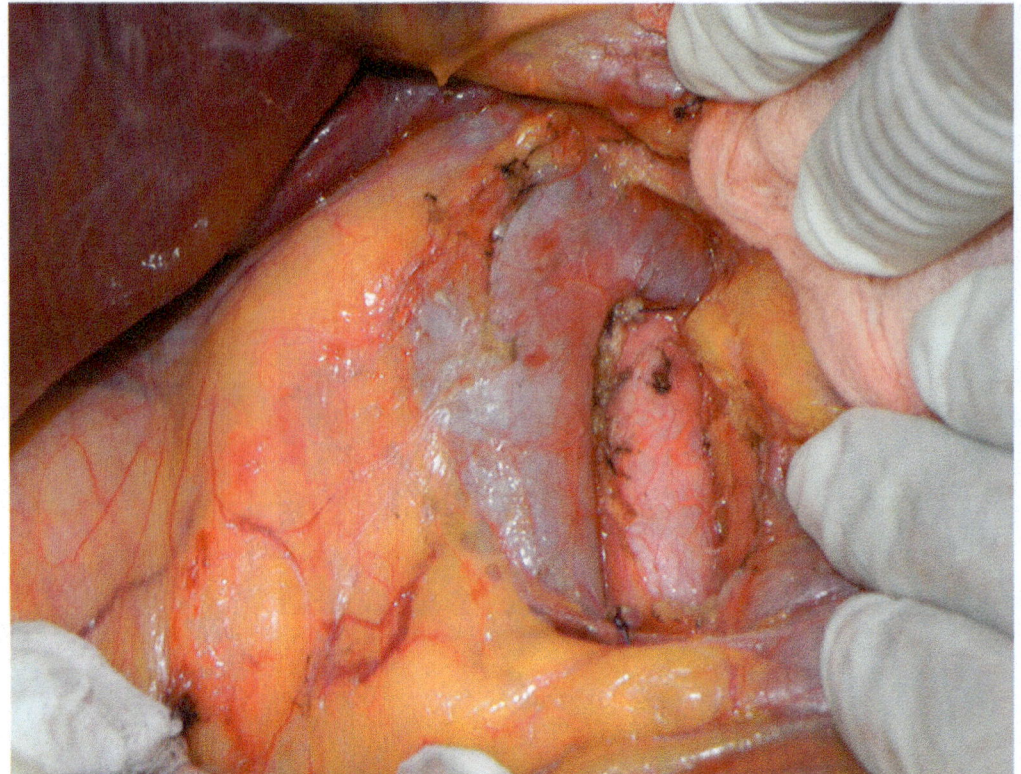

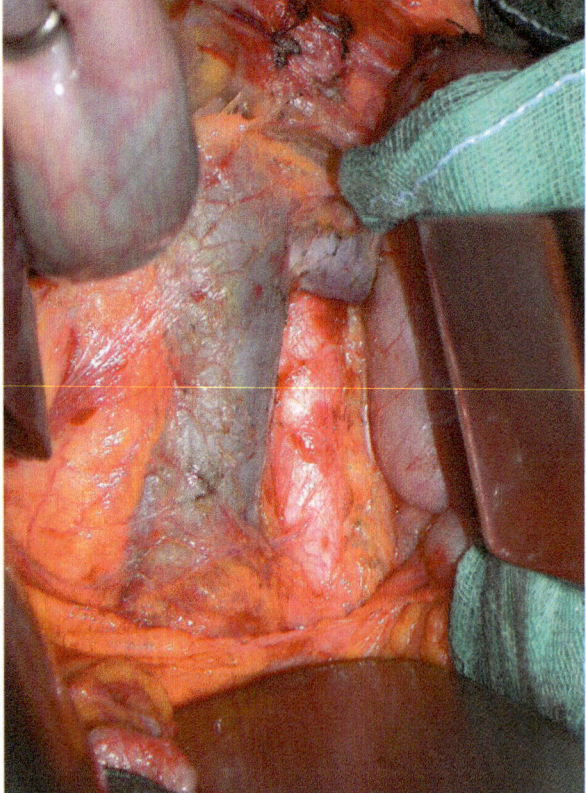

**Fig. 8.27, 8.28, 8.29, and 8.30** (continued)

# References

1. Nakajima T (2002) Gastric cancer treatment guidelines in Japan. Gastric Cancer 5:1–5
2. Japanese Gastric Cancer Association (2011) Japanese classification of gastric carcinoma: 3rd English edition. Gastric Cancer. doi:10.1007/s10120-011-0041-5
3. Japanese Gastric Cancer Association (2011) Japanese gastric cancer treatment guidelines 2010 (ver. 3). Gastric Cancer. doi:10.1007/s10120-011-0042-4
4. T. Waddell et al. (2013) Gastric cancer: ESMO–ESSO–ESTRO Clinical Practice Guidelines for diagnosis, treatment and follow-up. Annals of Oncology 24 (Supplement 6):vi57–vi63
5. NCCN Clinical Practice Guidelines in Oncology; 2015. Gastric Cancer. Version 3.2015
6. De Manzoni et al. 2013. The SIC-GIRCG 2013 Consensus Conference on Gastric Cancer. Updates Surg. 2014;66(1):1–6. doi: 10.1007/s13304-014-0248-1

# Special Cases

# 9

Emilio Feliciotti, Raffaella Ridolfo, Pierpaolo Stortoni, and Walter Siquini

E. Feliciotti (✉)
Department of Surgery,
"Ospedali Riuniti" University Hospital, Ancona, Italy
e-mail: feliciotti@live.it

R. Ridolfo
Division of General Surgery, Senigallia General Hospital, Senigallia, Italy
e-mail: raffaella.ridolfo@email.it

P. Stortoni
Division of General Surgery, "A. Murri" Hospital, Fermo, Italy
e-mail: pierpaolostortoni@libero.it

W. Siquini
Division of General Surgery,
"Madonna del Soccorso" Hospital,
San Benedetto del Tronto, Italy
e-mail: walter.siquini@sanita.marche.it

W. Siquini (ed.), *Total, Subtotal and Proximal Gastrectomy in Cancer: A Color Atlas*,
DOI 10.1007/978-88-470-5749-4_9, © Springer-Verlag Italia 2015

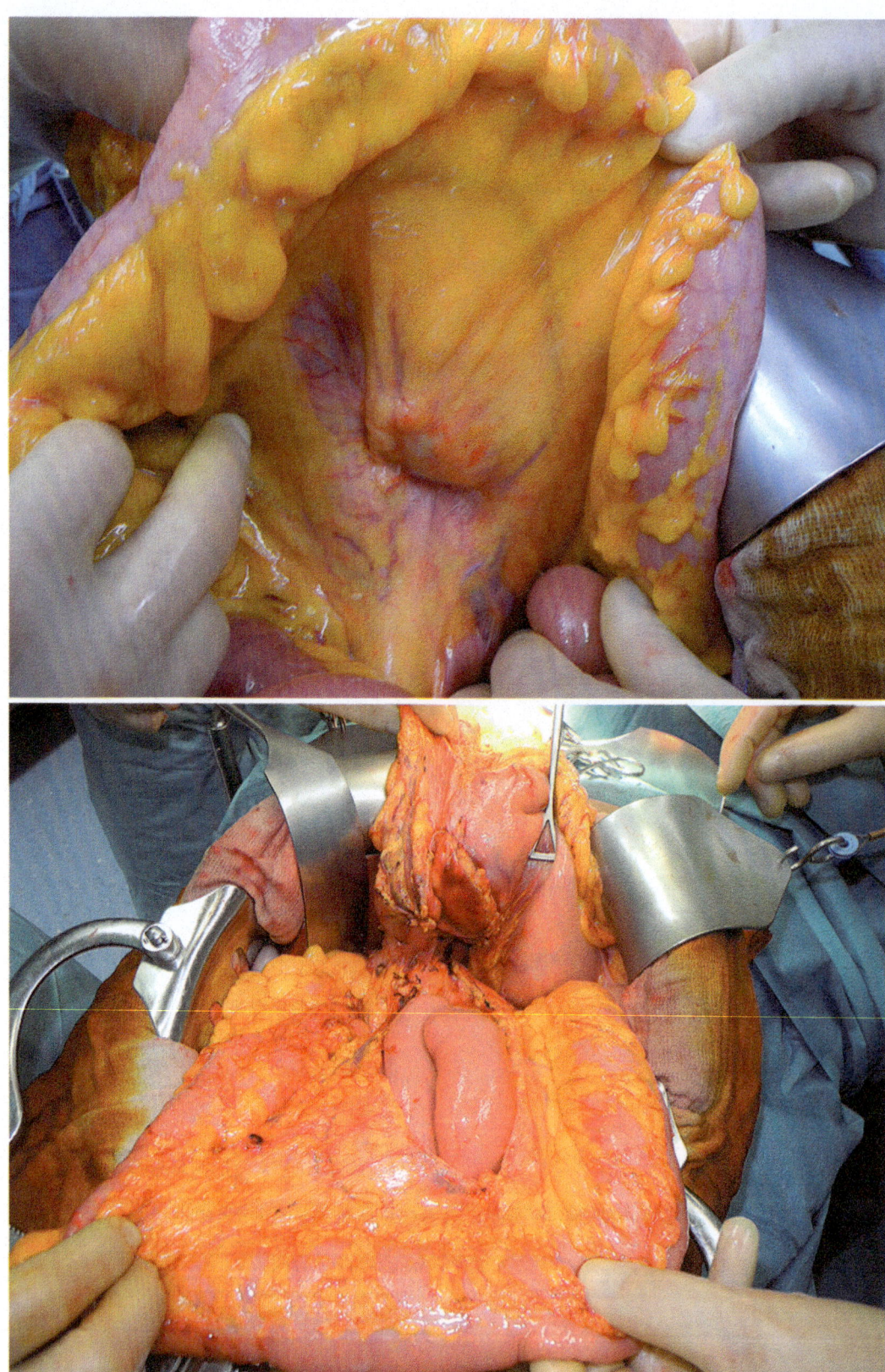

**Figs. 9.1, 9.2, and 9.3** A locally advanced gastric tumor infiltrating the transverse mesocolon without involvement of middle colic vessels. Subtotal gastrectomy with en bloc resection of mesocolic tissue was performed

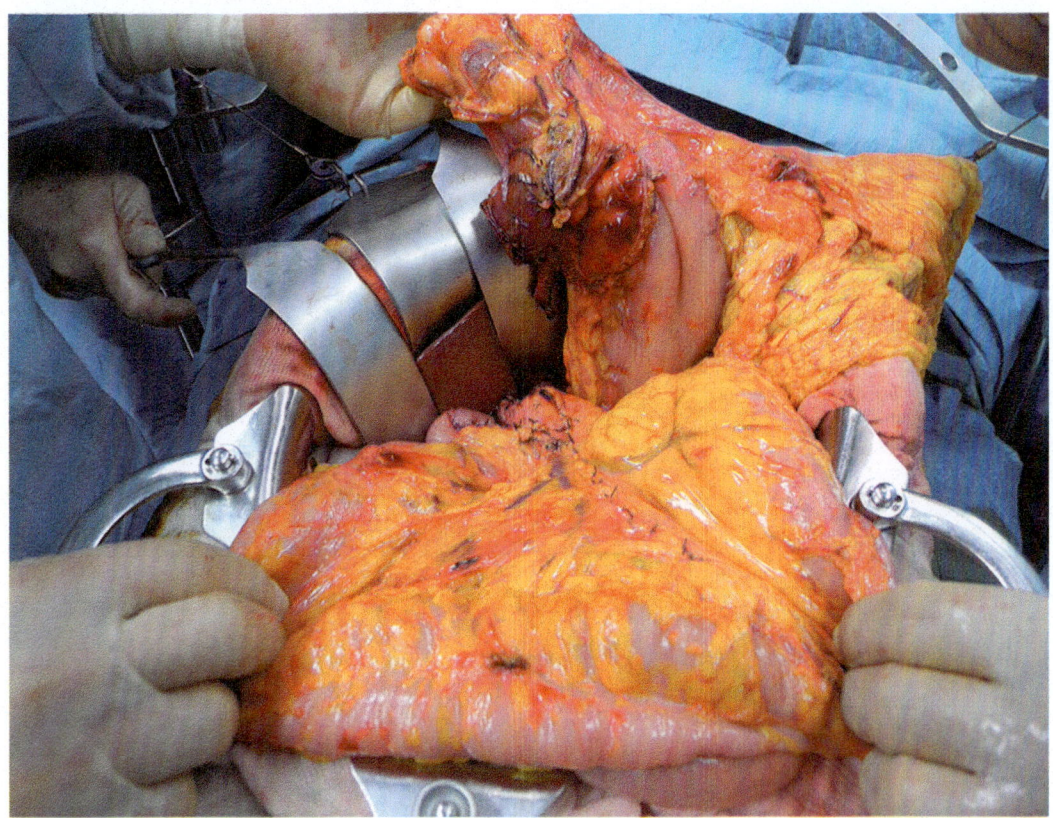

**Figs. 9.1, 9.2, and 9.3** (continued)

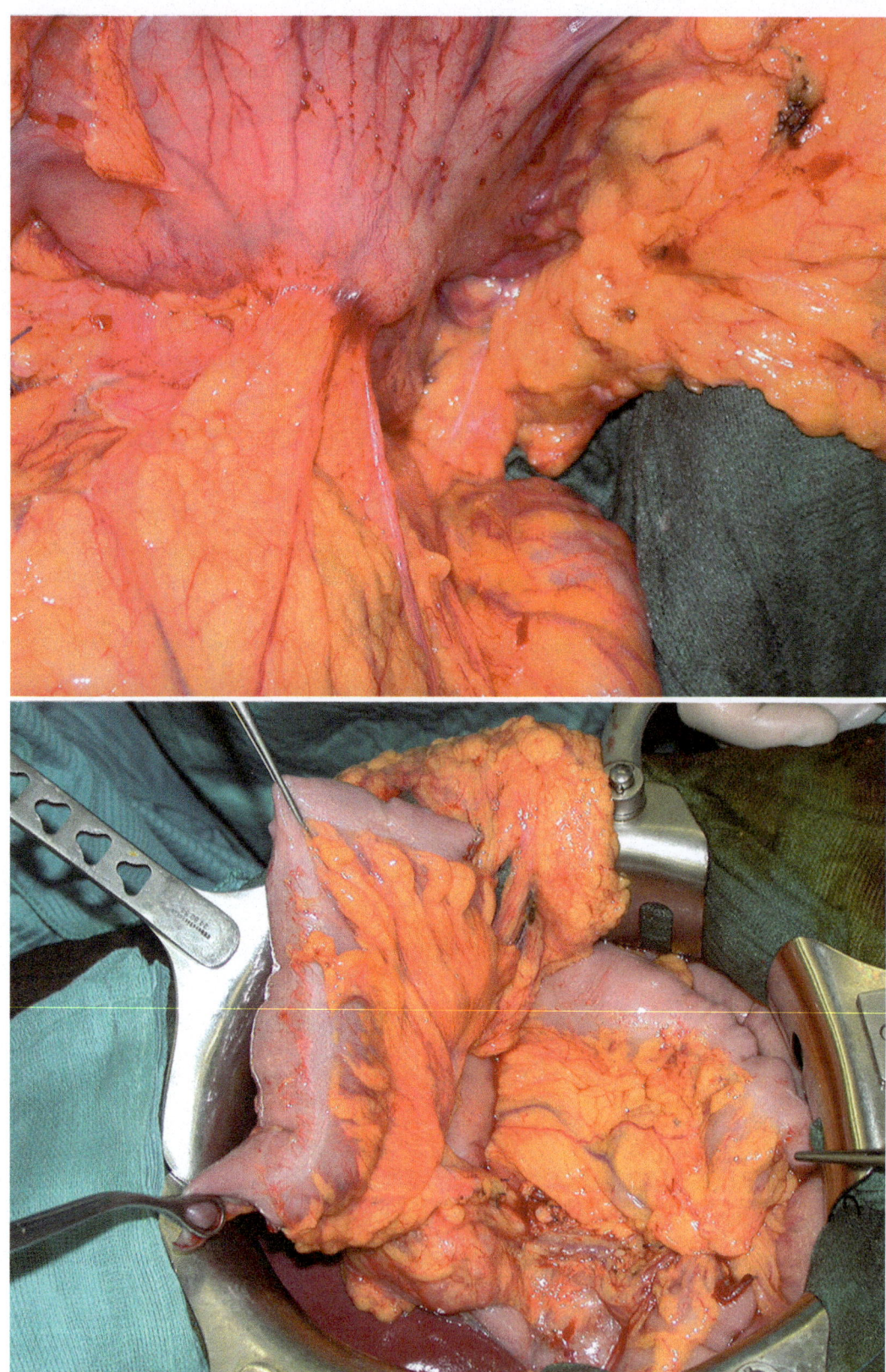

**Figs. 9.4 and 9.5** A similar case with involvement of middle colic vessels requiring en bloc segmental transverse colonic resection

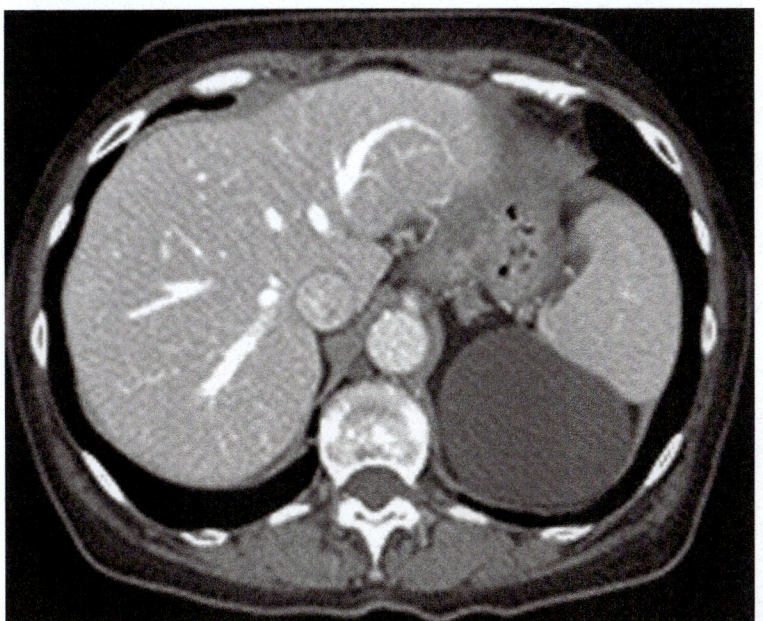

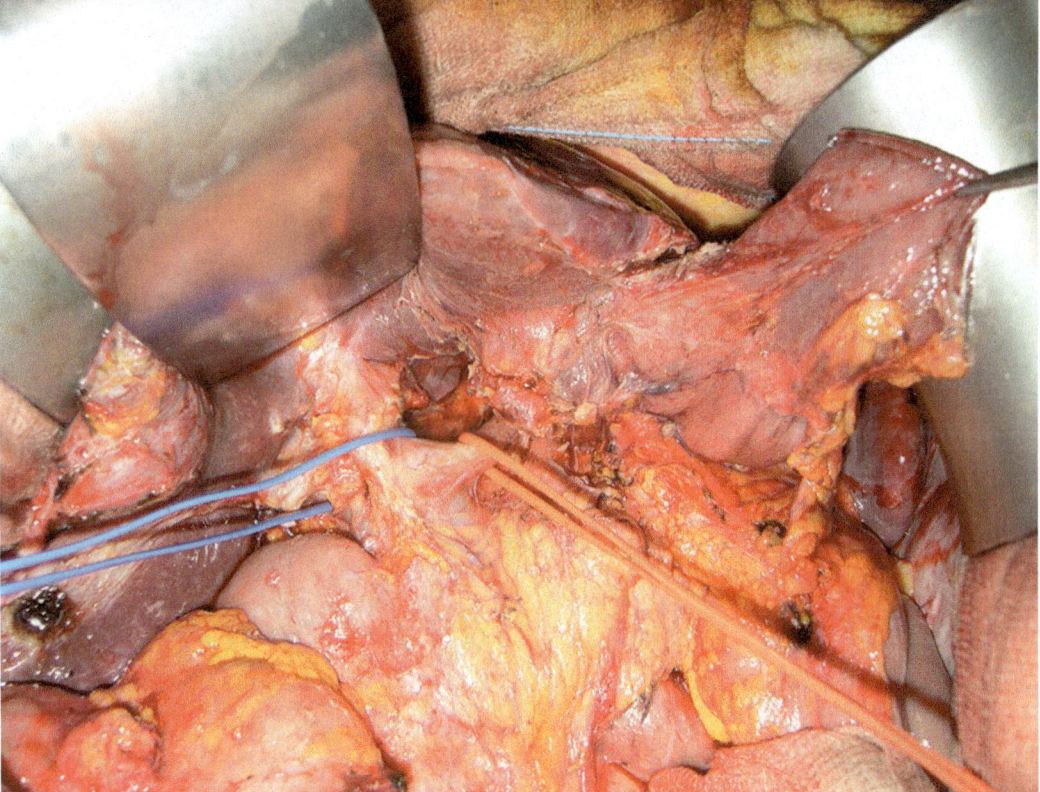

**Figs. 9.6 and 9.7** Nodal recurrence after subtotal gastrectomy and D1 lymphadenectomy infiltrating the S2–S3 liver segments and the gastrojejunal anastomosis

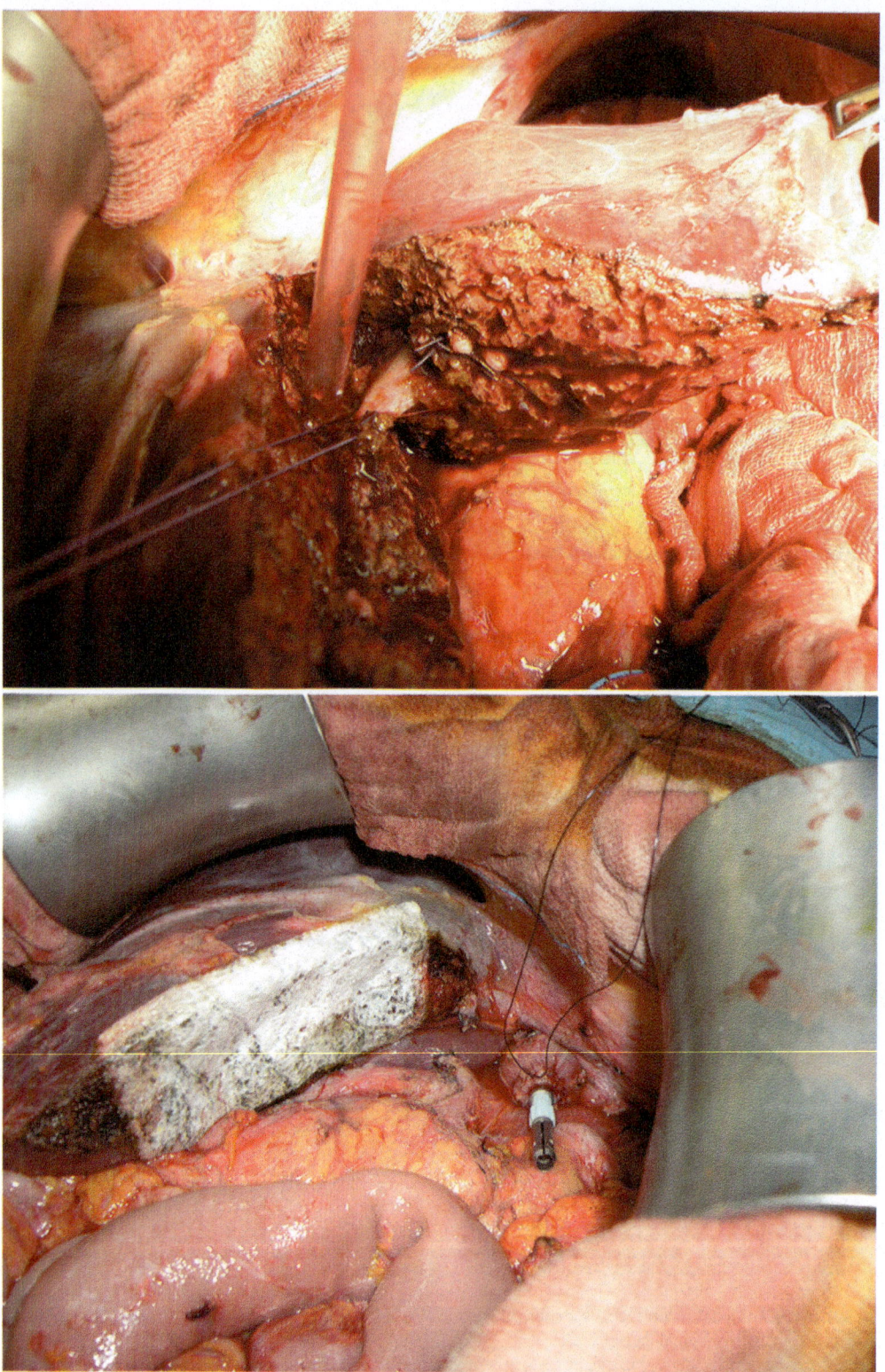

**Figs. 9.8, 9.9, and 9.10** Total gastrectomy with D2 lymphadenectomy and en bloc resection of the left lateral lobe of the liver. S2–S3 Glissonian pedicle transection. Hemostatic improvement achieved with TachoSil® on the hepatic resection surface

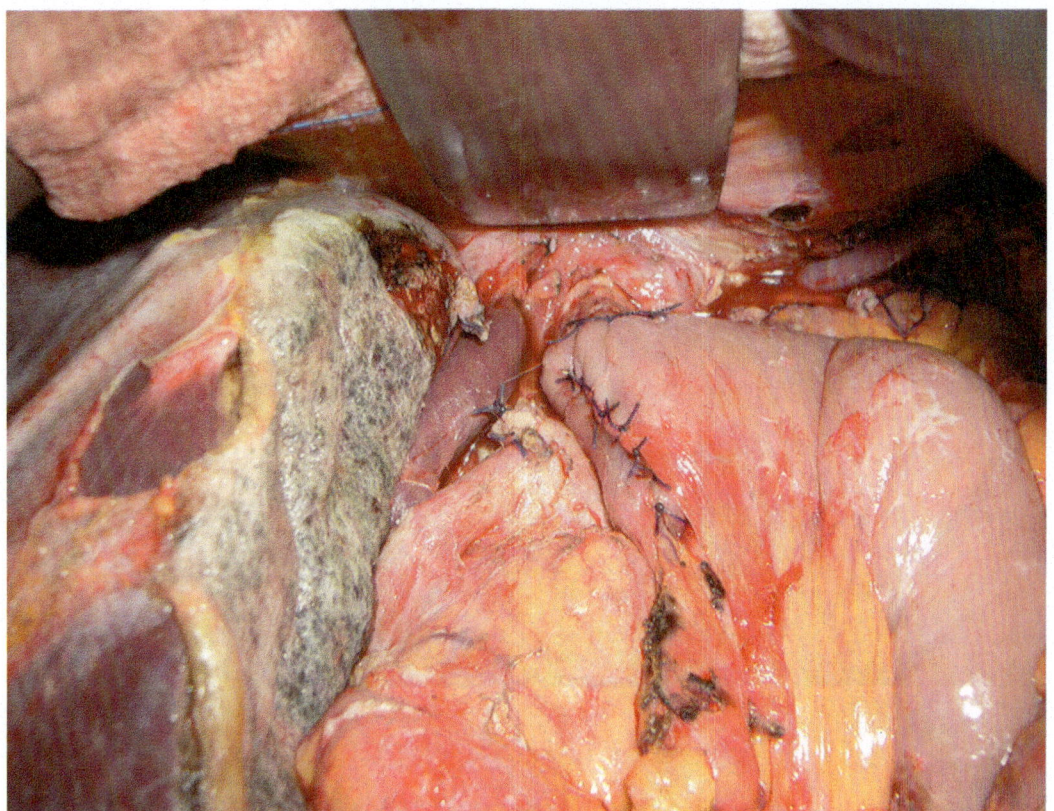

**Figs. 9.8, 9.9, and 9.10**   (continued)

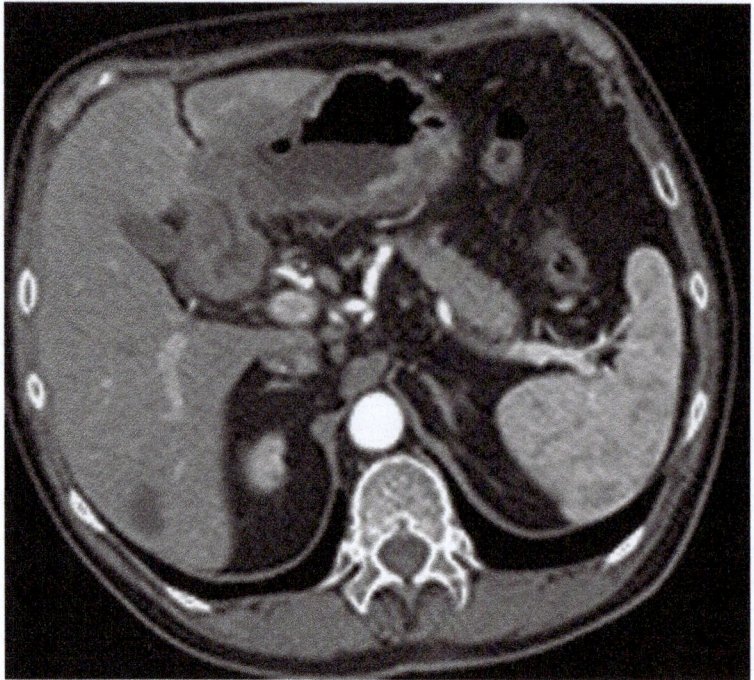

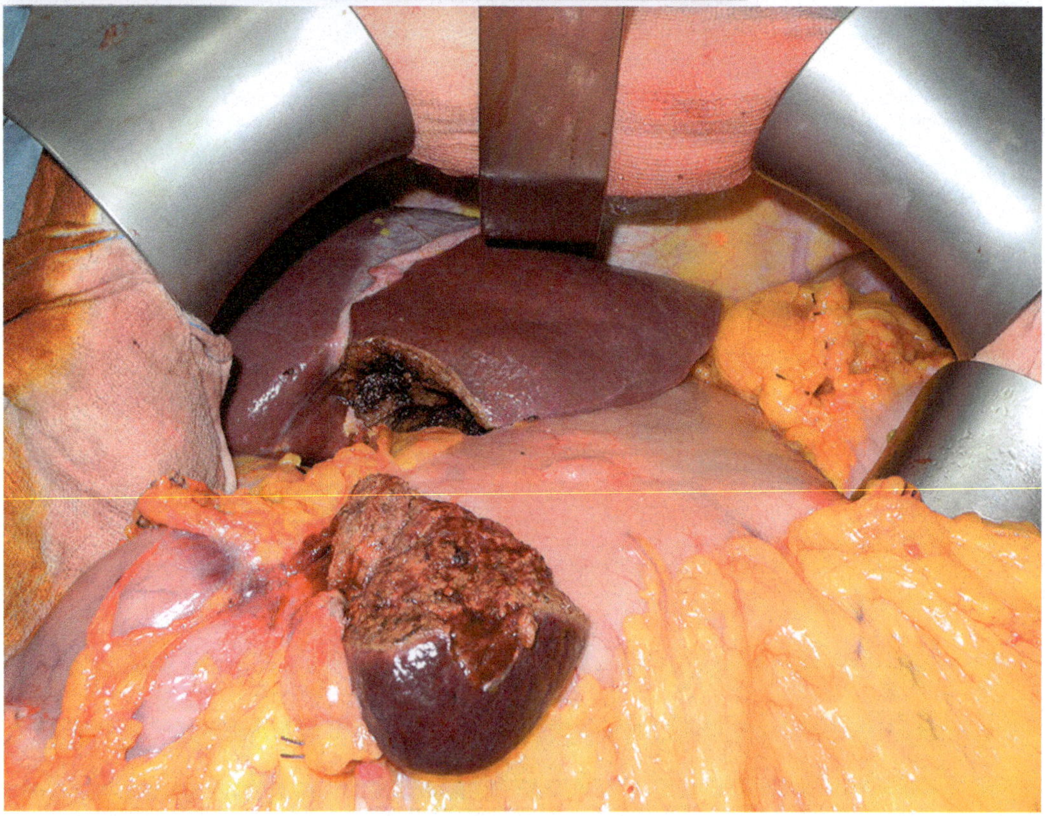

**Figs. 9.11 and 9.12** Preoperative CT scan shows antral gastric cancer infiltrating the third hepatic segment. Subtotal gastrectomy with en bloc S3 liver resection was performed

The manufacturer's authorised representative in the EU is Springer
Nature Customer Service Centre GmbH, Europaplatz 3, 69115 Heidelberg,
Germany. If you have any concerns regarding our products, please
contact ProductSafety@springernature.com

Printed and bound by CPI Group (UK) Ltd, Croydon, CR0 4YY
28/04/2026
02098457-0008